Krabi Krabong
The Tiger Sword of Thailand

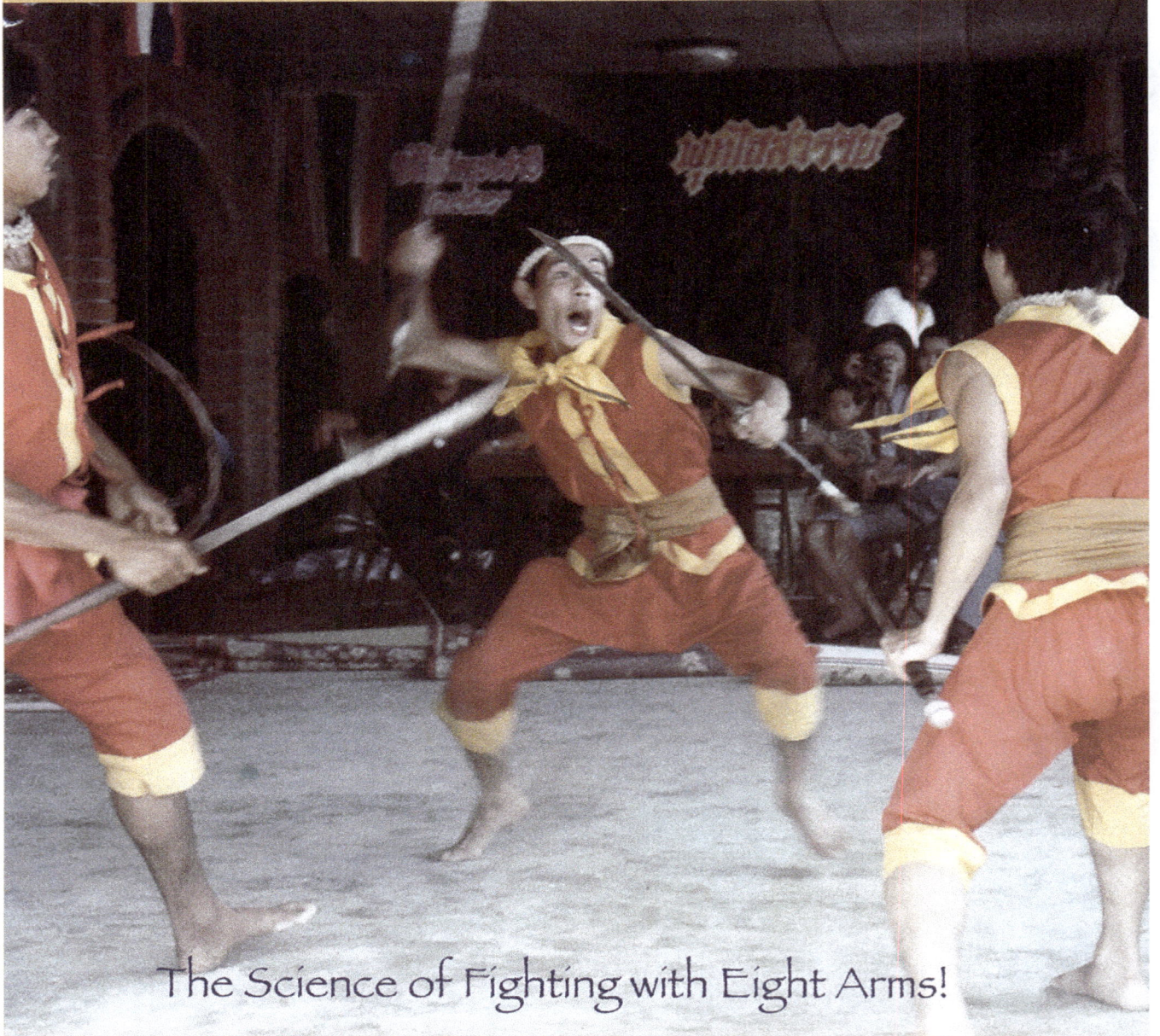

The Science of Fighting with Eight Arms!

Ajahn, Dr. Anthony B. James

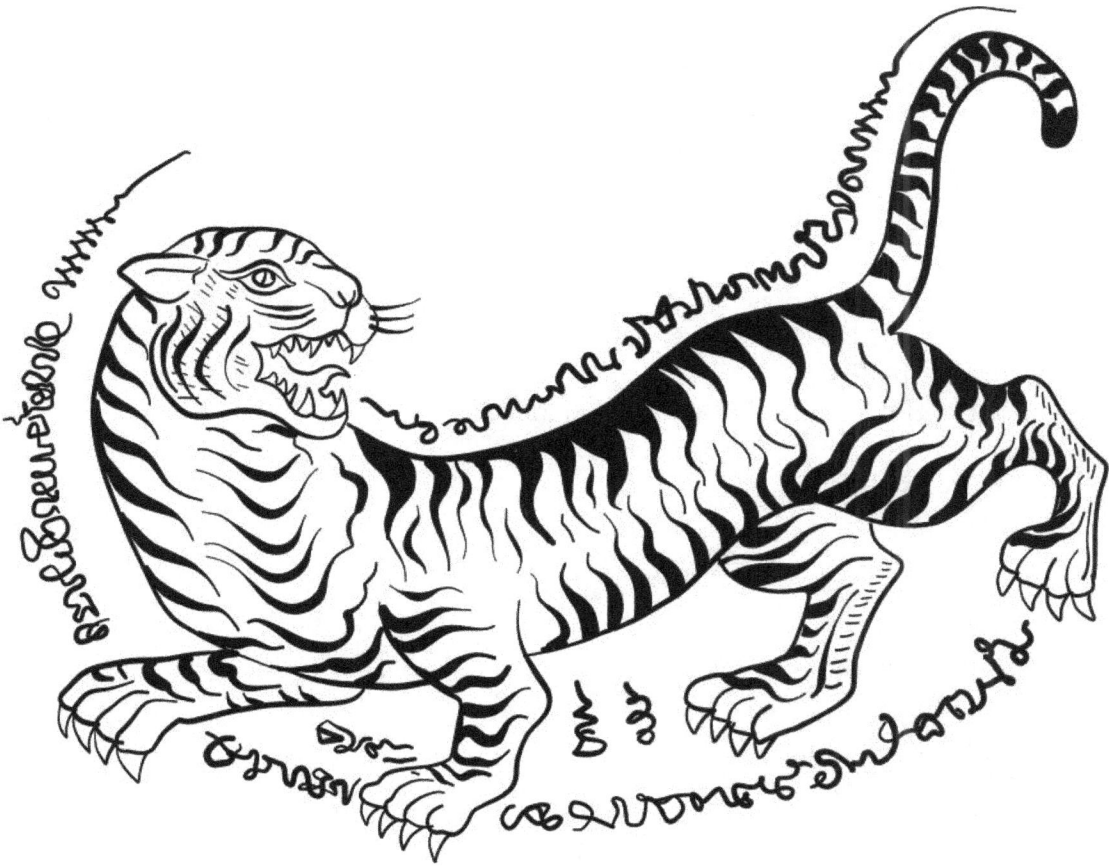

Krabi Krabong
The Tiger Sword of Thailand:
The Science of Fighting with Eight Arms!

Prof. Dr. Anthony James MSc.(Clinical Herbology), DNM(C), ND(T), MD(AM), DOM(Acu), DPHC(h.c.), PhD(IM), PhD(Hospitallar Medicine h.c.), DMM, RAAP, UTTS

Inquiries should be addressed to: Anthony B. James
c/o Meta Journal Press, NAIC INC.
5401 Saving Grace Ln, Brooksville, FL 34602 • 706 358-8646

nativeaic@somaveda.com
WWW.ThaiYogaCenter.Com

Printed in the U.S.A.
Cover Design: Arash Jahani (https://arashjahani.com/)
Inside Cover Illustration by Anthony B. James

Original art and photography by Anthony B. James
Typography by Anthony B. James
Design art and original design by Anthony B. James
Additional Images Licensed use under Adobe Stock Images
Additional Images Licensed use under Dreamstime Images

Revised Edition: ISBN: 978-1-886338-35-7

ISBN: 978-1-886338-35-7
52995 >

9 781886 338357

Special Thanks and Credit for this book to:

First and foremost, I dedicate this new book to GM Phaa Khruu Samaii Mesamarn who was my teacher and mentor in Buddhai Sawan Krabi Krabong arts and sciences. Additionally I also want to include in this dedication the other members of the Buddhai Sawan clan past and present including Maa Kruu Mesamarn, Ajahn Pramote Mesamarn and all the Buddhai Sawan crew who have and are also making sincere contributions to preserving the Thai and South-east Asian Fighting Arts and science.

There is no way this project could have come to fruition with out the aid and assistence of Dr. Julie Ann James, my wife. Julie has kept the ship afloat and helped create the space needed for such a huge and time consuming project.

SUGGESTED WAIVER

Please note that the author and publisher *of* this instructional book is not responsible in any way whatsoever for any and all injuries which might occur by reading and/ or following the instructions herein. Any or all of the material contained within may be under the auspices of local law. It is the reader's responsibility to be aware of his responsibilities under the law.

It is essential that before following any of the activities, physical or otherwise, herein described, the reader or readers should first consult his or her physician for advice on whether or not the reader or readers should embark on the activities described herein. Since the physical activities described herein may be too sophisticated in nature or difficulty, it is essential that a physician be consulted.

The material contained herein is the exclusive property of Ajahn ANTHONY B. JAMES and may not be copied or reproduced in any form whatsoever without the expressed written permission of the author. This material is presented for the author's students' primary use as an adjunct to actual class participation and is no substitute for competent personal instruction. Please see the Appendix in back of this book for some training sources and recommendations.

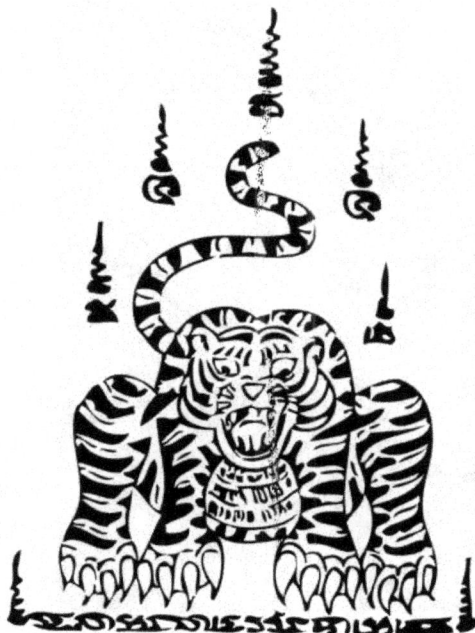

Author's Preface

Prof. Anthony B. James, *MSc.(Clinical Herbology), DNM(C), ND(T), MD(AM), DOM(Acu), DPHC(h.c.), PhD(IM), PhD(Hospitallar Medicine h.c.), DMM, RAAP, UTTS, MSGR./CHEV., Ordained Native Monsignor Native Bishop, Eastern Orthodox Catholic Church of the East in Brazil, Dean, Professor, Director of Education and Traditional Medicine.*

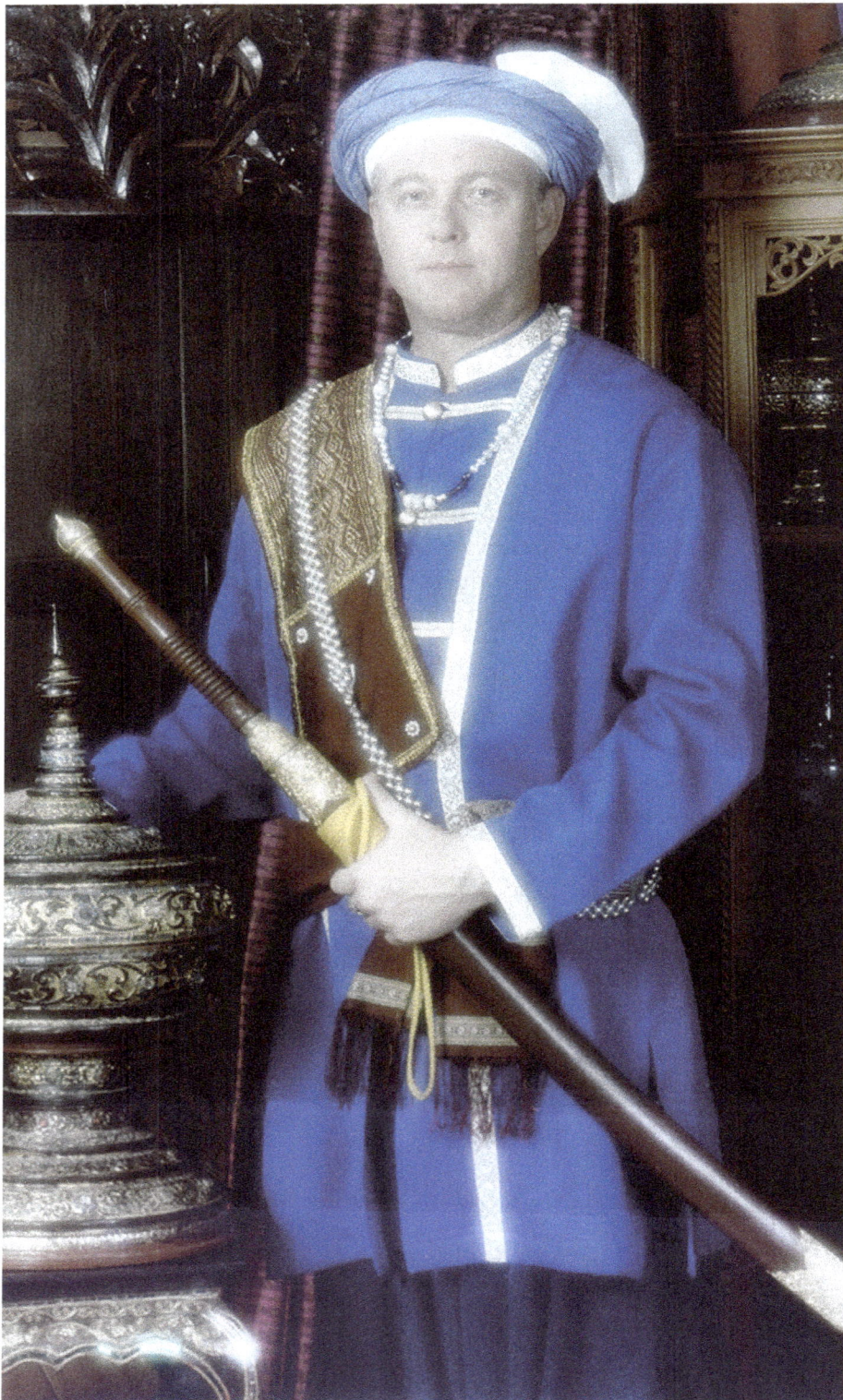

Ajahn (Gold Sash), Kruu Krabi Krabong

Buddhai Swan Sword Fighting Institute 1986

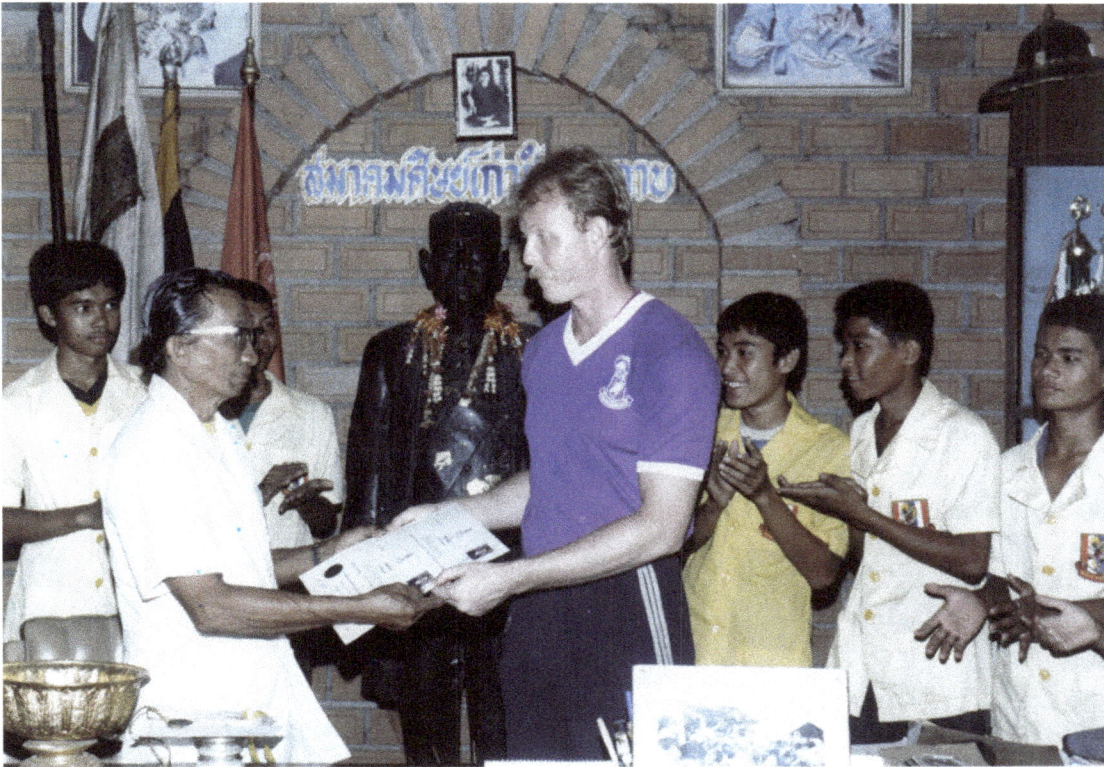

I have an extensive martial arts biography and history. My martial arts training and practice began at age eleven while living at Ft. McPherson, Atlanta Georgia at the base recreation center and gym (building 155). In 1966 there were many Vietnam Vets who were cycling in and out of "Ft. Mac" either for the base VA Hospital or the base Stockade where several famous prisoners were held. My family was there for the hospital as my father, disabled in Korean conflict, was a long-term patient there. I was one of the "Base Rats" i.e., children of both active and retired vets in service there who basically spent our time, when not in school, roaming the base… Rec center, the pool etc.

There was a group of Vietnam Vets, Non-coms and officers who would regularly be at the rec center. It was then and there I had my first   informal but regular training in self-defense and martial arts. I was a "puny" lad and I think they took pity of me as at that time I was susceptible to being bullied.

I never stopped! I am not listing my entire martial arts biography of training and accomplishment here. I will add some of it to the end of this project. I do want to say however, that long before I encountered the Thai Arts and specifically Buddhai Sawan Krabi Krabong system and Grand Master Phaa Kruu Samaii Mesamarn. I was already an expert teacher and practitioner of several different martial arts with multiple Black Belt and formal recognitions in teaching in several systems which did not use the "Black Belt" type of ranking (Colored Belt based ranking system).

I had been teaching and practicing Sijo Fong style *Wing Chun* Gung Fu, *Tang Soo Do Mu Duk Kwan*, American Karate (Lloyd Garrard, Joe Corley, Bill Wallace, Jeff Smith system) since the 70's. Transitioned to Danny Inosanto Style Kali and JKD as well as *Arnis de Mano*, Guro Jorge Lastra style *Lastra Maharlika*, GM Leo T. Gaje Jr. Filipino *Pekiti Tersia and Indonesian Pendakar Suyadi "Eddie" Jaffri style Pencak Silat* in 1981. 1981 is the year Khruu Alphonso Tamez, former teacher of the Inosanto academy, introduced me to both JKD (Bruce Lee fighting method) and BSKK.

Several years later, in 1986, I became the second non-ethnic Thai to be fully certified as a Buddhai Sawan, Kruu Krabi Krabong or traditional teacher of Thai sword in the Buddhai Sawan (*Pootaisawan*) lineage (After Kruu Alphonso J. Tamez, who was the first *"Falang"/ non-ethnic Thai* BSKK Kruu). From 1993 - 2008, Ajahn, Kruu Dr. James, Medical Doctor, Traditional Naturopath, Ayurveda

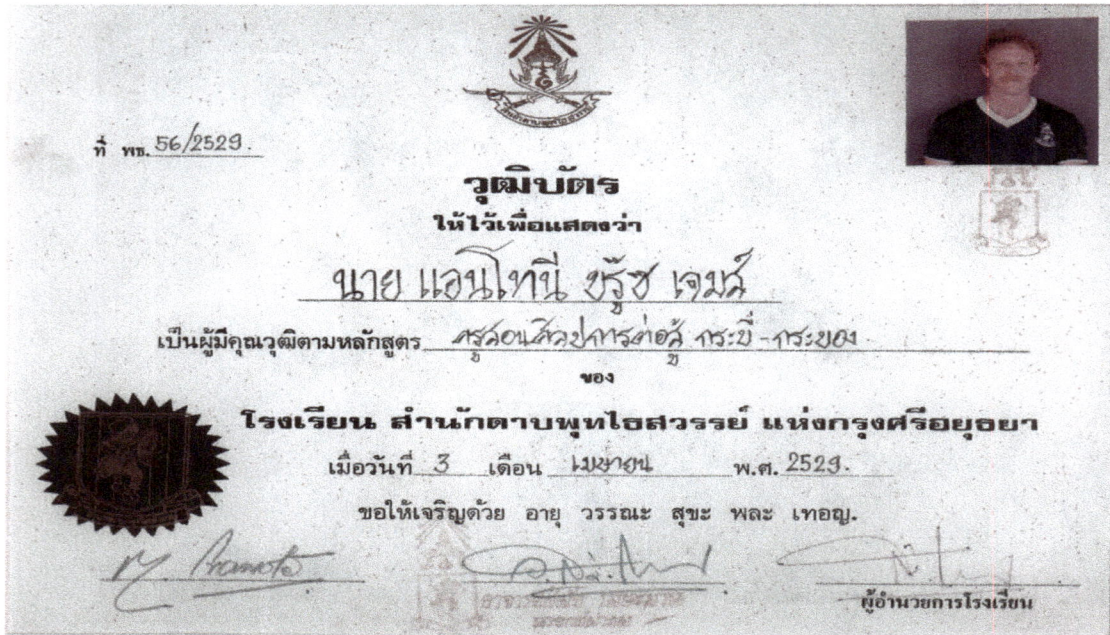

Clinician and professor of Oriental Medicine, served as President and Director of Education for The International Thai Therapist Association or ITTA from 1992 to 2008. Dr. James now acts as President and Director of Education and Clinical Services at the Native American Indigenous Church Inc. (NAIC) in Brooksville, Florida and is dedicated to preserving the unique heritage of indigenous, traditional medicine and healing sciences of Thailand.

Dr. James, has written over twenty books and hundreds of videos on Thai arts and culture, teaches both in the USA, South America, West Indies, Europe, India and Thailand. (Visit https://BeardedMedia.com and or Amazon.com for books etc. by Dr. Anthony B. James)

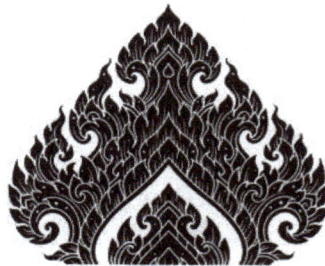

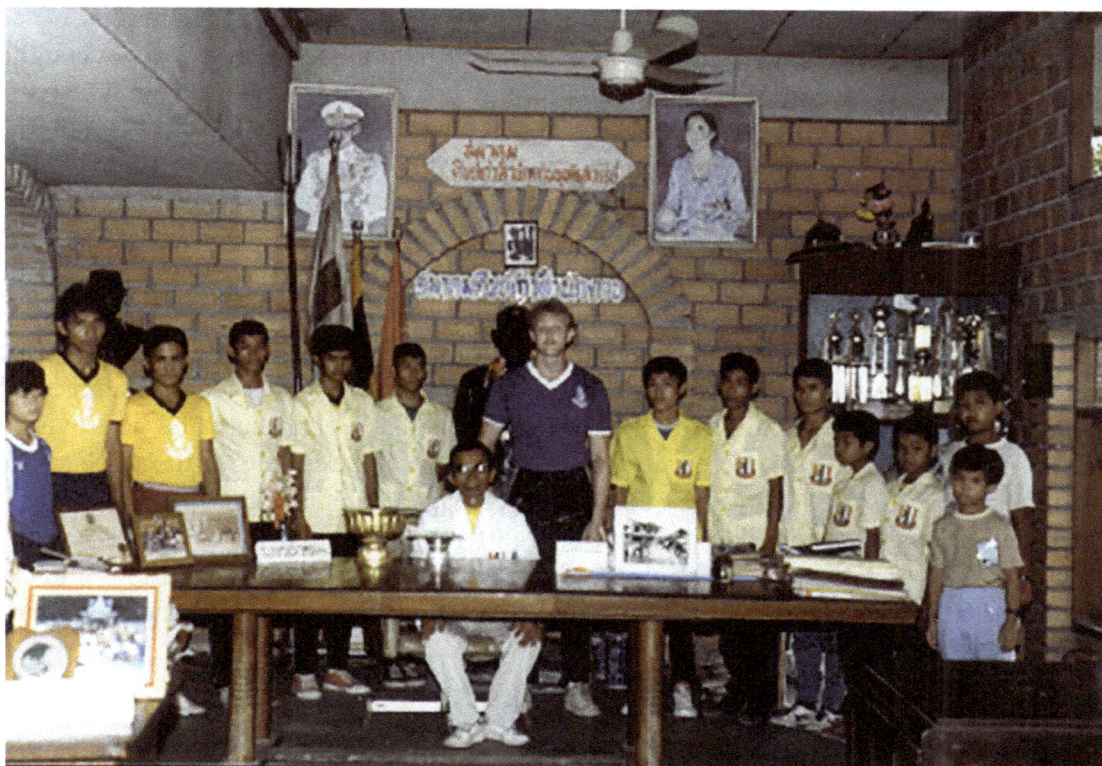

Buddhai Sawan Recognition as Kruu and group photo at Buddhai Sawan, Nongkam, Thailand

Furthermore, the effective fighting techniques derived from classic *Muay Thai* are now quite common as they have been integrated into the practices of almost all combative arts in modern times. Smart martial artist developed the attitude of "if you can't beat them… join them". What is not generally known is that Muay Thai is a safe, competitive sport, derived to a large degree from ***"Krabi Krabong, The Tiger Sword of Thailand: The Science of Fighting with Eight Arms"***

This edition *"Krabi Krabong: The Tiger Sword of Thailand: The Science of Fighting with Eight Arms!"*. is a revised and updated edition of the book *"Kabri Kabrong, The Tiger Sword of Thailand"*, Meta Journal Press, Atlanta Georgia published by me in 1984. I have added and updated most of the text and of course, most notably the title from *"Kabri Kabrong"* to *"Krabi Krabong"*. Since the 1980's the conventions of Thai Language transliteration to American English have been clarified in use. I now feel this is a better way to say the name.

It's been a bit of a struggle over the years as there is no exact way to say to translate many Thai words into American English! Regardless of how an English Speaker says it… *"Krabi"* or *"Kabri"*, we are still speaking of my experience in "The Tiger Sword" or "Science of Fighting with Eight Limbs" which I was trained in by Grand Master (GM) Phaa Kruu Samaii Mesamarn in particular and other notable Ajahn's and Master teachers such as GM Pramote Mesamarn and Ajahn Maa Mesamarn.

I acknowledge the other Ajahn's and teachers past and present in the Buddhai Sawan lineage such as Ajahn Alphonso Tamez, Ajahn Tony Moore, Ajahn Jason Webster, Ajahn Arlan Sanford, Ajahn Steven Wilson, Ajahn Pedro Villalobos, Ajahn Ralf Kusler, Ajahn Michael Delio, Ajahn Nut Mesamarn, Ajahn Jira Mesamarn, Ajahn, Guro Danny Inosanto (Inosanto Academy of Kali, Jeet Kune Do) etc.

Forgive me for missing any countries with active Ajahns's or active BS Ajahn's not listed or mentioned in this book, I have been diligently asking and researching who is active in our community for some time. Any omissions of qualified teachers are unintentional. If I am made aware of any oversights, I will commit to corrections in future editions. Forgive me for any errors and or omissions in my sharing of original Thai and other non-English language words, terms and concepts as the Native Southern American language speaker that I am! I have tried to italicize *non-English* words to show words that may have more than one translation and or transliteration.

I make no claim that this book an entirely finished or complete or perfect treatise on its main subject!

I ask for forgiveness in advance for all errors and or omissions. I have done much in the way of due diligence and in consulting with my own original handwritten notes and other learned sources where possible. I reached out to many teachers both in the US, Thailand and elsewhere and wherever possible have included their input with credit. If you find this text lacking, please feel free to make recommendations to be considered for future editions. I welcome, applaud and am open to doing what we can as a community together to secure the future of all Krabi Krabong traditions both traditional and or eclectic. Of course, as an "Ajahn" I am prejudiced to preserve especially the traditions and teachings of the Buddhai Sawan School of The Tiger Style of Krabi Krabong, of which I am most familiar.

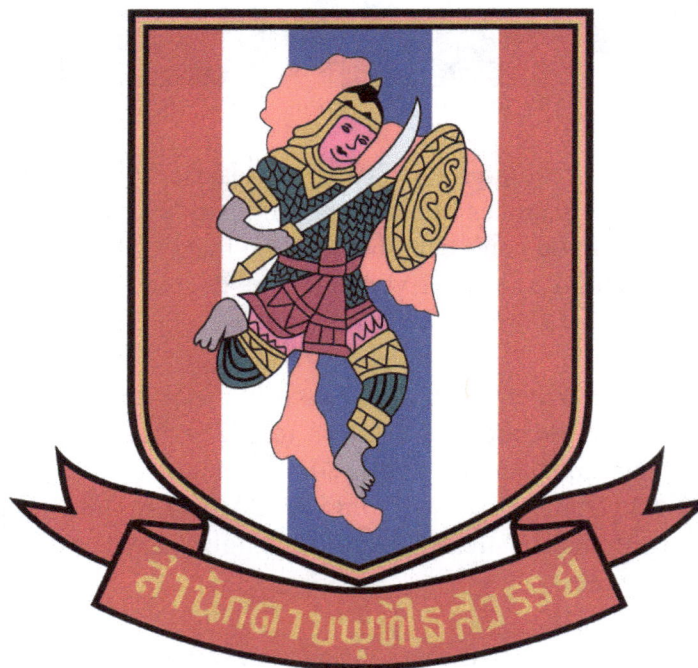

Thai Buddhai Sawan Krabi krabong Logo

Please note! *This Krabi Krabong textbook is not intended to be a Buddhai Sawan Krabi Krabong* **"How To"** *lesson plan! This book is intended to be a supplement text cover many bases from the history, the Thai culture and people in our school lineage and heritage to examples of the Thai martial arts and sciences we are working to preserve and pass on to future generations of both Thai and Falang alike! It is my personal story and journey, my relationship with this amazing traditional art and science as well as the people who cared enough to pass some of it on to me. Buddhai Sawan is uniquely "Thai" but as original and authentic cultural heritage of indigenous peoples of Thailand it also must be recognized and preserved as a valuable World Cultural Heritage!*

Table of Contents

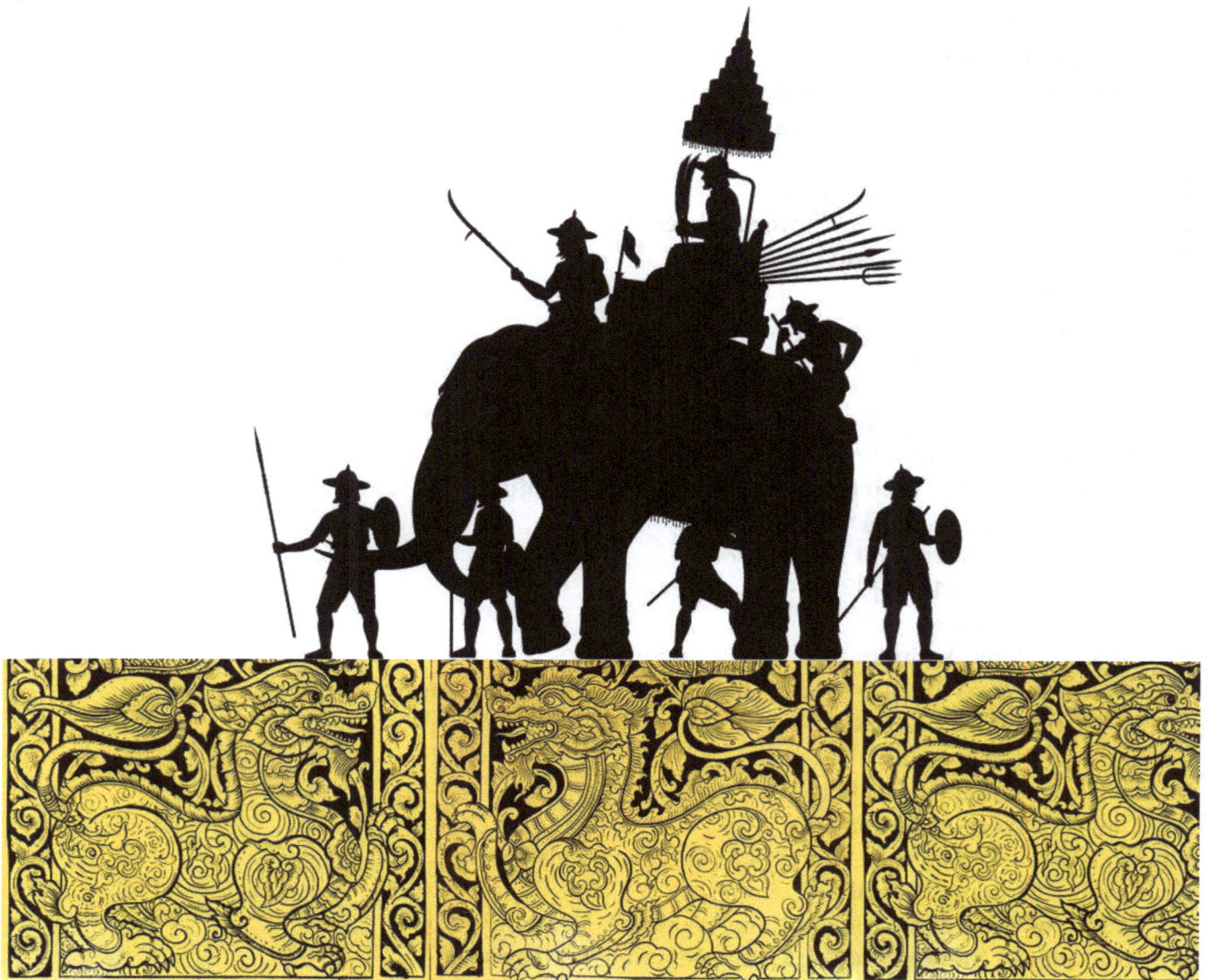

Traditional Tiger "Sak Yant Suea" Talisman Tattoo for Protection

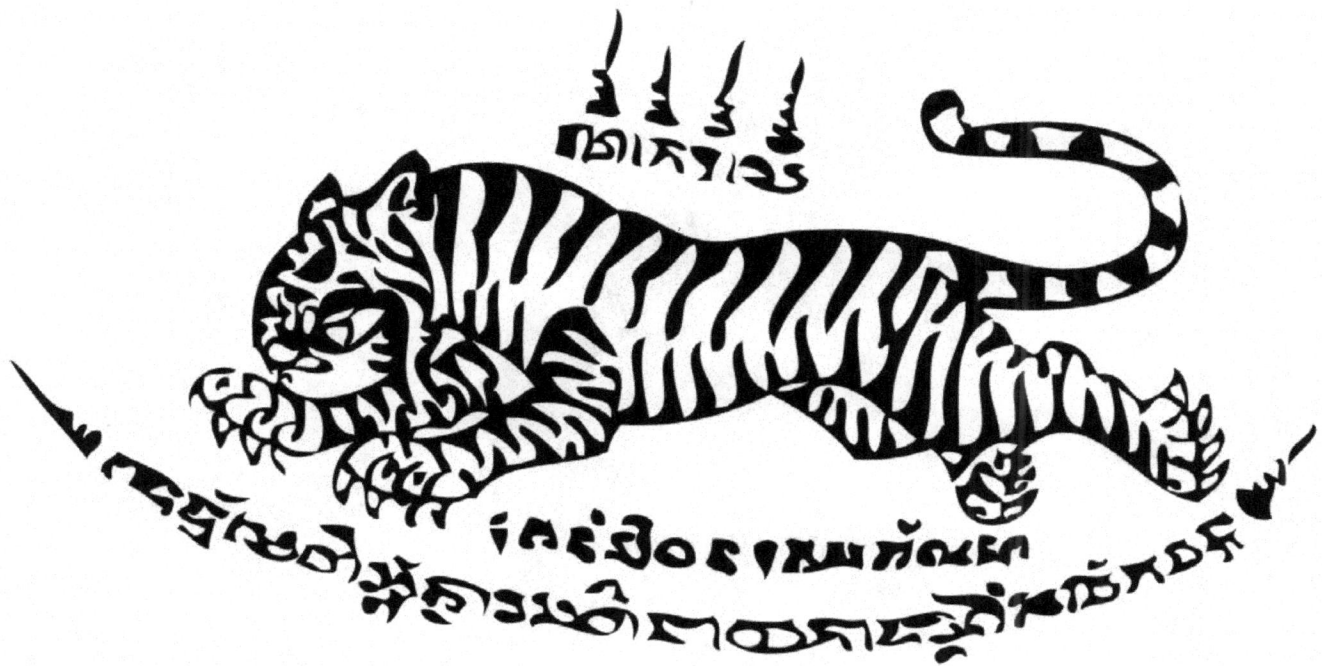

Maps of Thailand

THAILAND *is situated in the southeast part of Asia between 5 degrees north parallel, and 21 degrees north parallel, 97 degrees east latitude and 106 degrees longitude. It is bordered by the countries of Myanmar (Burma), Kampuchea (Cambodia), Laos and Malaysia. The terrain is quite diverse with sub-tropical lowlands bordered by the gulf of Siam in the south, the spacious great central plains of Menam Chao Phraya, and the craggy mountains of the Northern Highlands.*

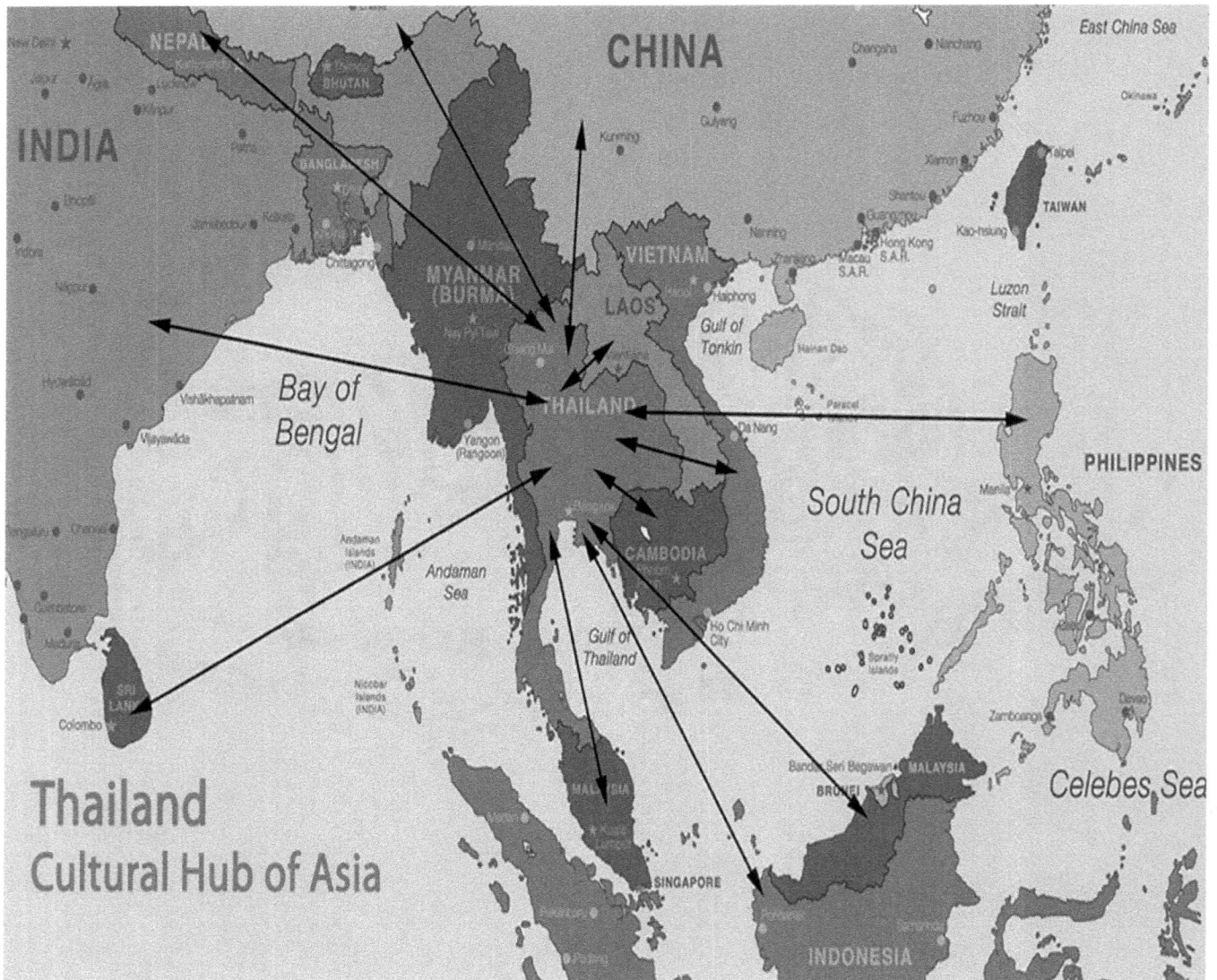

Note how centrally located in South and S.E. Asia the country of Thailand is not far geographically from India, China and the Philippines by land, river or ocean.

When we speak of the origins of "Krabi-Krabong", in particular the "Buddhai Sawan" style, we have to consider the trade routes, historical migrations, multi-ethnic cultural influences which in the past were from West to East- India to Japan (Nippon) to Philippines and from North to South from Tibet and China to Malaysia and Indonesia and back!

Krabi Krabong is not only or just literally only the "***The Tiger Sword***" or "***Science of Fighting with Eight Limbs***", or simply the "Eight Limbs". Could not we just as easily refer to the eight (8) primary indigenous ethnic cultures or the eight countries of origin or the eight systems originally organized under the "Tartarian- Tartaria" which eventually became Europe, Asia, Asia Minor, South East Asia etc. to be assimilated over many, many centuries into cohesive systems of warfare arts with a common spiritual focus tying them together?

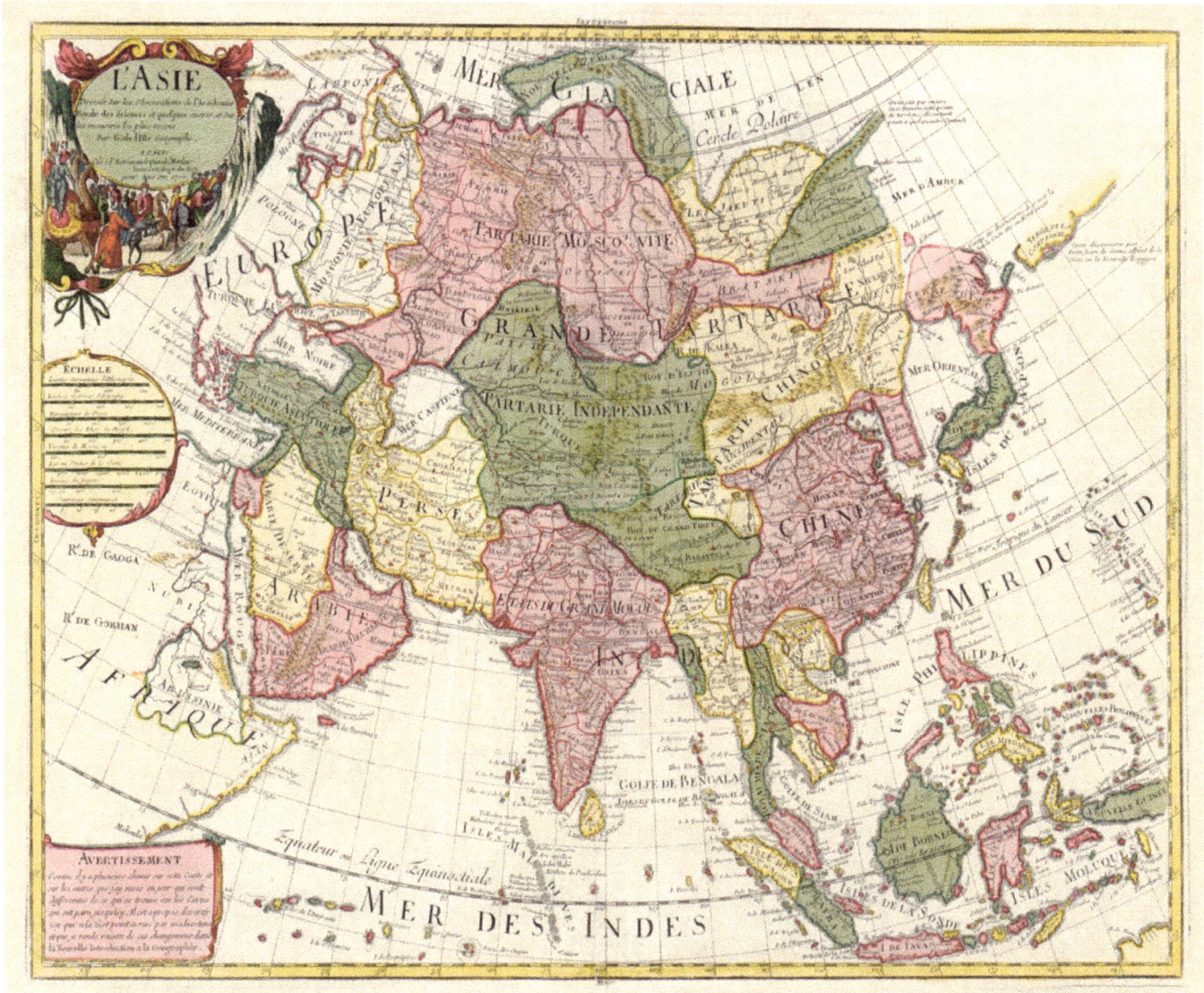

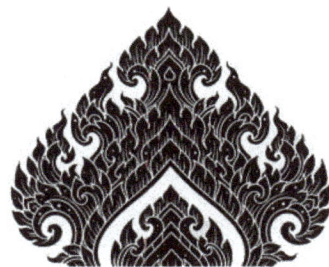

Origins of the Thai people

In this text we will be referring frequently to the country of Thailand... Please note that the country's name was originally Siam. The name was changed from Siam to Thailand officially in 1933. There is some controversy and differing opinions as to the historical origins of the Thai people who came to found and or establish the country of Thailand. Formerly the country was called Siam, a designation which likely originated with the Portuguese, who were among the first westerners to visit the region.

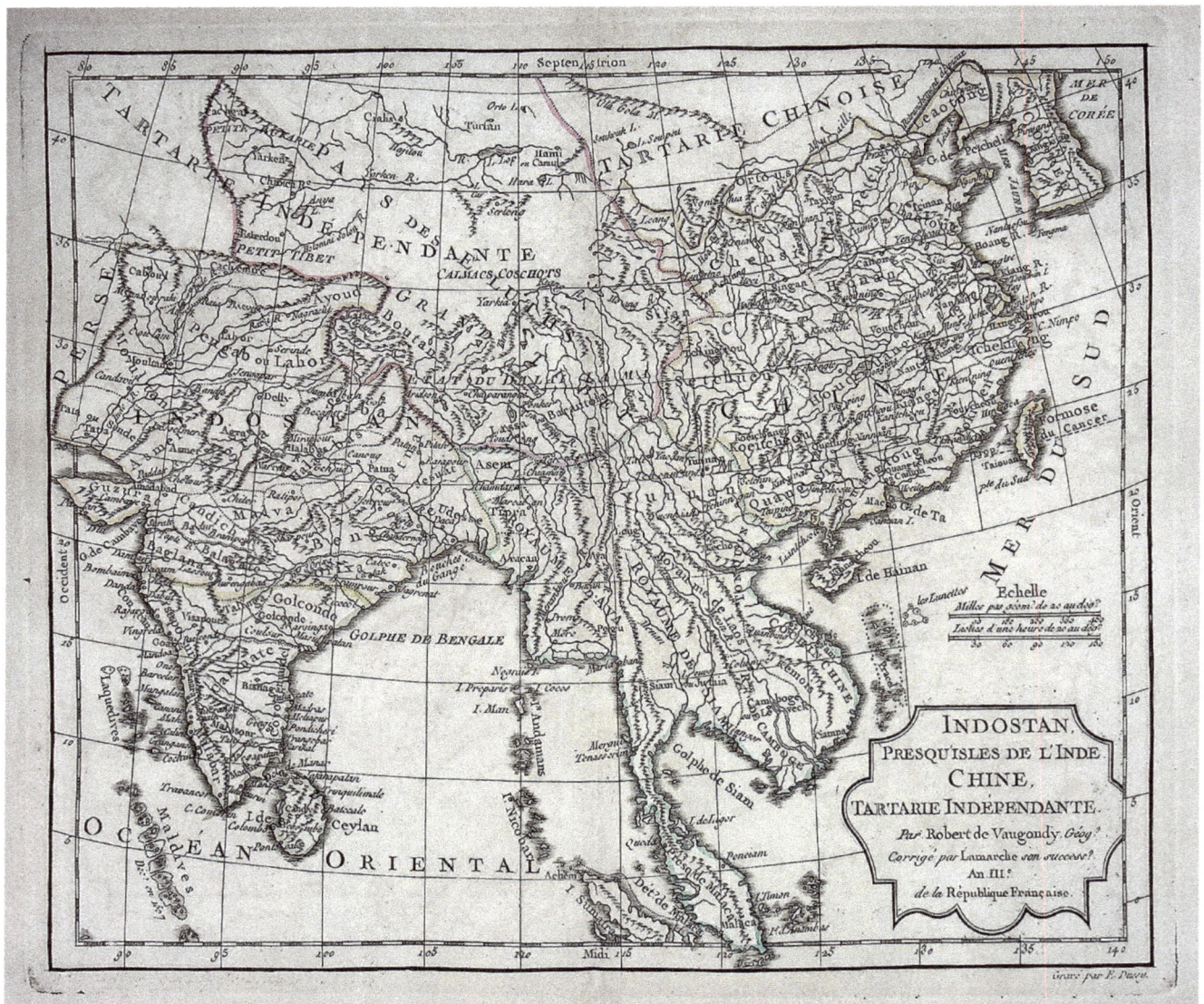

Indostan, Indo-China, Independent Tartaria Map. 1794 edition by Robert de Vaugondy/ Delamarche, from "novel Atlas Portatif", posthumously published. Vaugondy was appointed geographer to the King Louis IV in 1760. Hand colored Copper plate engraved on velum, published in Paris, original in private collection of author.

Some historians estimate that the origin of the Thai people is in the north of what we today call Siberia. In a later period, these people immigrated in a southerly direction and eventually settled in China in an area from the Huang Ho River downward. About 2,500 years before the Buddhist Era (about 4,500 years ago) displaced Chinese people crossed the Thien Cham Mountains and began to infiltrate the basin of the Huang Ho River. They met the "Ai Lao" or "Thai" people there. The Chinese called these people "*Tai*" and or "*Ai-Lao*" meaning powerful and prosperous. The Thai themselves have always preferred to refer to themselves as "*Meung Thai*".

Recently, this migratory theory has been challenged by the discovery of prehistoric artifacts in the village of *Ban Chiang* in the *Nong Han* District of Udon Thani province in the Northeast [28]. There is evidence of bronze metallurgy going back 3,500 years, as well as other indications of a far more sophisticated culture than any previously suspected by archaeologists. Based on these discoveries a new origin theory has been proposed: the Thais may have originated here in Thailand and later scattered to various parts of Asia, including China.

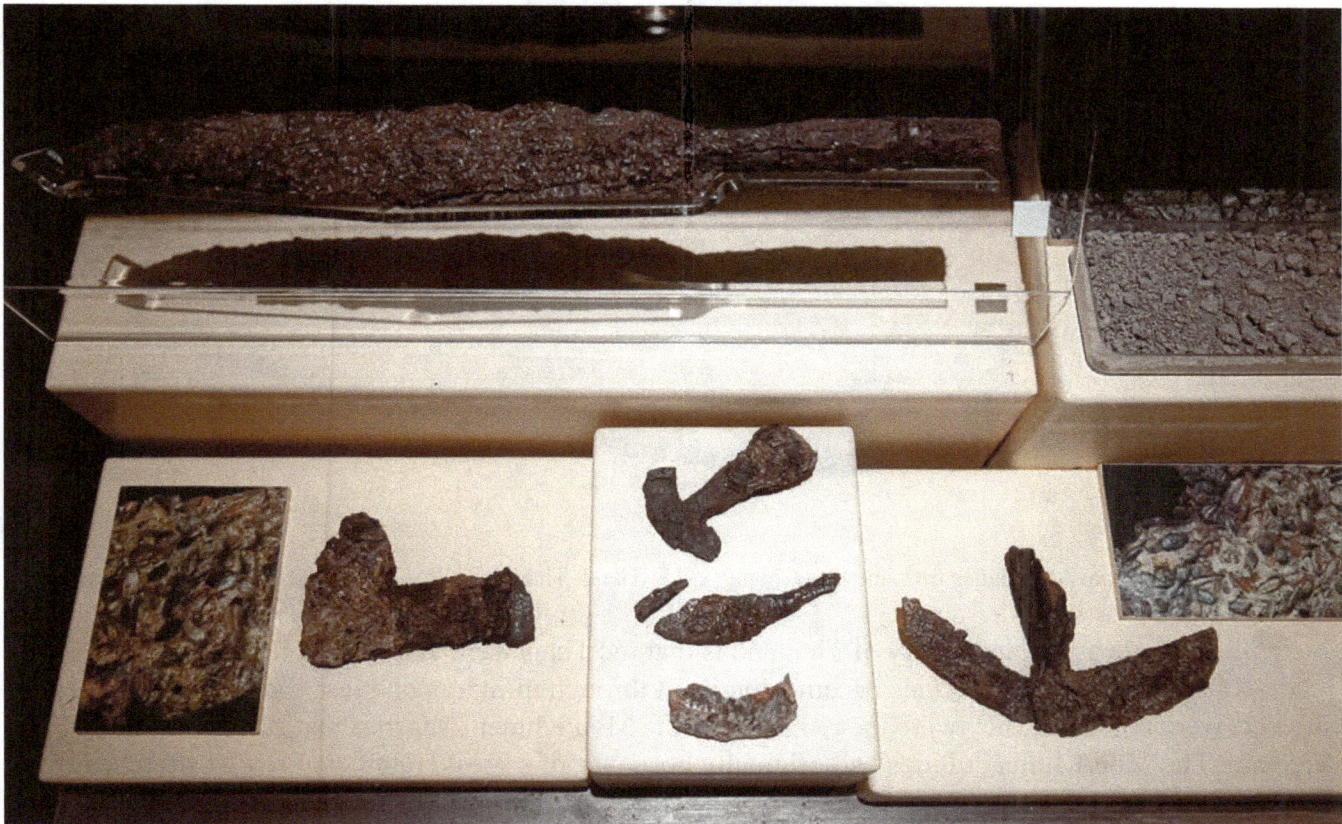

Prehistoric Thai Weapons from the Ban Chiang, Udon Thani, Thailand - World Heritage, archaeological site

When you consider the Ban Chiang weapons? Especially pay attention to their shape! The oldest swords, possibly some of the oldest intact bronze age swords known to exist, are medium length, long handled and double edge... Thick at the base/ hilt and full tang... These were no toys! Based on their antiquity, they could predate Chinese, Indian and proto-european (Etruscan, Greek, Roman, Indian, Egyptian etc.) construction and technology for making metal, bladed weapons!

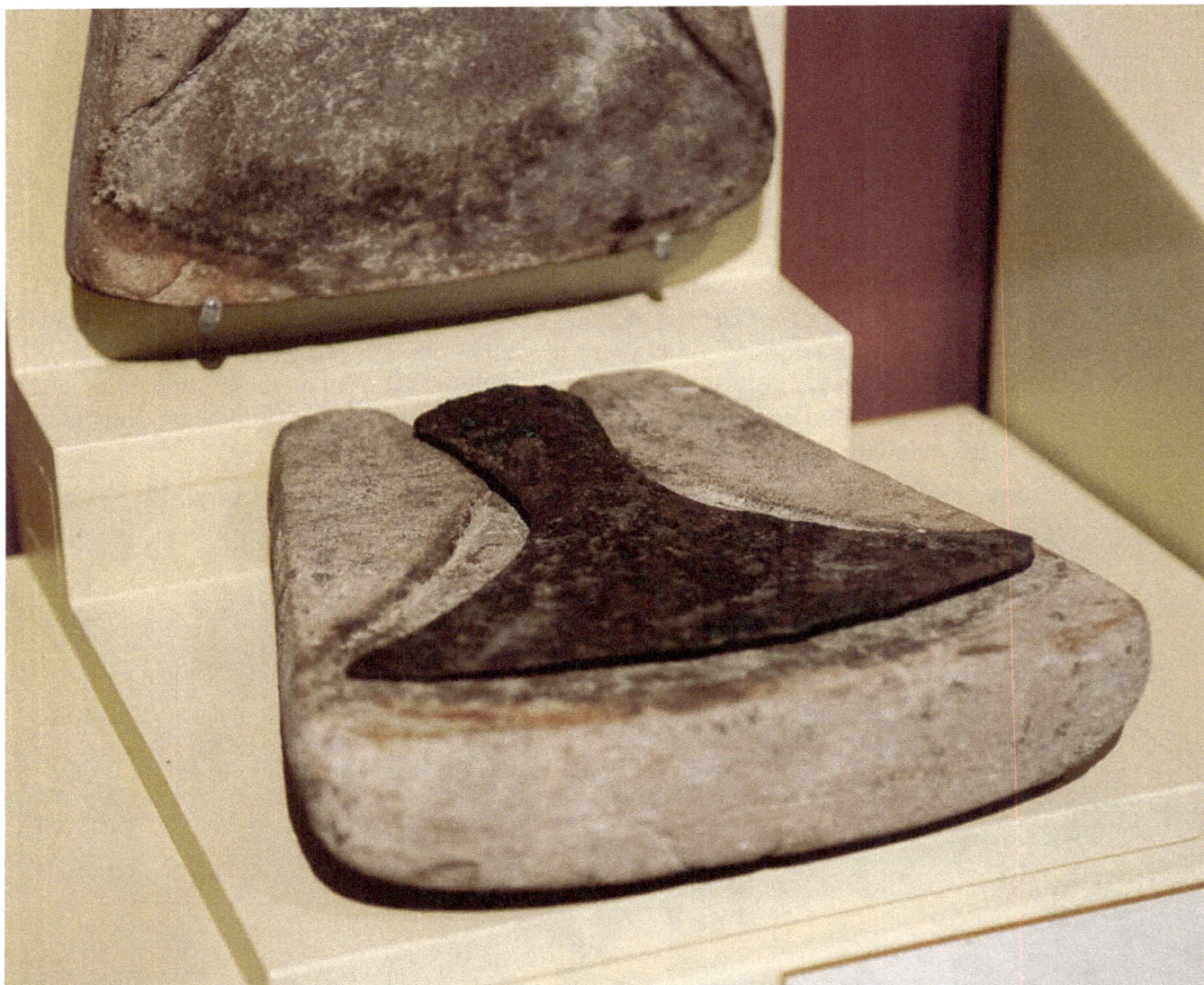
Prehistoric Thai Axe Blades from the Ban Chiang, Udon Thani, Thailand - World Heritage, archaeological site

A significant note about the history of Thailand is that the Thais were not the first inhabitants of Thai land. Although over time the Thais became dominant through military conquest, the majority of their subjects were not Thai. They were the remnants of the Mon/Khmer dynasties that ruled from India to Vietnam. The Mon/Khmer cultures had originally been part of a great Hindu empire that stretched from Tibet to the Philippines by way of South and Southeast Asia. Historically this Hindu empire dating back to the lifetime of the Buddha (500 BCE) was known as the Majapahit (Maharlika) empire (Virgil Apostal: Way of the Ancient Healers). Thai rulers in their expansion and southward migration gradually adopted many of the ways and cultures of the people they came to rule.

According to researchers (Braun and Schumacher: Traditional Herbal Medicine in Northern Thailand: White Lotus 1994) [2] "The Thai Court followed a pattern of adopting (and adapting) the Indianized culture of the people they conquered. During the Ayutthaya period Indian influence thus became firmly established in many domains: the concept of divine kingship replaced the original Thai version of feudalism; Indian Law - The Code of Manu - became the model for Thai law; The astrologers surrounding the king were Hindus; the alphabet was modeled after the Indian (and Khmer alphabets); Indian literary genres and metrics were introduced and of course Buddhism became the national religion.

However, the main Thai migration became in earnest around 200 b.c., when the Han dynasty of China began their wars of expansion. Out-gunned and out-numbered, the Ai-Lao fought fiercely and were for quite some time able to maintain a relatively autonomous region in what today we call Yunnan Province, China…

Still today, when traveling in Yunnan a traveler can still hear the Thai Language spoken there! The longevity of the Thai people in that region against wave after wave of invading armies was mostly due to their reputation of being greatly skilled warriors.

They were eventually overcome with the region being integrated into the Chinese Szechuan empire. Most of the ethnic Thai refugees chose to leave, to migrate their entire society south, rather than be under submission to the foreign invaders.

I want to say that in my opinion this whole invasion, war and refugee situation was traumatic to the survivors and their children. This in some ways explains the ferocity with which later generations would fight to maintain their independence and freedoms… To be THAI!

The "*AI-lao*" eventually divided up into three branches: The Shans who mainly settled into what we now call Myanmar (formerly "Burma"), The "*Ahom*" who continued their migration east to what is not called Kampuchea (formerly Cambodia) and Vietnam (now Republic of Vietnam), and the : "*Lao-Thai*" who took up residence north of the "Mighty Mekong" river in what today is named after them… the country of Laos.

The Thai people who stayed behind, still in Sichuan (Szechuan China), eventually created the independent Kingdom of *Nanzhao*. *Nanchao* and greater China continued to be in a state of war for over 100 years. They fought mostly as enemies but over time eventually fought as allies against the Tibetan tribes to the west who were also migrating south along the Mekong. One of these originally Tibetan tribes, the "Burmans' ' eventually became the Thais' worst enemy.

By the end of the 9th. Century a.d., the now isolated kingdom of *Nanzhao* was dismantled and absorbed into the Chinese empire. It was also around this same time that new Thai states were forming in Laos and Siam. (The term "*Siam*" is derived from the Sanskrit word for GOLD. This indicates a long traditional association of Thai with Gold!

The new Thai States now had only to contend with the hill tribes and indigenous aboriginals. The most entrenched local culture they had to deal with was that of the previously mentioned Mon/ Khmer civilization, famous in today's historical narrative as the original founders of Angkor and Angkor Wat Temple in Cambodia (*Campochia*).

Khmer/Mon/Sumatra/Majapahit Cultural Influence

The influence of the "Indianized" Khmer/Mon culture in all aspects of traditional life in much of the central and western regions of Thailand should not be underestimated. Most aspects of life reflected this influence including the colloquial traditional medicine practices of the era. For a little over 300 years Mon/Khmer and Sumatran cultures were the dominant cultures of the region. Khmer culture was a Vedic culture, revering the Hindu art, culture, and text of classical India including the practice of traditional or classical Ayurveda.

According to the World Health Organization (WHO) Legal Status of Traditional Medicine and Complementary/ Alternative Medicine: The use of traditional medicine is documented in the stone inscription of the King *Chaivoraman* (around 1182-1186) who ruled the Khmer Kingdom (Thai/ Cambodia) which is in the northeastern part of Thailand. Traditional medicine was used in 102 hospitals which, at that time, was called *'Arogyashala'*.[25] [31] "

It can be inferred that Khmer doctors practiced Ayurveda and Vedic medical astrology (Jyotish). Remnants of this ancient Indian Ayurveda practice may be seen today in the *Anantasuk* TTM (Anantasuk School of Thai Traditional Massage) practice of medical astrology (Anantasuk Korosot) as taught at the Wiangklaikangwan Industrial College TTM curriculum in Hua Hin, Thailand.

From the 9th to the 11th century, the central and western area of Thailand was occupied by the Mon civilization called *Dvaravati*. The Mon share the same lineage as the Khmer and settle in southern Burma later. The influence of *Dvaravati* includes *Nakhon Pathom, Khu Bua, Phong Tuk*, and *Lawo* (Lopburi). *Dvaravati* was Indianized culture, Theravada Buddhism remained the major religion in this area.

After 1157 CE [25] (Chockvivat, Chuthaputti, Chamchoy), Mon heavily influenced central Thailand. Khmer cultural influence was brought in the form of language, art and religion. The "Sanskrit '' language entered Mon-Thai vocabulary during the Khmer or *Lopburi* Period. The influence of this period has affected many provinces in the north-east such as *Kanchanaburi* and *Lopburi*.

The Architecture in *"Angkor"* was also constructed according to the Khmer style. The Khmer built stone temples in the northeast, some of which have been restored to their former glory, those at *Phimai* and *Phanom Rung* and further cultures are stone sculptures and stone Buddha images. "Politically, however, the Khmer cultural dominance did not control the whole area but exercised power and cultural influence through vassals and governors." [32] Sumatra/Sumatran culture, a Buddhist culture until the 1300's when it became officially Muslim, controlled or ruled southern Thailand and especially peninsular and coastal Thailand.

Originally called the *Melayu* Kingdom (*Malayu, Dharmasraya* Kingdom or *Jambi*), it was absorbed by the Kingdom of Srivijaya. Sumatra was a vassal state in the *Majapahit* (*Magadha- Maharlika*) Empire which stretched from Sumatra to New Guinea.

The "Indianized" Sumatran/*Majapahit* culture and trade were factors in early Thai history from the Ayutthaya and Bangkok periods first because these were the culture and belief systems of the indigenous people who lived there before being assimilated into the Thai Kingdom and secondly due to trade and exchange.

The common traditional medicine of the *Majapahit* was Ayurveda and their famous martial arts were based on *Kalaripayattu* (Malaulat language: South India- Kerala dialect). Thai Kings, traders and military would have encountered all of them. The vast *Majapahit* Empire controlled the seas and trade routes of the Asian, SE Asian, Malaysian, and Indonesian archipelago all the way to the Philippines. Keep in mind trade is a two-way system and ancient trade always included medicine and medicine practices.

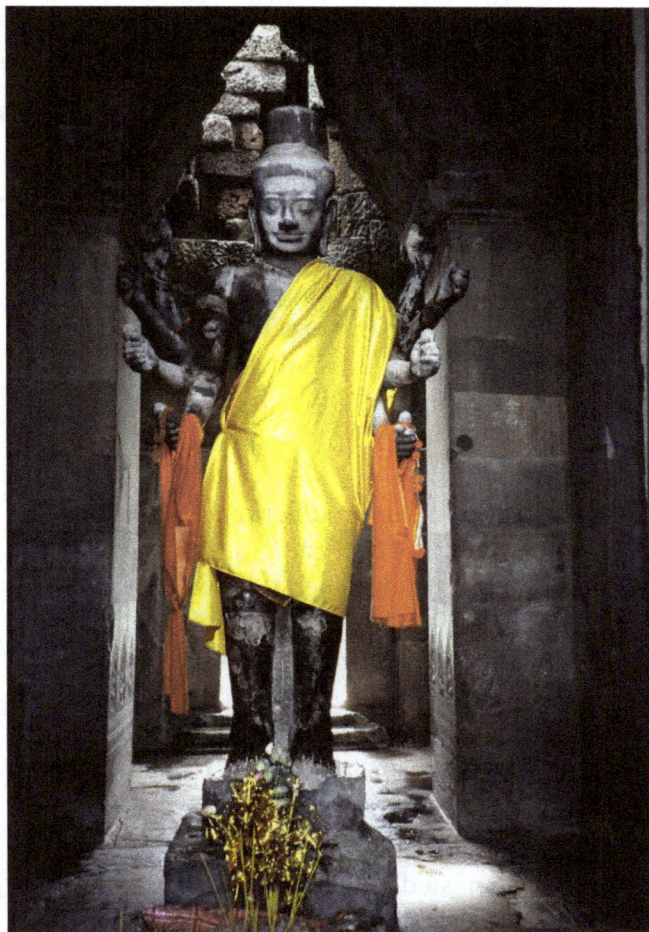

The history and research I have given here is far from complete! My intention is to give a background and context for the birth and development of the Royal Thai Traditional Medicine and Healing system (Indigenous, Traditional Thai Medicine: Indigenous, Traditional Thai Massage: ITTM) which we simply call the Southern or Royal style.

Image is of the Hindu deity "Shiva" from Angkor Wat Campochia (Cambodia)

The Mon/Khmer cultures had originally been part of a great Hindu empire that stretched from Tibet to the Philippines by way of South and Southeast Asia.

Historically this Hindu empire dating back to the lifetime of the Buddha (500 BCE) was known as the Majapahit (*Maharlika*) empire (Guro Virgil Apostal: "Way of the Ancient Healers").

The *Magadha-Majapahit*- Javanese Kingdom of the 6th. Century A.D. were the largest, strongest and wealthiest empire in South and South-east Asia stretching from Northern India South and East to as far east as Vietnam, Malaysia, Indonesia to the Philippines and of course entirely covering Thailand (*Siam*).

The "*Khymers*" had elite royal troops called the "*Nayers*" who were a significant element of their "*Shatria*" or warrior caste. Following the Aryan Indian Martial Ancient Martial Arts teaching of "*Kalaripayattu*" passed through many generations and survives today mostly in South India, Kerala. The "*Nayers*" would have been trained from childhood to be masters of combat arts including psychological, mental, emotional as well as physical warfare using every conceivable type of weapon…

both naturally found such as in animal parts like teeth and claws to found objects such as sticks and stones. Their arsenal of weapons included many types and configurations of shields, bladed weapons long and short, throwing weapons, archery and ballistic slings of similar complexity to that of the s ophisticated Chinese armies of the same day.

Battles between the migrating *"Ai-Lao"* and the *"Khymers"* began roughly in the 11th century. The AI-Lao were successful in displacing the ruling elites of the Khymer and in 1238 managed to capture and control two of the main *"Khymer"* cities and created the first seed nation which was called *"Meung Thai"* or "Land of the free".

In 1253 the Northern Thai kingdom of *Nanzhao* was invaded by the Mongol armies of Kublai Khan, routing the remaining Thai and forcing a new wave of southward migration. As the newcomers arrived in huge numbers, swelling the ranks of the predecessors, the now "Thai" Kingdom grew quickly and began to spread its influence and dominance of the region. Northern Thailand and most of Laos was united under the banner of the Lanna Kings which established the first official kingdoms in *Sri Satchanalai* and then *Sukhothai* in modern Golden Triangle region of Northern Thailand…Chiangrai Province. In and around 1350 a.d., the Thai capital was moved from *Sukhotai* south and west to *Ayutthaya* where Prince U-Thong established a firm site, capital of Siam for 400 years before being conquered by the Burmese.

Please note: The Thai did not entirely abandon their original Chinese influenced heritage, according to Braun and Schumacher and other sources (Andaya, Reid, Wyatt, Wood). The Thai Kings up to this last century, looked to the emperors of China for official recognition. They maintained relationships formally through tributes made to the Chinese court and through trade. Large numbers of Chinese have always been part of the great migrations into Thailand bringing with them their cultural identities.

We can see the Chinese influence in *Wat Raja-Orasarem* (Korat) and in *Wat Po* (Ayutthaya/ Bangkok) temple design. *Wat Raja-Orasarem* is literally a Chinese style temple built according to Feng Shui principles with eight sides, large circular doors, Chinese style mosaic decorations throughout and a grand multi-tiered pagoda right in the middle. Wat Po is adjacent to the Reclining Buddha statue, an actual Taoist shrine and large guardian statues in the Chinese style posted at all entrances and exits. *Wat Raja-Orasarem* is allegedly the first temple built by the Thai people and the way to Thonburi after the sacking of Ayutthaya by the Burmese, officially ending the Ayutthaya period. The temple *Wat Orasarem* is also famous for its stone medical inscriptions

There is a strong indication of Chinese Martial influence in Thai Traditional Martial arts. Many of the traditional weapons and accoutrement ("a soldier's outfit usually not including clothes and weapons, usually used in plural, also referring to items of traditional armor and uniforms for dress, parade or combat) of the Krabi Krabong arsenal to this day are referred to by their original Chinese names. These original Chinese derived practices were found, alive and well, in the **Buddhai Sawan Sword Fighting Institute (*Hall of Revivals National Culture* – Nongkam & Ayutthaya Thailand)** in the South, but more common in the Krabi Krabong schools of the North.

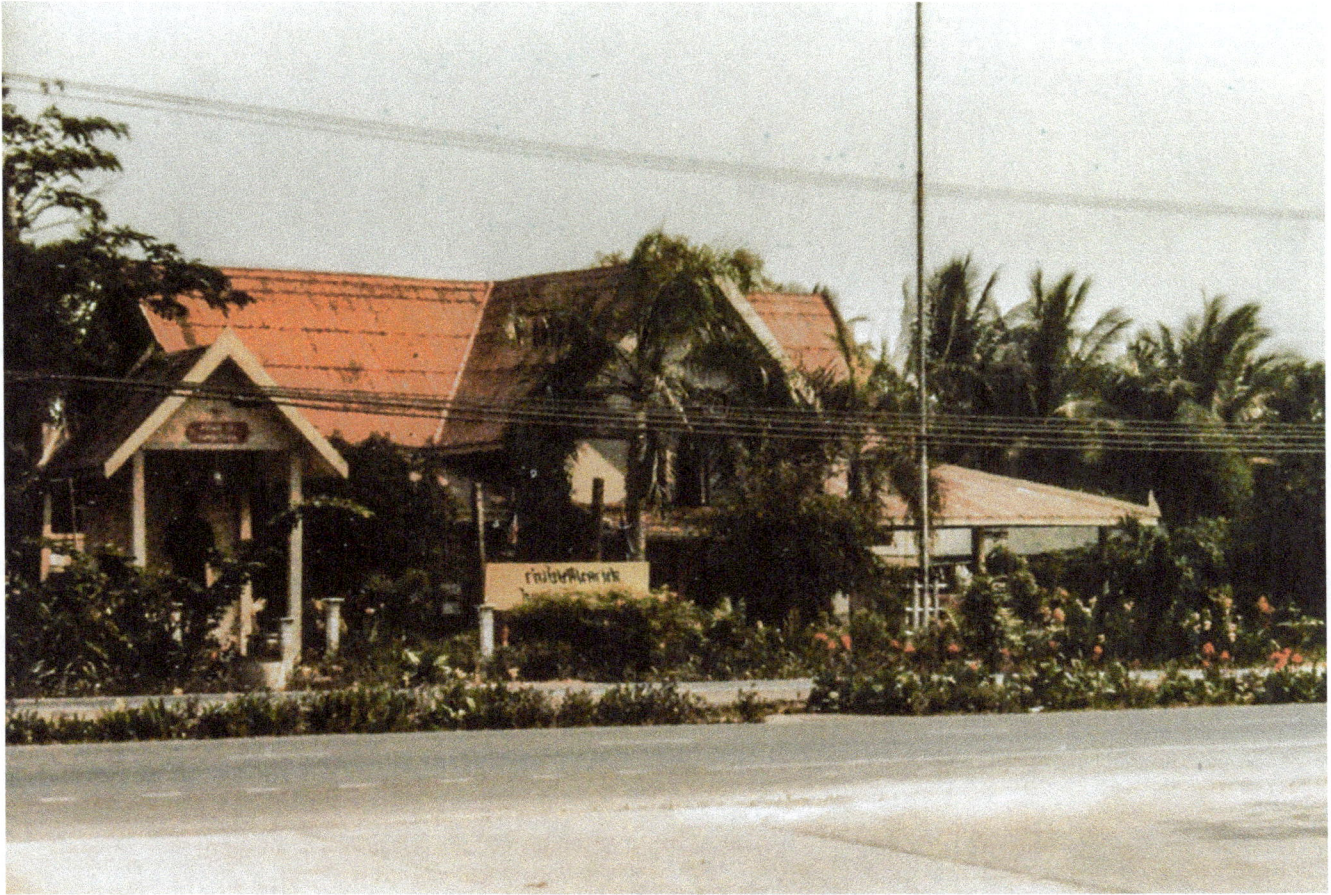

Buddhai Sawan Hall of Revivals National Culture Center and Thai Sword Fighting Institute:
5/1 Phetkasem Rd. Nongkam, Thailand. Photo Circa 1982.

The Thai's apparently split up into two main groups as they traveled along the southern part of China. One group eventually settled in the area of what is now Northern Thailand establishing the "*Lanna*" kingdom (Chiang Rai- Chiang Mai).

The second group settled further south and after being conquered by the Khmer (Angkor: Kampuchea) founded the kingdoms first of *Sri Satchanali* and then **Sukhothai**.

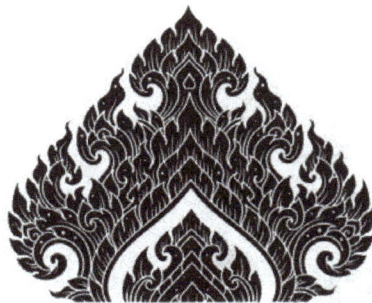

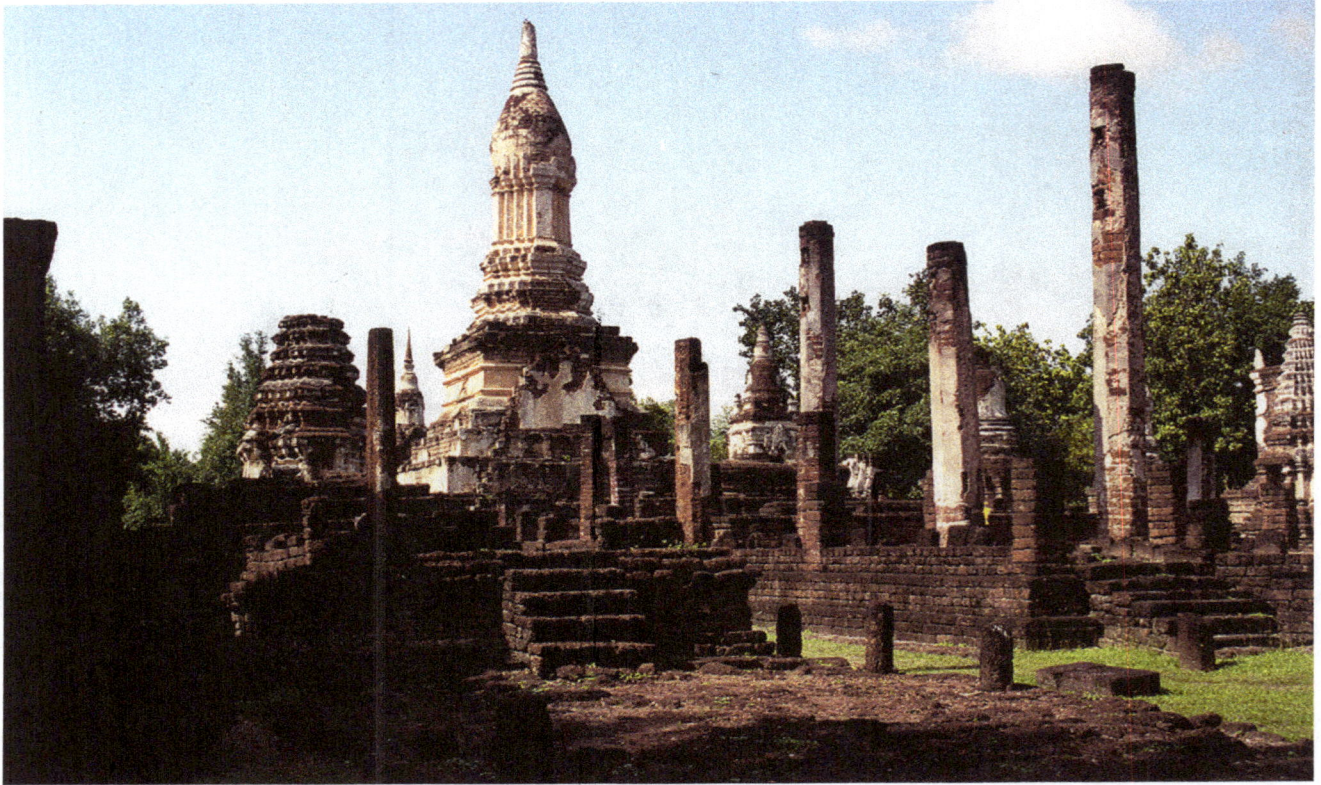

Wat Chedi Chet Thaeo "The Temple of the Seven Rows" old city Sri Satchanali

According to "Wiki"… "Prior to the 13th century, Thai migrated into upper Chao Phraya valley and established a town named Chaliang (Thai: เมืองเชลียง), which means "City of Water" on the bank of the Yom River. Chaliang gradually developed into an important trade center between China and Khmer Empire. The Chinese called the town "Chengliang". The town enjoyed a substantial autonomy under Khmer until 1180, during the reign of *Pho Khun Sri Naw Namthom* who was the local ruler of Sukhothai and Sri Satchanalai, Khmer general *Khomsabad Khlonlampong* started to take control directly and introduced prohibitive taxes. In 1239 *Pho Khun Bangklanghao* and *Pho Khun Pha Mueang* decided to rebel and declare independence from Angkor and captured Chaliang. Chaliang then became part of the Sukhothai Kingdom." (https://en.wikipedia.org/wiki/Si_Satchanalai_Historical_Park)
The Thai united and set up a large territory which they called "*Narn Chao*".

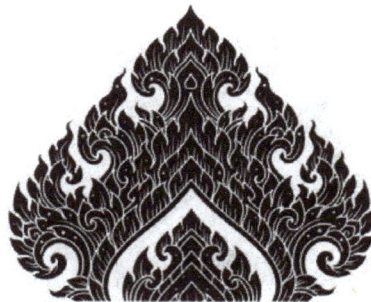

They controlled this area from approximately 648/B.E. 1192 to 1253/B.E. 1797, for a total of about 600 years. The Chinese continued to press the Thai people until finally a famous Chinese emperor, *Ng Quan Lee Cho* or Kublai Khan, lead a large army against the *Narn Chao* and conquered the territory. Most of the Thai's fled further South, although there are still ethnic Thai people in the area of Yunnan China today.

The remaining Thai people settled in the area in which they now predominate and set up independent kingdoms (*Ngoenyang, Sukhothai, Chiang Mai, Lanna*) much like those of India of the same period.

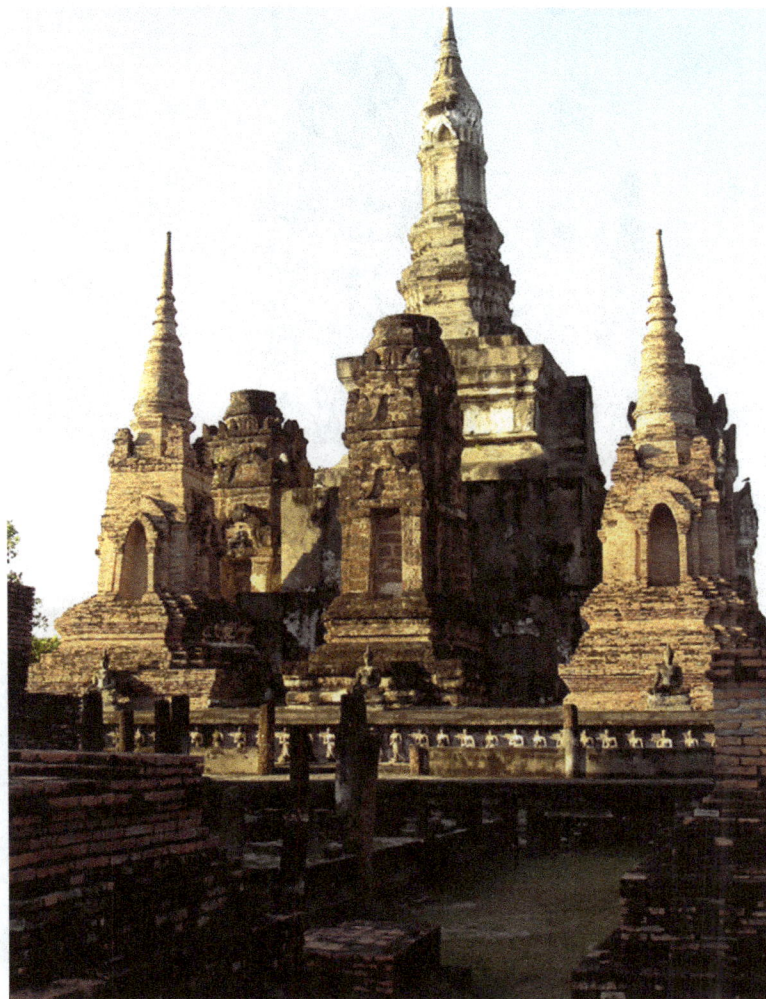

Wat Mahatat "Phra Chedi Mahathat, Phumkhao Ban"Sukhotai, Thailand

These kingdoms were assimilated into the kingdom of *Ayudhya* (*Ayudthaya/ Ayutthaya*) around 1369/B.E. 1913.

Krungthep Dvaravati Sri Ayudhya

Krungthep Dvaravati Sri Ayudhya was the Capital of Thailand for 417 years under 33 kings of the *Ayudhya* Dynasty. At its peak, this Capital was larger and cleaner than contemporary European capitals. *Ayudhya* was founded on an island bordered by the *Joburi* River on the North, the *Pasak* River on the East, and the *Chao Phya* River to the West and South.

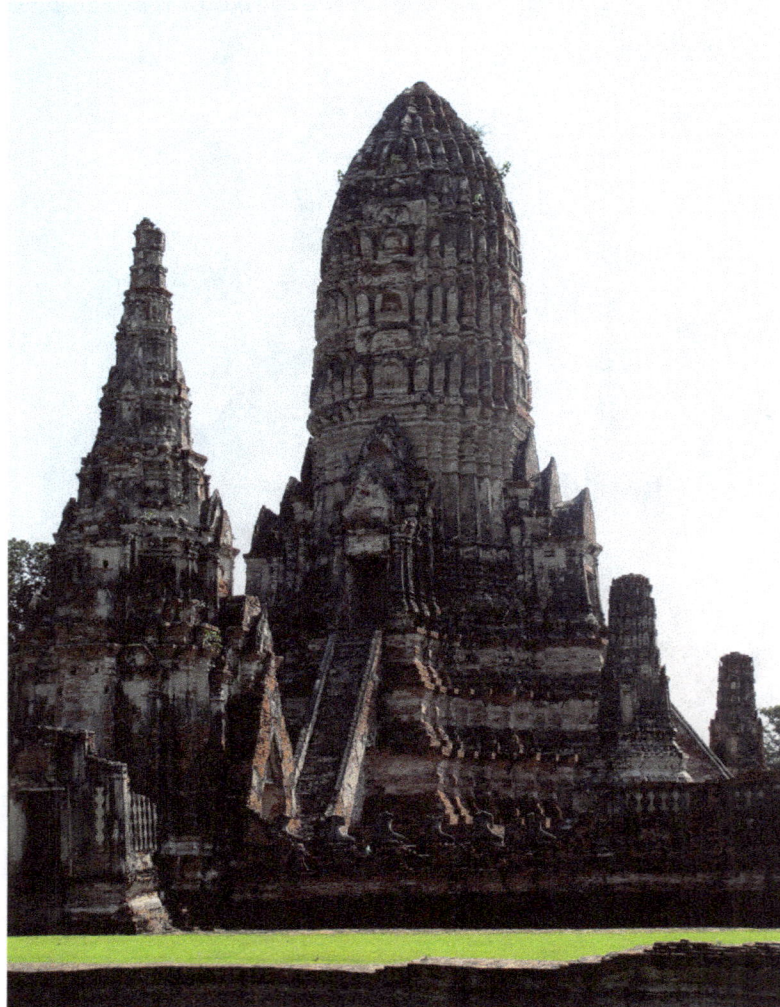

Wat Chaiwattanaram, "Prang", Ayudthaya, Thailand

At its peak, this capital was larger and cleaner than contemporary European capitals. Ayudthaya was founded on an island bordered by the Lopburi River on the North, the Pasak River on the East, and the Chao Phraya River to the West and South.

In the 11th century A.D., before the Thai settled there, existed a small outpost settlement formed and named *Ayudhya* by the Khmer who dominated this region of the "*Menam Chao Phraya*" river. *Ayudhya* was of some importance because it formed a boundary with the U-Thong (a vassal State under the *Sukhothai* - the first integrated Thai kingdom called the "Cradle of Thai Civilization"). The first King of *Ayudhya* was *Somdej Phra Ramathibodi*. The kingdom was ruled in succession by 33 kings for 417 years, from A.D. 1350 to A.D. 1767.

The *Ayudthaya* kingdom was ruled in succession by 33 kings for 417 years, from A.D. 1314 to A.D. 1767.

When the original buildings of the new capital were completed in A.D. 1353, the first Ayudthaya King U Thong ``Ramathibodi'' (A.D. 1314 to A.D. 1369) constructed *Wat Phutaisawan (Phootaisawan)*, "The Temple of the Brave and Free Buddha's Heart" on the site of his first residence at *Wienglak Ayudthaya*, next to the riverbanks of the Chao Phrya river. This area became known as *"Wienglak"* (the place of iron) neighborhood. It was a center for the manufacture of steel and weapons and in particular knives, spears and swords. Even today, one can travel through the Wienglak streets and see the many shops and foundries where weapons including swords are still made in a traditional manner.

On the grounds of *Wat Phutthaisawan*, King U Thong established his swordsmanship school. It is this wat or temple which became the home and training ground for the Krabi Krabong Fighting Arts. These Arts were practiced by the monks as a form of meditation and physical exercise and the monks, themselves, were responsible for training the royal family and the military. Essentially, this tradition continues to the present day under the authorizations of the various Ajahn's in several different countries.

The arts and sciences taught and passed down through generations, enabled Thailand over a period of four centuries to eventually become the greatest military power in S.E. Asia and the only nation in the region to avoid colonization and colonial domination by the western powers of the 16th. 17th. And 18th. Centuries.

The period of settlement in the old capital of *Ayudthaya* is significant, in that it was marked with numerous altercations and battles with the neighboring country of Myanmar (Burma). Battles mean training of warriors for battle in the systematic martial arts of *Krabi Krabong & Muay Boran*.

Similarly, *Wat Chetuphon* (*Wat Po*- later rebuilt in Bangkok during the re-establishment of the sovereign Thai Nation... **Wat Pho** (Thai: วัดโพธิ์, pronounced [wát pʰōː] (🔊listen)), also spelled **Wat Po**, is a Buddhist temple complex in the Phra Nakhon District, Bangkok, Thailand. It is on Rattanakosin Island, directly south of the Grand Palace.[2] Known also as the **Temple of the Reclining Buddha**, its official name is ***Wat Phra Chetuphon Wimon Mangkhalaram Ratchaworamahawihan***[1] (Thai: วัดพระเชตุพนวิมลมังคลารามราชวรมหาวิหาร; pronounced [wát pʰráʔ tɕʰêːt.tù.pʰon wíʔ.mon.maŋ.kʰlaː.raːm râːt.tɕʰá.wɔː.ráʔ.máː.hǎː.wíʔ.hǎːn]).[3] The more commonly known name, Wat Pho, is a contraction of its older name, *Wat Photharam* (Thai: วัดโพธาราม; RTGS: *Wat Photharam*).[4]) (Wiki: https://en.wikipedia.org/wiki/Wat_Pho#:~:text=Wat%20Pho%20%28Thai%3A%20%E0%B8%A7%E0%B8%B1%E0%B8%94%E0%B9%82%E0%B8%9E%E0%B8%98%E0%B8%B4%E0%B9%8C%2C%20pronounced%20%5Bw%C3%A1t%20p%CA%B0%C5%8D%CB%90%5D%20%28lis-ten%29%29%2C,Rattanakosin%20Island%2C%20directly%20south%20of%20the%20Grand%20Palace.)

... was also established as a teaching center for traditional healing and medicinal arts. In addition to the Chinese influence which the Thai brought with them and the integration of the Indian culture via the Mon/Khmer cultures they conquered, there was significant and continuous migration, trade and exchange directly between all of the neighboring states and cultures such as India, Burma, Malaysia, Indonesia, Cambodia, Laos and as far away as Persia and Japan.

The *Ayudthaya* period as it is called is often referenced as the Golden Age with much growth and prosperity.

However, *Ayudthaya's* wealth and Gold gilded temples were envied both by the Burmese to the west and the remaining Khymer/ Javanese empires to the south. At Wat Buddhai Sawan the collected teachings of generations of "Warrior Monks' ' and their lineages were brought together and collected in a manual of arts called the *"Chupasart' '*. This written codification of these arts, adopted by and under the patronage of the Thai Kings created a standardization and cohesion of the arts for many centuries to the present day.

The Martial Arts teachings associated with *Wat Buddhai Sawan* (*Wat Phootaisawan*) were forged on the battlefields of generations and were at the same time practical and functional. Because of the sources being under authority of the Buddhist temple system, mind, spirit and inner development were emphasized from day one as well as the character of practitioners being considered an important aspect of overall fitness for battle.

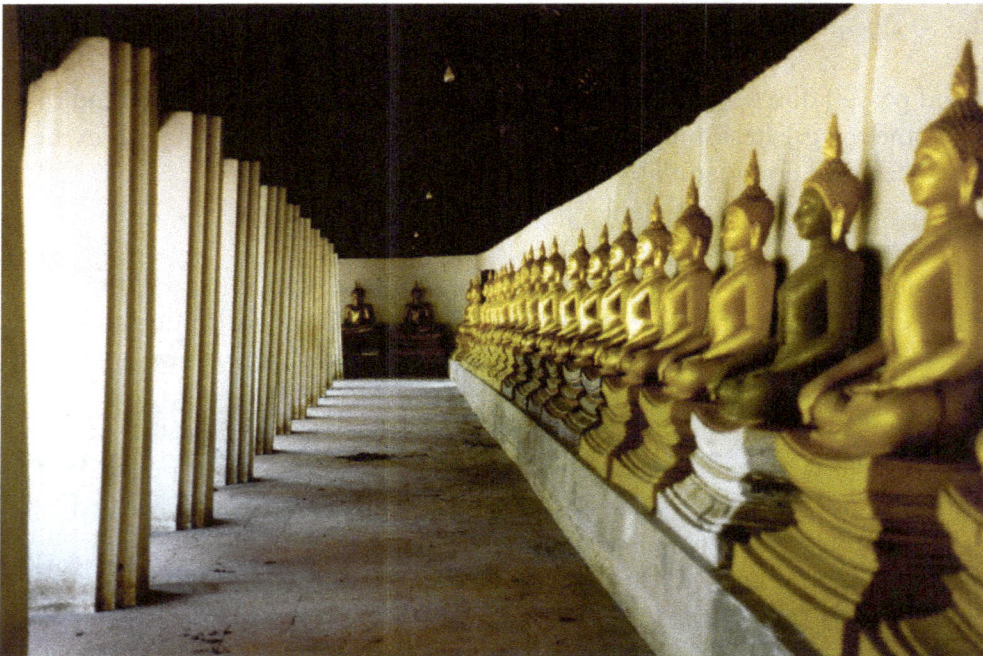

One of the Buddha galleries at Wat Buddhai Sawan "Prang", Ayudthaya, Thailand

The *Ayudthaya* period also marks the founding and construction of the famous *Wat Buddhai Sawan*, on the banks of the *Chao Phrya* river, with its classic Vedic style "Prang" in an inner courtyard and training area, surrounded by the magnificent famed "Buddha gallery, which provided the *Ayudthaya* Kings and their retinue with Spiritual, Martial and medical training and advice.

Burma (Myanmar) was certainly one of the primary sources of cultural influence with a periodically contentious and warlike relationship. The period of settlement in the old Capital of *Ayudhya* is significant in that it was marked with numerous altercations and battles with the neighboring country of Burma.

The Burmese captured the capital of "*Siam*" (As it was called in B.E. 2112) and took most of the population as prisoners back to Burma in captivity. For a time, Siam became a vassal state of Burma.

Around 1582 a.d./ B.E. 2126, The captive Thais, led by the self-declared Thai King *Narasuan*, revolted against the Burmese. King *Narasuan* had become famous for being a great boxer or fighter of the Buddhai Sawan style. King *Narasuan* and the Burmese Crown Prince allegedly met in single combat, mounted on elephants (Elephants = Heavy Cavalry. Heavy cavalry was for royalty!).

They dueled fiercely and King *Narasuan* defeated the Burmese Crown Prince. The Burmese army was defeated and routed by *Narasuan's* militia.

This was the genesis of the freedom for the enslaved Thai people and the restoration of an independent Thai lands and kingdom.

Monument to Naresuan, The Black Prince, Thailand

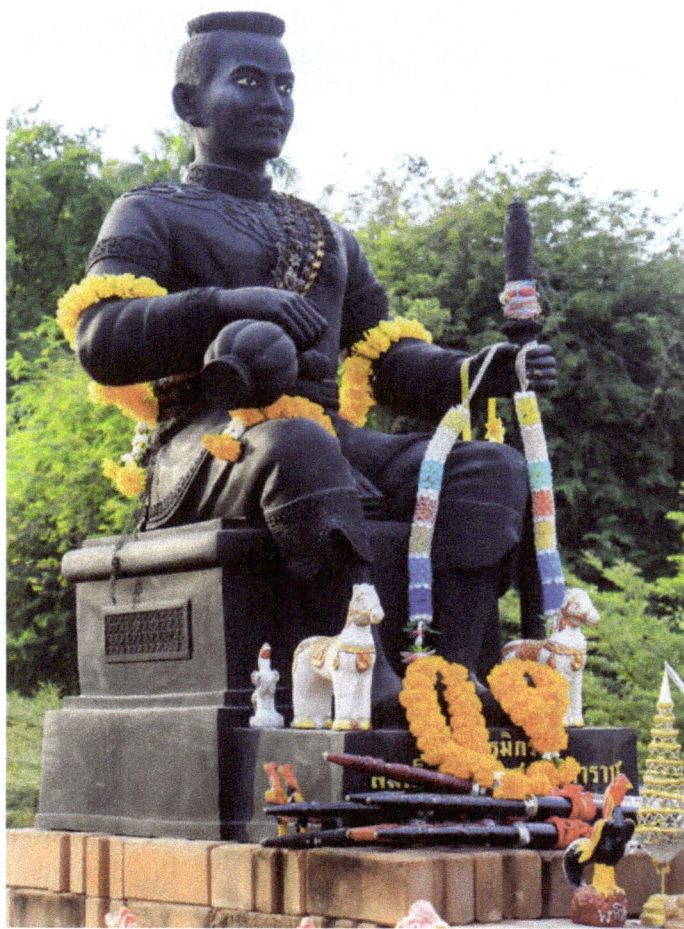

Many of Thailand's greatest or best-known historical warriors, both men and women, spent time at *Wat Phootaisawan* (*Buddhai Sawan*) which was not only a martial training center, but know as an educational center for religious ceremony, medical treatments and a meeting place, famous as inspiring the cultivation of personal discipline for all circumstances of life.

The *Phootaisawan* Buddhist monks were known to serve the functions of teacher, doctor, priest and warrior sometimes interchangeably. These practices continued there until the sack and destruction of Ayudthaya by the Burmese in 1767 A.D.

After this war and for a time after the temple and school fell into disuse and disrepair.

Prince Naresuan was and still is, Thailand's most notable and most famous martial artist. Prince Naresuan was a Thai Royal captive/ hostage in Burma while growing up. During the time in captivity, he was educated in the Burmese fighting arts of "*Thaing*" (Concepts of Martial Arts and personal development incorporating Buddhist Yoga practices of pranayama, meditation and principles of "yielding force" (characteristically shared by modern martial arts such as Tai Chi Gung, Wing Chun Kung Fu, Aikido, Jiu-jitsu and or Judo).

The term "*Thaing*" in Burmese loosely translates into "total Combat" (*Burmese Martial Arts… https:// www.burmalibrary.org/en/burmese-martial-arts*), or "*Bando*" (combat fighting arts originally developed by the Gurkha minority centuries before), "*Banshay*", "*Naban*" (Burmese wrestling), "*Lethwei*" (Burmese Kick Boxing counterpart and in some descriptions the precursor to Muay Boran/ Muay Thai), and Shan style "*Thaing Byaung Byan*".

According to G.M. Dr. U Maung Gyi (Burma/ USA) & Burmese Bando Grand Master related to me in person at the Bando Nationals Port of Prussia, PA 1986: "*No nation has a monopoly of the sunlight*" & "Bando Philosophy "*No system is completely unique. No system is completely independent from external and internal influences. Every system evolves over time by integration, modification and restructuring, resulting in what we then call "uniqueness." Overtime, this unique system will also change.*" (*Myanmar Martial Arts: https://www.burmalibrary.org/en/myanmar-martial-arts*)

Apparently, the ' 'Black Prince '' as he is sometimes called took this Burmese philosophy to heart in applying these principles to freeing the captive Thai people and reconstitution of a nation and heritage which remains today's one of the world's treasures.

There is a mausoleum and statue of the "Black Prince '' there to commemorate. I originally learned of this place not far from the *Phitsanulok* River from GM Samaii as he once described a pilgrimage there in commemoration of the Black Prince's contribution to the legacy and traditions, an aspect of the origins story of *Buddhai Sawan*.

It is also Prince Naresuan who is credited with emphasizing the development and practice of the empty hand arts strongly in conjunction with the weapon-based systems. The methods of attack and defense previously used exclusively in empty hands applications were modified to emulate the combat methods used with weapons. At the time a shocking and unique concept in SE Asian fighting arts. Pre-arranged fighting "duets" were taught and practiced widely.

These "duets" became military drills for readiness for battle and as to gain non-lethal combat experience in peace time to cultivate confidence and a strong spirit. The Black Prince is known to have emphasized public demonstrations and contests/ competitions to engage the public to show they were now strong and not weak. Out of this we eventually see the formation of *Muay Boran/ Muay Thai* as serious training without the occasional, infrequent, lethal consequences of training with "live" blades during peacetime.

GM Phaa Kruu Samaii Mesamarn once told me "… the purpose of "*Muay Boran*" was if you were in combat or war and dropped your weapon, that you should negotiate to live long enough to either get it back or take up a new one!"

We call *Muay Thai*, Thai Boxing a sport safe for babies. It is now taught in all Thai schools from elementary schools to college. However, it is devastatingly effective and sometimes described as BRUTAL… It is, however, no match for Krabi Krabong's deadly efficiency.

The Black Price is recorded to have passed away in 1590 while leading an army against the Burmese. I will reference later the beautiful mausoleum built to honor Prince Naresuan in Phitsanulok city. It is considered a pilgrimage site for *Buddhai Sawan* practitioners and teachers.

Another great fighter referenced in our *Buddhai Sawan* lineage from *Ayudthaya*: early 1700's, Thai King *"Pra Chao Sua"* the "The Tiger King". King *"Suriyenthrathibodi"*, King Sampet VIII (1703a.d.- 1709a.d.). He was noted to be a great and prolific fighter. There are stories of him traveling around the Thai countryside in disguise, without his usual royal retinue of attendants, fighting as a peasant in local or regional fairs and seasonal gatherings! The rules of the ring, observed in Muay Thai contests today, were originally formulated by him. The exceptions being instead of "Ropes binding the fist and arms" we now use safety gear such as Boxing gloves and mouthpiece. (https://en.wikipedia.org/wiki/Suriyenthrathibodi)

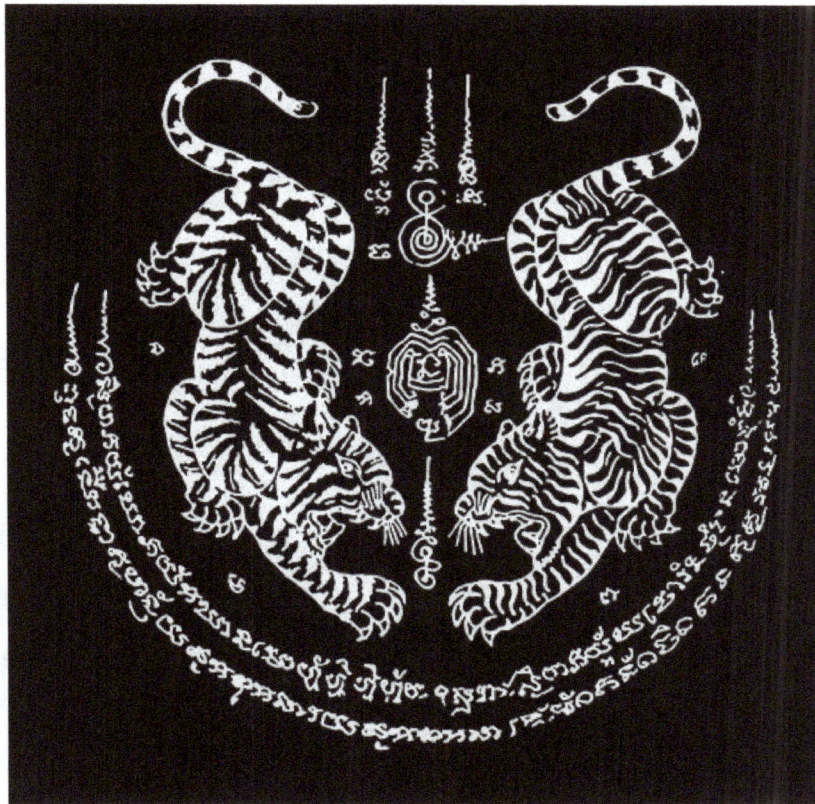

A traditional Tiger "Sak Yant Suea". A sacred tattoo of twin tigers for strength, power, protection and conviction, as well as authority over one's subordinates. Thai warriors-soldiers-fighters have adorned themselves with these types of protective symbols for centuries to present day.

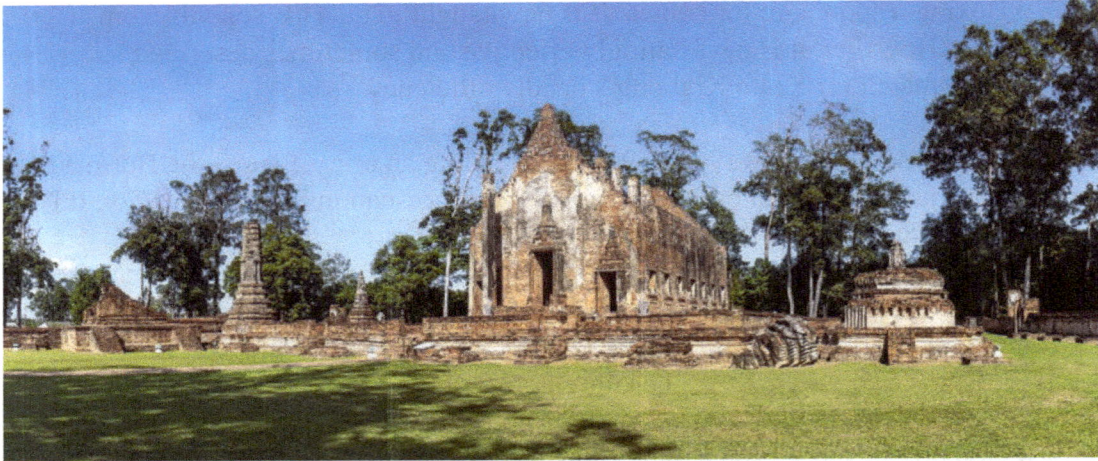

"Wat Pho Prathap Chang", Pho Prathapchang District, Phichit Province, Built by King Sampet VIII

King Sampet VIII is also revered for having codified and documented the traditional hand to hand combat fighting methods known as "*Mae Mai*" of the Thai Royal bodyguards- elite units known as the **"Tanaileuak"** equivalent to Japanese Samurai or modern special forces. He commissioned text in written form. These text have been preserved and recreated in various forms to the present day.

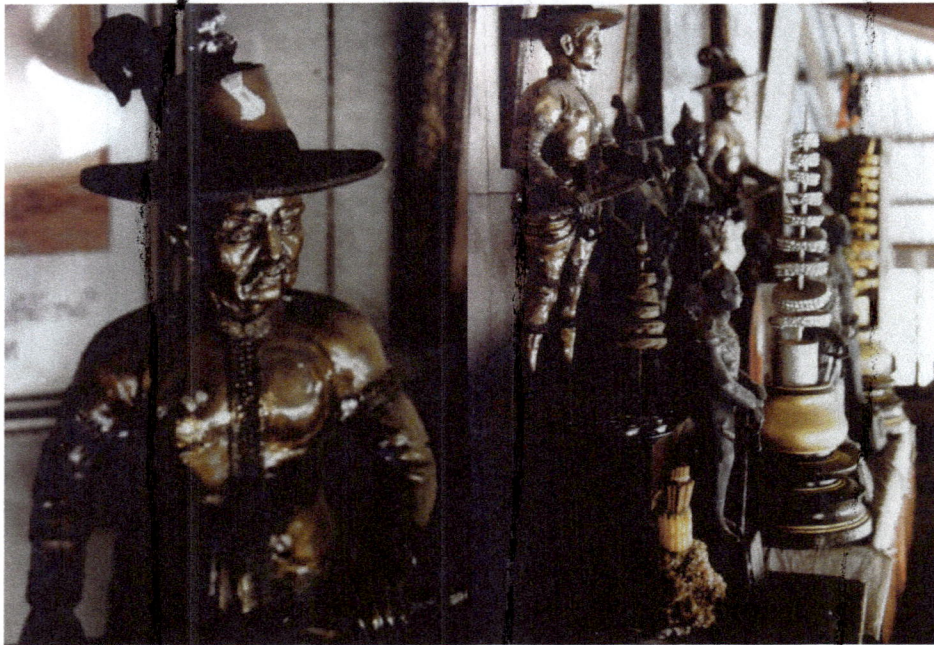

"Pra Chao Sua" the "The Tiger King", Shrine at Buddhai Sawan Institute, Nongkam

Thai rulers in their expansion and southward migration gradually and continually adopted many of the ways, architecture, customs, clothing styles, medicinal practices, martial arts and foods of the people they came to rule.

According to researchers (Braun and Schumacher: Traditional Herbal Medicine in Northern Thailand: White Lotus 1994) [2] "The Thai Court followed a pattern of adopting (and adapting) the "Indianized" culture of the people they conquered. During the Ayutthaya period Indian influence thus became firmly established in many domains: the concept of divine kingship replaced the original Thai version of feudalism; Indian Law - *The Code of Manu* - became the model for Thai law; The astrologers surrounding the king were Hindus; the alphabet was modeled after the Indian (and Khmer alphabets); Indian literary genres and metrics were introduced and of course Buddhism became the national religion.

The Indian medical classic text, the "Sanskrit lang. *Charaka Samhita*" became the basis for institutionalized Thai Ayurveda practices and education.

It is said, there was one king of the Ayutthaya period, whose entire personal retinue of bodyguards were Japanese Samurai! [7] This is part of the Buddhai Sawan history of the development of the Thai Martial Art Krabi Krabong which includes the use and techniques appropriate for the Katana and the Thai equivalent the "*Maha Deo*" or "Two Handed" Great Sword.

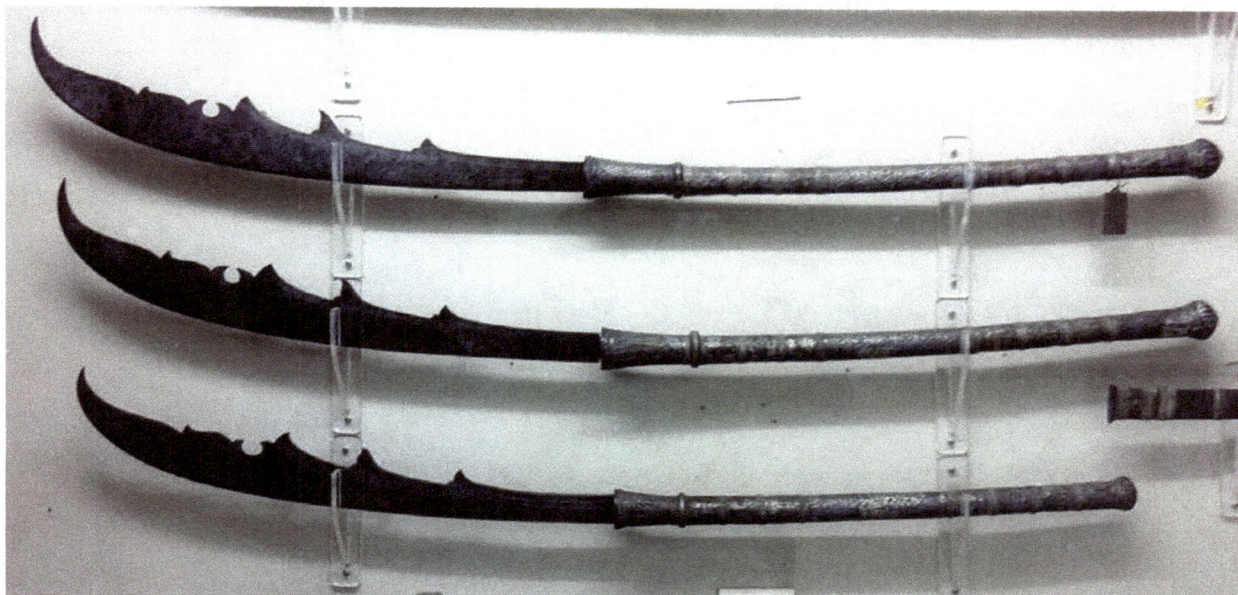

Dhap Naa Look Ka – Sukhotai National Museum, Sukhotai World Heritage Site: (Long handled, long blade, leaf shaped, semi-rounded in scabbard) Popular with Royalty. Blade sometime forged with appearence of a flame or flames. These amazing weapons may also be known as "*Dhap Sri Gun Chai Dha*".

I personally saw the examples of these great swords both in Phaa Kruu Samurai's personal collection and in the weapons collection of the National Museums in Bangkok and in Sukhothai. The latter are so massive that I can hardly imagine the size and strength of any Thai warrior giant, strong enough to wield them in practice, much less in combat. In years past the weapons were openly displayed in the "sword room" and not behind glass.

In the 80's a very close inspection was not only possible, but with permission, it was possible to actually hold the swords! They were old, used, pitted and massively deadly in appearance. These old swords were of great variety of blade shape and handle design and construction with some utilitarian and relatively small and other massive and ornate with much in the way of forged details such as the heads of god like or demon like figures and the blades being the breath being blown from the head at the hilt or handle!

Phaa Kruu Samaii Mesamarn once gave a lecture on the Japanese influence in Thai Sword fighting and in Thai healing arts saying the Budo arts and Japanese (Chinese) Amma were influential beginning during the Ayutthaya kingdom period. Some of the Samurai allegedly returned to Japan where we suspect they shared the Thai teachings of medicine and martial arts as well.

Two possible examples of Japanese Cultural Influence

1) The "Extraordinary meridians" of Japanese Shiatsu Anma (Sensei Massanauga/ Sensei Ohashi Schools), which are virtually identical to the depictions and stated functions of Thai Sen Lines. I corroborated this in discussions with Japanese Shiatsu & Amma Master, Dr. Do An Kaneko, PhD, a researcher, University of Tokyo in 1989 and 1991.

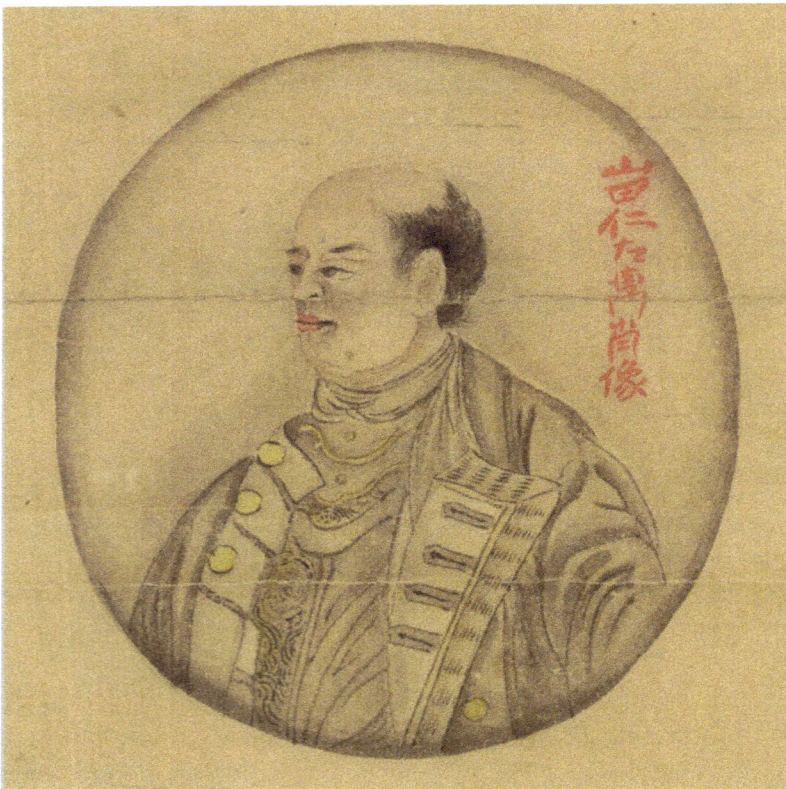

"Yamada Nagamasa Sensei ''', a Samurai, was first famous as a warrior and later in life as a merchant.

2) Historical accounts of Japanese merchants and Samurai in Ayudthaya from the Twelfth century through the fall of the old capital[8] [9] [10] [11]. ("Thai-Japanese Relations in Historical Prospective" (1988), edited by Chavit Khamchoo and E. Bruce Reynolds; and "From Japan to Arabia: Ayodhya's Maritime Relations with Asia" (1999), edited by Kennon Breazeale.) From Japan, besides historical material, come numerous tales narrating the adventures of *Yamada Nagamasa* (ca. 1585-1630), the most prominent Japanese figure in the history of *Ayudhya* [7].

(Yamada-Nagamasa-Portrait-Shizuoka-Sengen-Shrine By Unknown - Tokyo National Museum, https://www.tnm.jp/modules/rblog/index.php/1/category/1?lang=ja&start=105 , https://4travel.jp/travel-ogue/11265067, Public Domain, https://commons.wikimedia.org/w/index.php?curid=103666669)

There was a vibrant Japanese enclave in *Ayudthaya* for hundreds of years. There were also many accounts of commerce and communications, trade and exchange between the Thai Kings and Japanese Shoguns." It is estimated that the Japanese district, in its heyday in 1620, counted 1,000 to 1,500 inhabitants [29], making *Ayudhya's* ("*Baan Ippun*"), "*Nihonmachi- Nihonjin-machi ''enclave* (https:// en.wikipedia.org/wiki/Japanese_Village_(Ayutthaya)) the second largest in population of the Japanese enclaves in southeast Asia. (https://en.wikipedia.org/wiki/Yamada_Nagamasa)

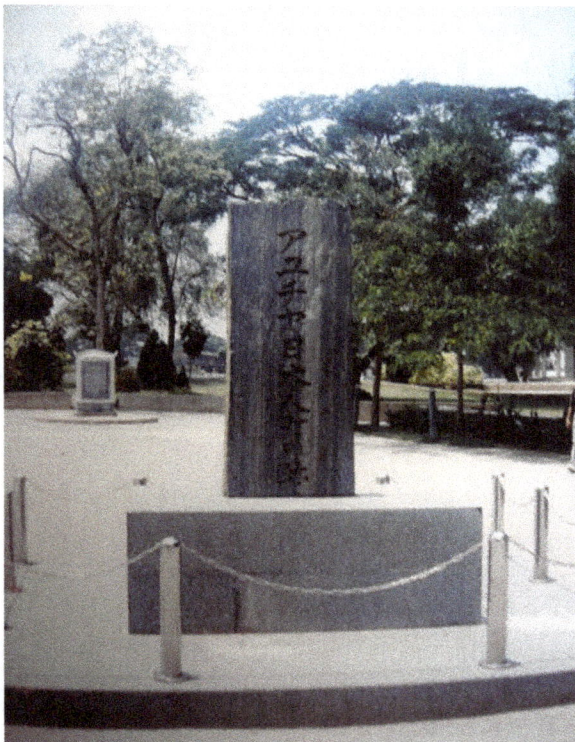

Ayutaya Japanese Town Monument marker: Ayudthaya: licensed under the Creative Commons Attribution-Share Alike 3.0 Unported, 2.5 Generic, 2.0 Generic and 1.0 Generic license.

To the present day you will see ancient and famous Japanese weapons: *Katana, Daisho, Yori* etc. in the Royal Museum Weapons Armory in Bangkok. Thai Kings in Royal Regalia wear and/or hold a Japanese sword decorated in the ornate Thai style.

Question? Do you think there are remnants of Japanese influence, Japanese Budo arts and Samurai fighting systems reflected in traditional Krabi Krabong? Phaa Kruu Samaii said emphatically, Yes! That is why there was a protrait of O Sensei Moryai Ushiba hanging in the school. Not to mention the Japanese Jiu-Jitsu we practiced as taught by Ajahn Pramote Mesamarn. As I was a Black Belt in Japanese Gobudo Jiu-Jitsu before I first went to Thailand?

Ajahn Pramote and I with Phaa Kruu Samaii had many discussions about this idea of Japanese influence.

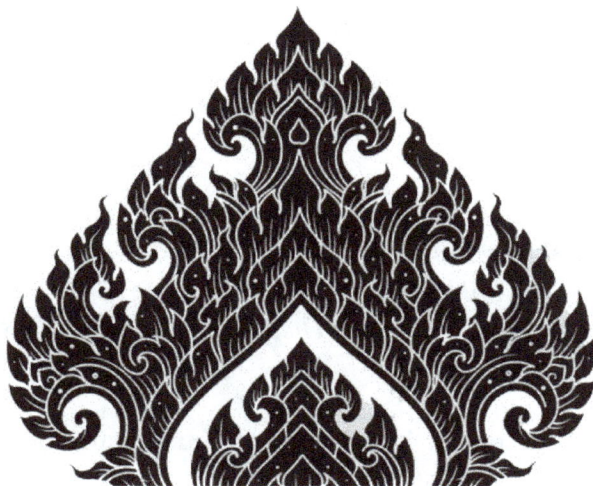

When King Thaksin shifted the capital of Thailand to Thonburi, the Buddhai Sawan (*Phootaisawan* Temple) traditions went with him.

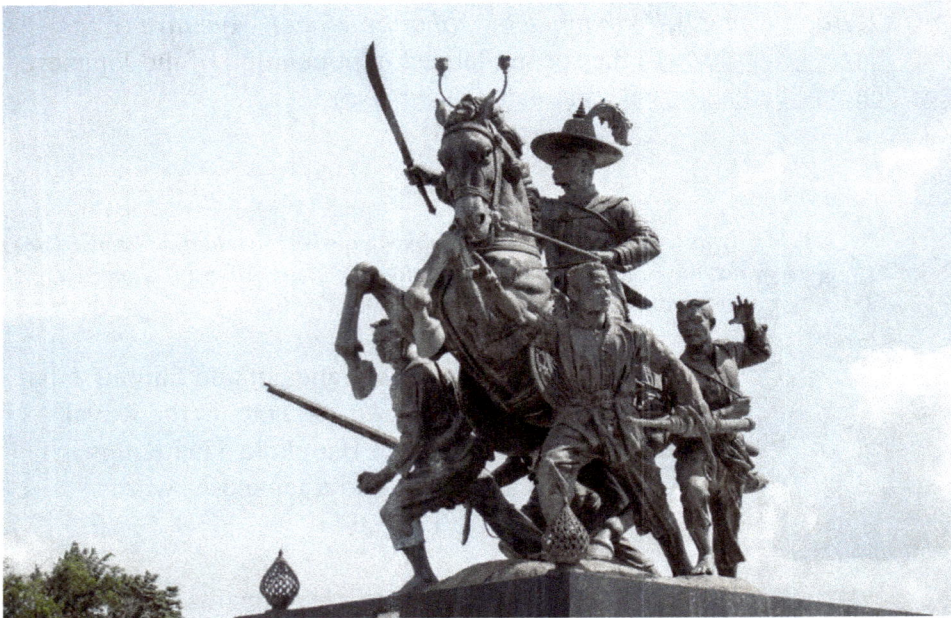

Monument to King Thaksin

Thailand continued as an independent State from this time, the sacking of the capital *Ayudthaya* to the present day.

In 1781/B.E. 2325, King *Phra Buddha Yodfa Chulaloke* ascended the throne as the first King of the Chakri Dynasty. King *Phra Budda Yod Fa ChulaLoke* (**King Rama I**: *Phra Bat Somdet Phra Paramoru-racha Mahachakkriborommanat Phra Phutthayotfa Chulalok*) ascended to the throne as the first king of the Chakri dynasty. Thailand (Siam) continued as an independent state from this time in history to the present day where it is currently under the Patronage of H.M. King *Maha Vajiralongkorn*, tenth king of the Chakri dynasty.

The capital of Thailand in the present time is "*Krungthep*" or Bangkok, where the king resides in the Grand Palace next to the famous temple "*Wat Phra Kao*" commonly known as the temple of the Emerald Buddha. King *Phra Budda Yod Fa ChulaLoke* (King Rama I) is buried at *Wat Po (Bangkok)*.

This king was also celebrated as the founder of "*Rattanakosin*" (now Bangkok) as the new capital of the reunited kingdom.

The full traditional name of Bangkok is quite long! 168 characters! "*Krung Thep Mahanakhon Amon Rattanakosin Mahinthara Ayuthaya Mahadilok Phop Noppharat Ratchathani Burirom Udomratchaniwet Mahasathan Amon Piman Awatan Sathit Sakkathattiya Witsanukam Prasit*". Thai people actually call their Thailand's capital city 'กรุงเทพมหานคร' (*Krung Thep Maha Nakhon*) or 'กรุงเทพฯ' (*Krung Thep*) instead of Bangkok.

This "Royal Style '' is what I was introduced to by GM Phaa Kruu Samaii and other teachers of note Pichai, Colonel Chatchai (now General Chatchai!). Every day, every morning after breakfast, before we would train in earnest, we would line up and practice the "Morning Meditation" and the morning Yoga warmups rituals. These were sometimes simple, sometimes complex with emphasis to be different daily depending on the training to be the focus for the day.

In addition to the Yoga vinyasa (Thai *Reussi Dotan* or Reishi Yoga) and asana practice to build strength and flexibility, we did specific "*Reishi*" Hand Yoga to work on dexterity and strength to be able to wield weapons, long and short, long enough to practice, and or to be able to practice without injury. The hand exercises also included using all the different weapons as conditioning tools themselves... such as in "wagging" swords, and "twirling" and "Finger Spinning" "*Plong*" (poles and long staffs) and "*Hau Kwan*" (Large bladed spears and polearms meant to be wielded from the carriage of War Elephants).

Long Handled, massive and heavy weapons as seen in GM Phaa Kruu's private collection, would typically have been carried on a War Elephant and or Horse Cavalry in battle.

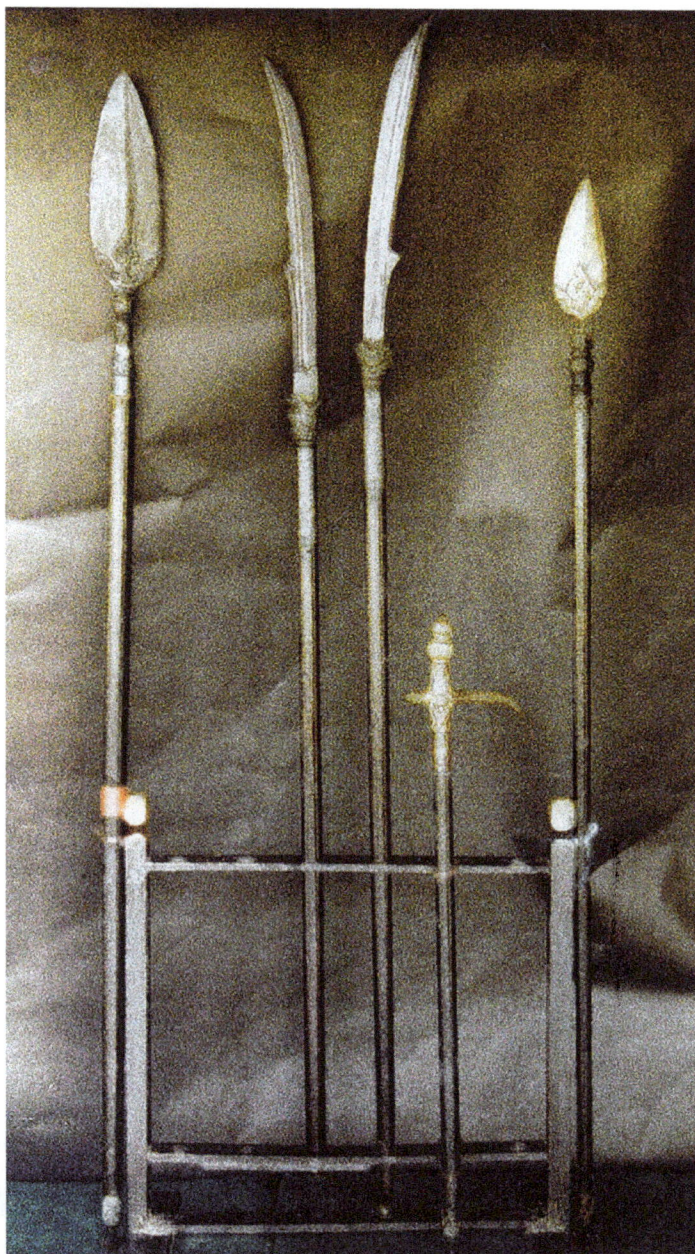

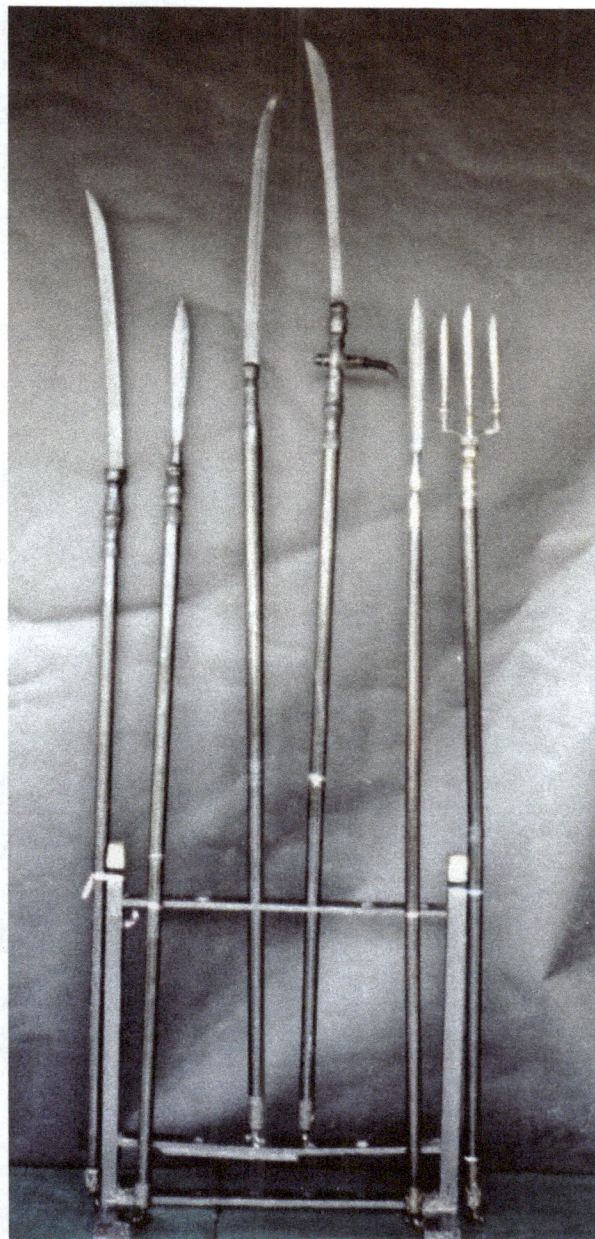

Wat Buddhai Sawan Sri Ayudhya

The original home of Krabi Krabong

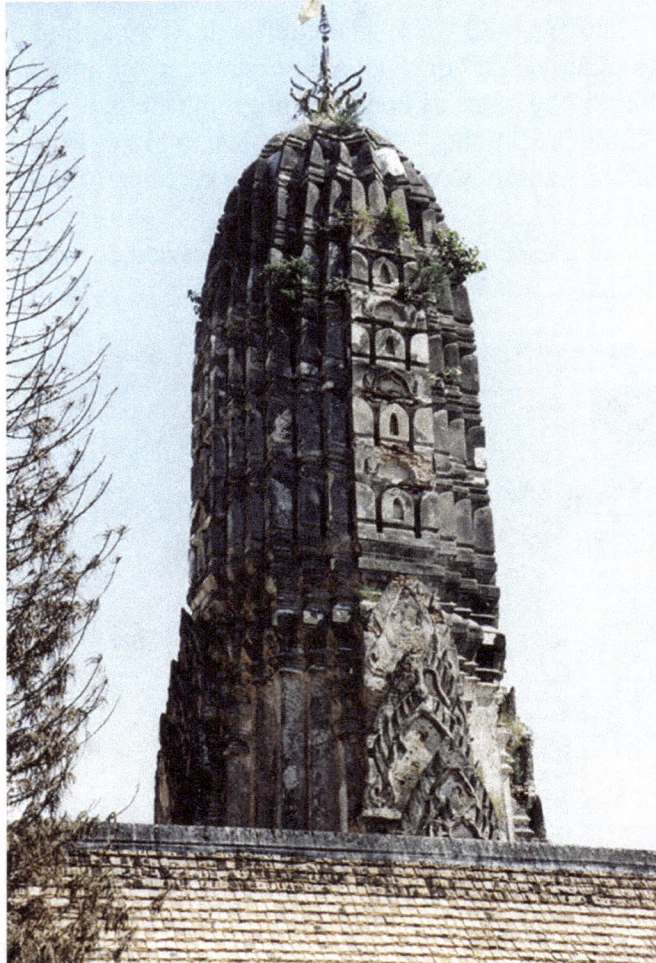

The central "Prang" in the main courtyard.

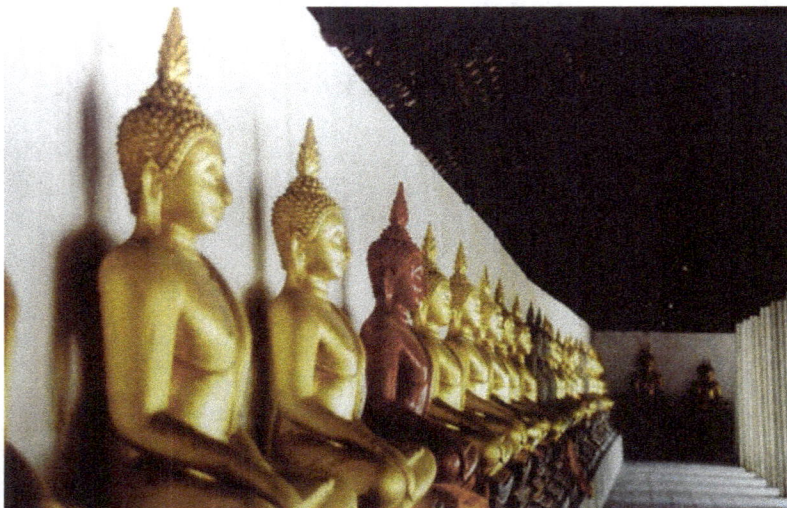

One of the Seated Buddha Galleries… Red Buddha.

A little known and seldom visited corner of the old Ayudthaya city, the aged sires of Prang and Chedi belonging to *"Pra Wat Buddhai Sawan"* rise, covered by the jungle growth. Although still used today by initiates, this sacred place is seldom seen by tourists.

When we speak of the old Thai monks who developed and perfected Krabi Krabong, this is the actual location where this work took place.

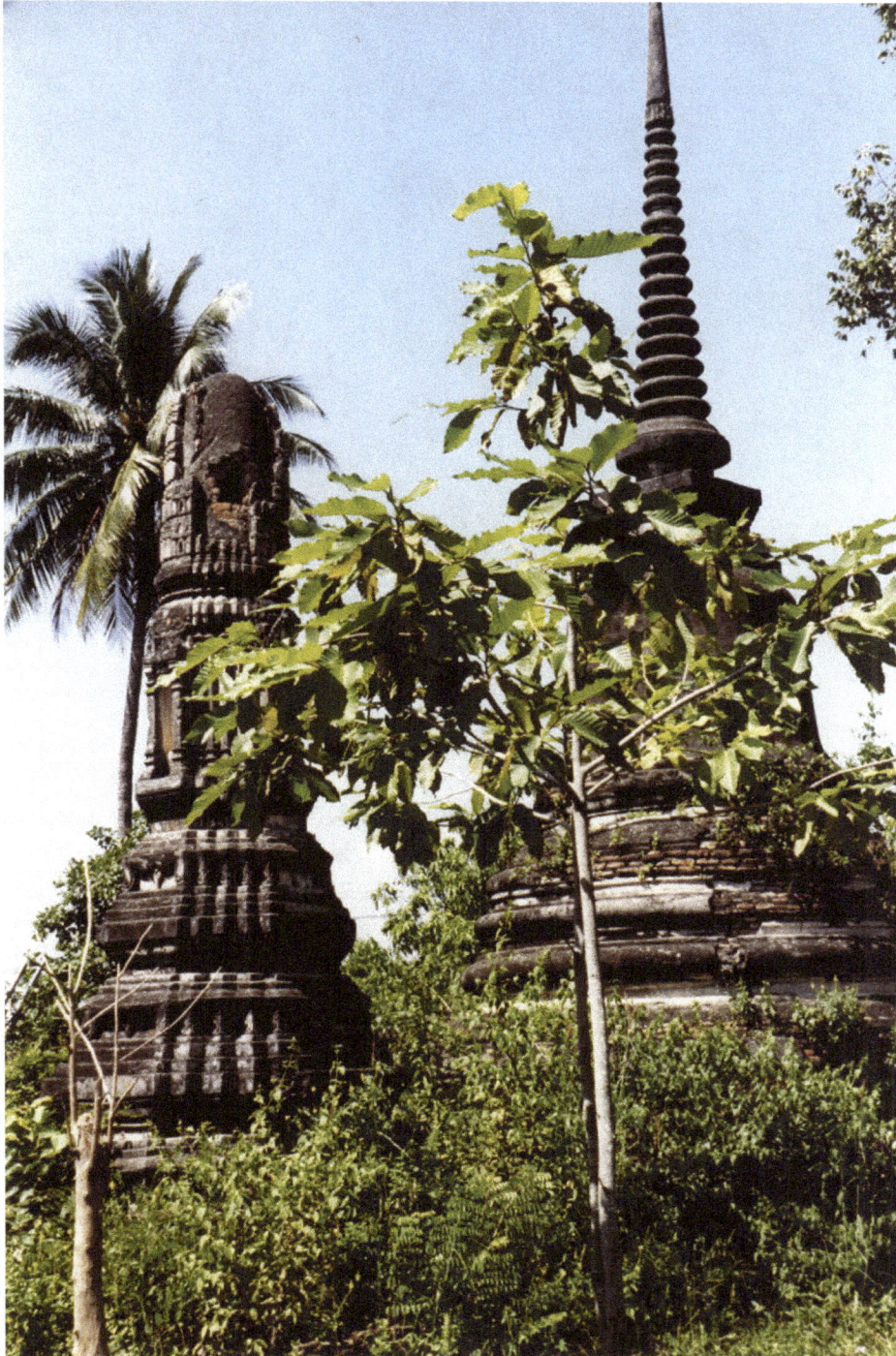

The Buddhai Sawan Chapel (Phootaisawan Temple)

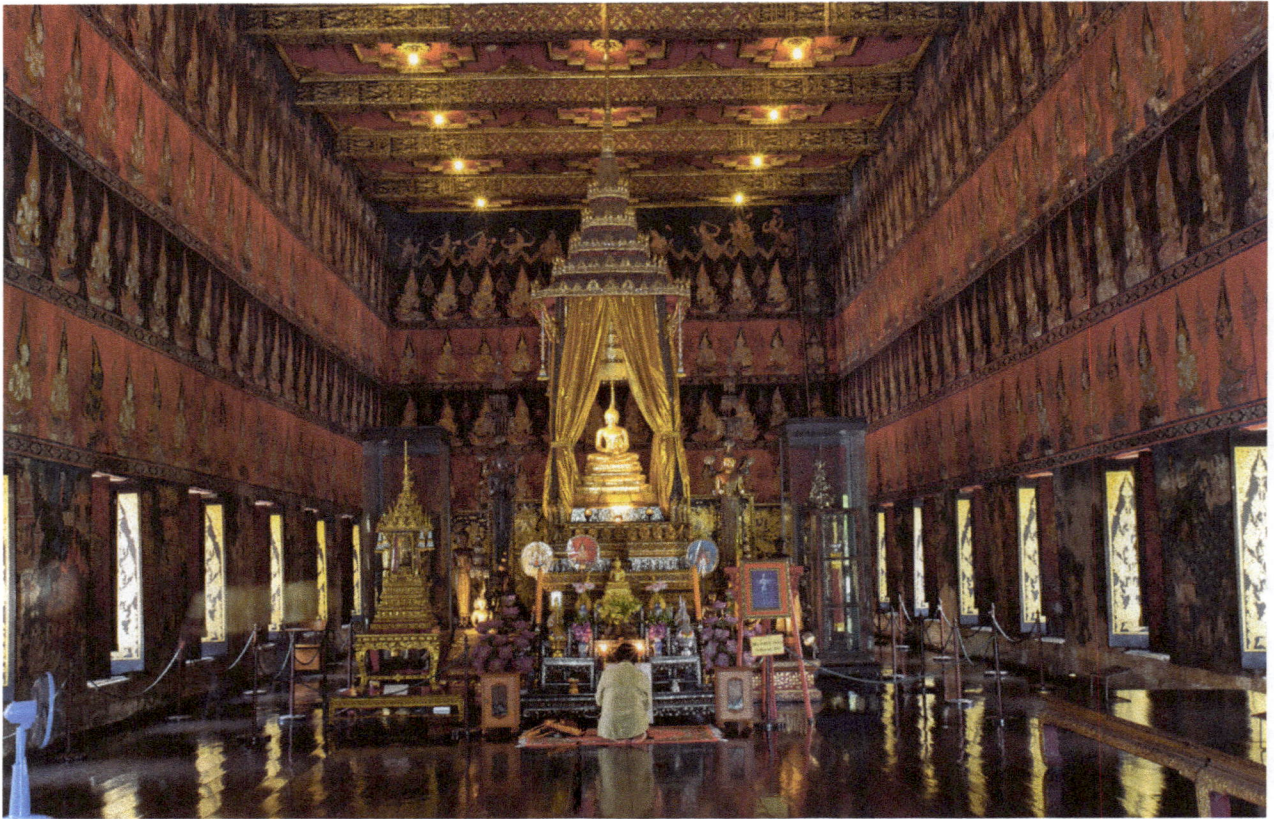

The Buddhaisawan (Phutthaisawan) Chapel interior

"One of the buildings of the Bangkok National Museum, was once the private chapel for the Wang Na, the former palace which stands in the center of the museum compound. During the Reign of King Rama I (1782 – 1809), the position of the "Prince of the Wan Na '' was occupied by the King's younger brother, who served as a general. From one of his northern campaigns, he brought back the famous *Phra Buddha Sihing* image. The *Buddhaisawan (Phutthaisawan)* Chapel was built in 1795 to house that image.

After this prince's death, the image was installed in the Temple of the Emerald Buddha for a time, before being returned and re-installed in the *Buddhaisawan* Chapel where it has remained ever since.

The interior of this little chapel is amazing! It is decorated from the floor to the ceiling with painted frescoes of the Buddha's life and significant events from his birth to his death. The paintings on the four walls. These are the oldest murals in Bangkok. (*Mrs. Dorothy H. Fickle: The Life of the Buddha Murals In The Buddhaisawan Chapel National Museum, Bangkok. Department of Fine Arts, Hardback Edition,1972.*)

During my time with GM Phaa Kruu Samaii we visited the *Buddhaisawan* Chapel to pay respect several times. This chapel, *Wat Buddhai Sawan* in Ayudthaya and the Phitsanulok mausoleum/ monument to Prince Narasuan were considered very important and to be acknowledged in our traditional lineage.

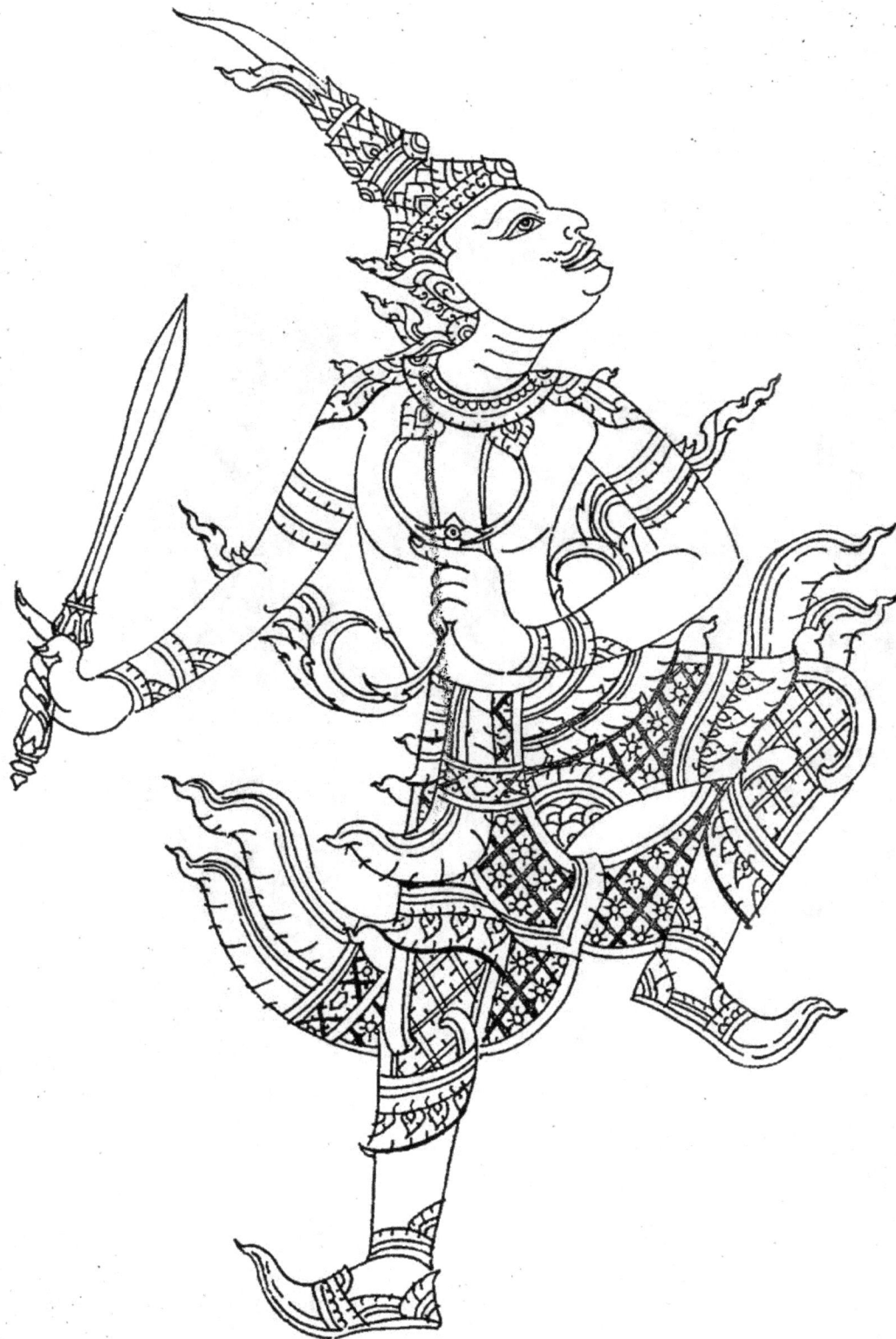

Classic depiction Rama from the Ramayana Epic Dancing with Leaf shaped sword.

The Modern Era of Buddhai Sawan

Buddhai Sawan Institute of Swordsmanship and Traditional Culture (Buddhai Sawan) was created in homage to the original traditions of the historical temple. It was the life work of GM Samaii Mesamarn (known as the Father Teacher or *Phaa Kruu*). He dedicated his life to preserving the ancient arts of the Thai people.

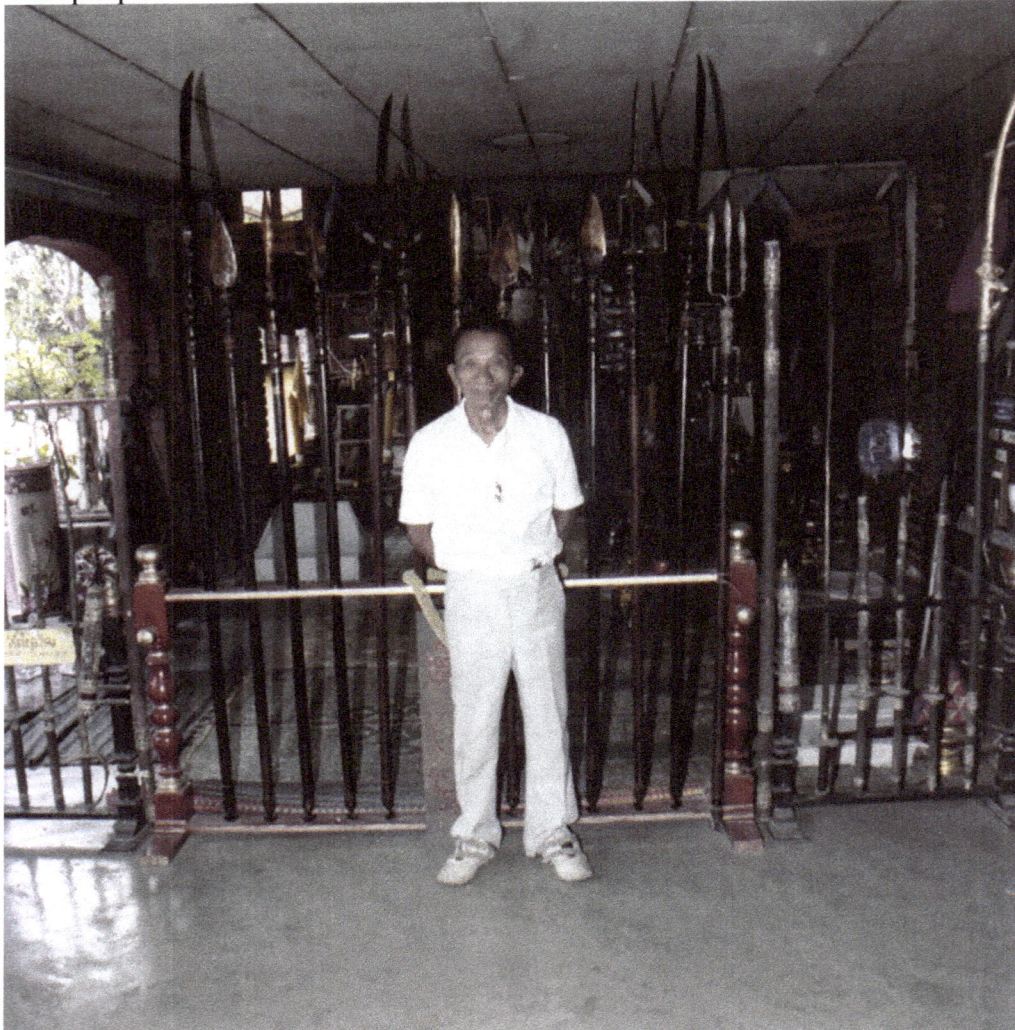

Grand Master Phaa Kruu Samaii Mesamarn at The Buddhai Sawan Institute, Nongkam, Thailand 1983. Phaa Khruu Samaii in front of "Hau Kwan" collection at Buddhai Sawan Institute, Nongkam. This image gives some scale as it can be seen some of these weapons are eight feet in length or longer.

Grand Master (GM) Phaa Kruu Samaii was born in 1914, near *Ayudthaya* and was first exposed to BSKK (*Buddhai Sawan Krabi Krabong*) by his father who worked for a Thai government countryside development agency. His path from a young age was following the tradition of integrating the old with the new. He attended college and was awarded the very first Education degree to be issued to a Thai person. The curriculum of physical education included, at that time, Japanese Judo, Jiu-Jitsu and Aikido as the education system had obviously been heavily influenced by both traditional Japanese culture from the Ayudthaya period but more recently by the Japanese occupation of Thailand before and during World War II. Additionally, he excelled in Olympic sport of western fencing, boxing and gymnastics as well as Thai traditional martial arts of Muay Thai, Muay Boran and Buddhai Sawan Krabi Krabong.

Early students would have seen the large painting of Japanese Sword Master (Kenjutsu) Sensei Morei Ushieba, O Sensei, founder of Aikido hanging on the wall at Buddhai Sawan Nongkam. Phaa Kruu Samai's oldest son Phaa Kruu Pramote Mesamarn continues the family emphasis on Jiu-jitsu today in addition to Buddhai Sawan Krabi Krabong, operating Pramote Gym in Bangkok. Promote Gym has been formally recognized as the oldest school of Japanese Jiu-Jitsu in Thailand.

Historical accounts of Japanese merchants and Samurai in Ayudthaya from the Twelfth century through the fall of the old capital[8] [9] [10] [11]. ("Thai-Japanese Relations in Historical Prospective" (1988), edited by Chavit Khamchoo and E. Bruce Reynolds; and *From Japan to Arabia: Ayodhya's Maritime Relations with Asia*" (1999), edited by Kennon Breazeale.) From Japan, besides historical material, come numerous tales narrating the adventures of Yamada Nagamasa (ca. 1585-1630), the most prominent Japanese figure in the history of Ayudhya" [7].

Phaa Khru Samurai's most influential professor at this time was Ajahn *Nerk Thephussadin na Ayudthaya whi in* and around 1935 devised- developed an extensive curriculum in Krabi Krabong based on his father Kruu Lem's teachings combined with his own research and practice. His goal and dream were that one day the traditional arts would be taught in every school in Thailand to every child. Ajahn Nerk's dream was realized!

Phaa Khru Samaii Mesamarn World War II

Of course, during the war, most Thai people had a bit to keep track of more than diaries! However, we did learn some of Phaa Kruu's story of his life during the Japanese occupation. During the second world war Phaa Kruu opened and operated a dorm or group house for students and others displaced by the air raids and bombings. The bombings were from all sides! There were air raids by both the Japanese and the Allied armies. It was also during this time that Phaa Kruu opened the first "Bar" in Thailand for foreigners (*falang*), the "Moonlight Bar". The Moonlight Bar was frequented by foreigners… mostly Japanese military and civilian infrastructure people. Both the bar and the dorm were integral to his support and intelligence gathering as a member of the "*Seri Thai* '' resistance movement (https://military-history.fandom.com/wiki/Free_Thai_Movement) or the wartime underground insurgency dedicated to liberating the Thai People, driving off the Japanese invaders and to rescuing allied (American and Australian) prisoners of war.

Many of these thousands of prisoners, being used as slave labor building highways and bridges for the Japanese, had been captured in the Philippines and force marched from there, via Indonesia, Malaysia to Thailand and eventually all the way to Burma. WW2 military historians refer to this period as the CBI Theater (*China, Burma, India War Theater: (https://cbi-theater.com/menu/cbi_home.html*). Even in today's world we see remnants of the CBI conflict (in the founding of the "Flying Tigers" (https://cbi-theater.com/pm-tigers/pm-tigers.html & https://en.wikipedia.org/wiki/Flying_Tiger_Line). in 1989 Federal Express merged Flying Tigers into its operations, and the Flying Tigers name passed into history.

Phaa Kruu received recognitions and awards for his freedom fighting actions during the war. As for the bar? Well now they are infinite in number and variety!

After the War

After the end of the war, Phaa Kruu went back to teaching Buddhai Sawan Krabi Krabong to any and all in a small temple annex opposite the Grand Palace, near what became the Royal Thai Ministry of Defense (Thai Pentagon). He also worked at this time as a photographer and Muay Thai teacher and match promoter… one of the first!

In 1946 he established the non-profit Buddhai Sawan Institute of Swordsmanship and Thai Culture.

In the early days, Phaa Kruu Samaii worked in cooperation with other Ajahn's and teachers who were from the same era and education system. Many knew each other from their college days. Ajahn Arimeta and other student teachers. The post war time was a period of intensive collaboration to try to preserve and save as many traditions as possible. Many individuals including Phaa Kruu worked together to create a national system of Krabi Krabong which could be taught nationally in the Thai school system. This system is heavily based on the work of the aforementioned Krabi Krabong master Ajahn Nak.

Eventually, there was a schism between Phaa Kruu Samaii and Ajahn Arimeta which resulted in which Ajahn Arimeta going North to his family's traditional home in Chiangmai, where he continued to develop his style of Krabi Krabong system incorporating the traditions of the Lanna Kingdom (Chiangmai/ Chiangrai). The Ajahn Arimeta's Lanna style of Krabi Krabong continues to the present time and is very influential in the North.

Phaa Khru Samaii saw the warrior heritage as a way to draw on this heritage, built for survival… for life and death before, during and after combat to create a peacetime training and discipline suitable for everyone including children. He wanted to instill in them a sense of pride in both themselves and in their traditional culture. He wanted these teachings to contribute to the children's developing sense of self and identity as uniquely "Thai", i.e., powerful and prosperous!

Phaa Khru Samaii saw the integrative Krabi Krabong system as a way to enrich the lives of Thai Children's lives by encouraging the development of personal discipline of spirit, mind and body. I believe this is why he encouraged students such as myself to pursue practices of spirituality, personal discipline and ethical ways of being irrespective of our daily practices.

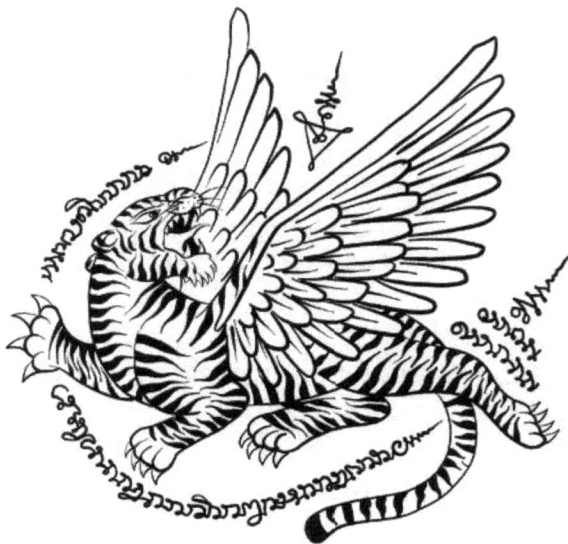

Ajahn James Receives Guidance from Phaa Kruu Samaii on his path.

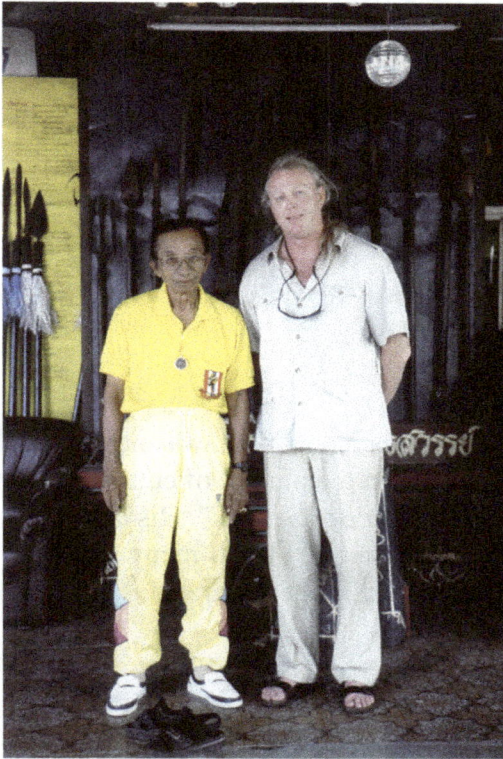

GM Pramote Mesamarn working with Kruu James

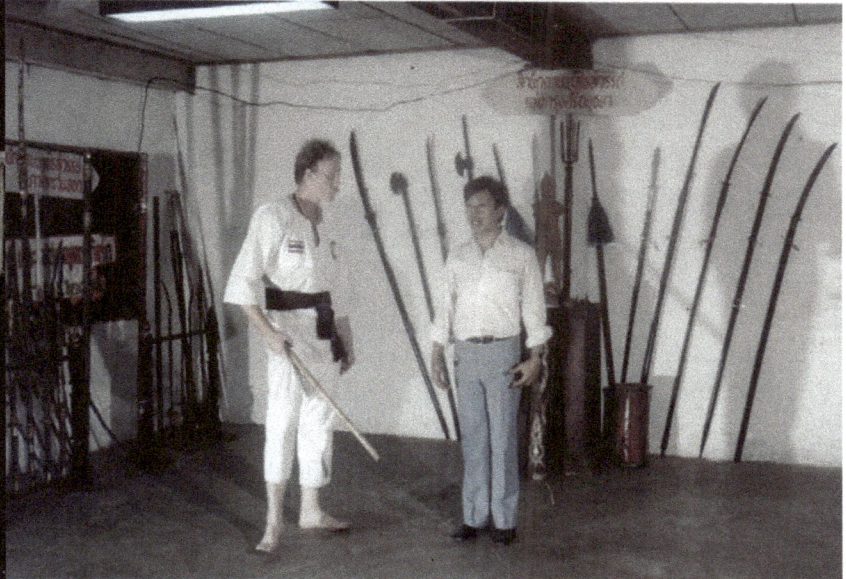

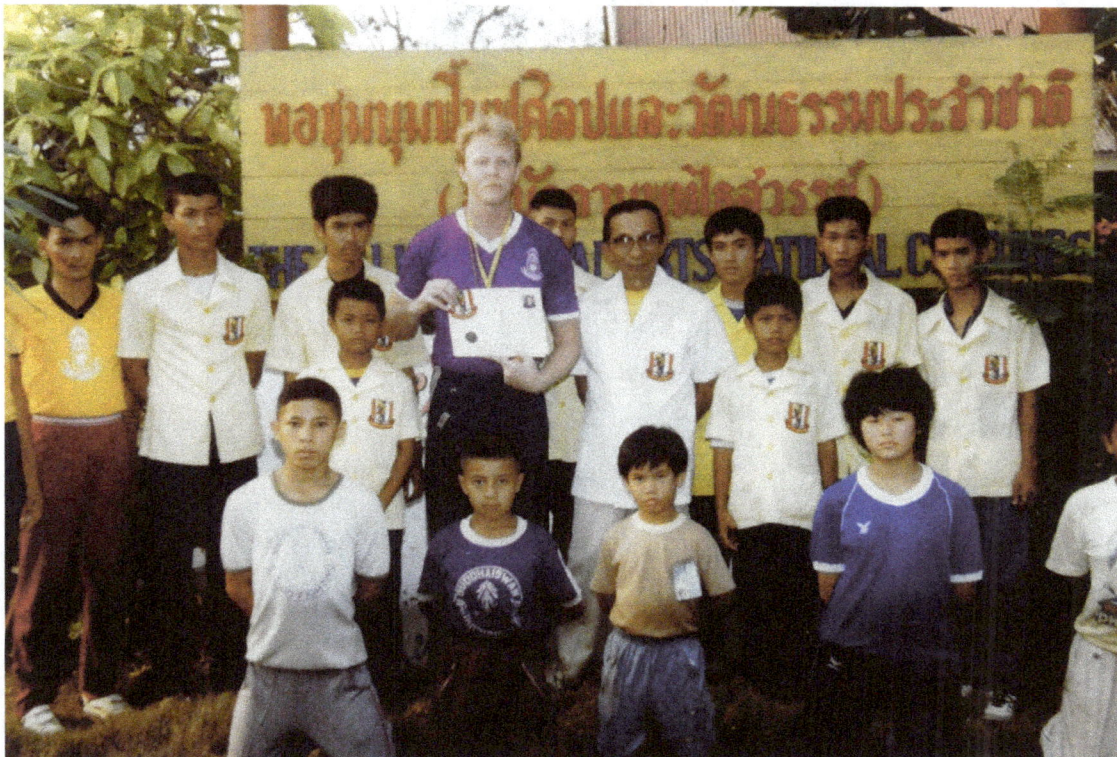

Buddhai Sawan Khruu Certification from Phaa Kruu's hand. (1984)

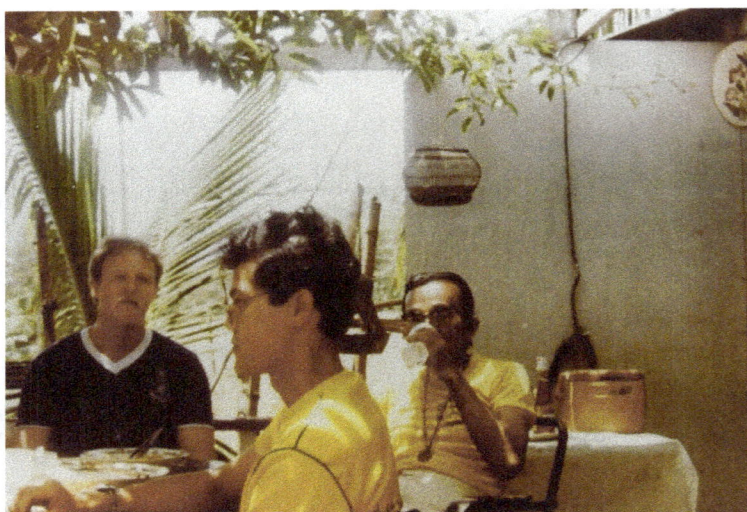

Ajahn James enjoying breakfast with Phaa Kruu and Pitchai

I believe this is at the core of why Phaa Kruu eventually told me, that my personal path, was not just in the mastery of "martial arts, sword fighting, combat and competition" but in the pursuit of cultivation and mastery of the traditional Thai healing arts *"Ryksaa Thang Nuad Phaen Boran Thai"*. His direct quote to me was in response first to a question… "Do you want to be a master?". I knew many masters of this time in several different countries and in several different traditions… I knew it was possible for someone like me to become a master teacher. I answered "yes"…

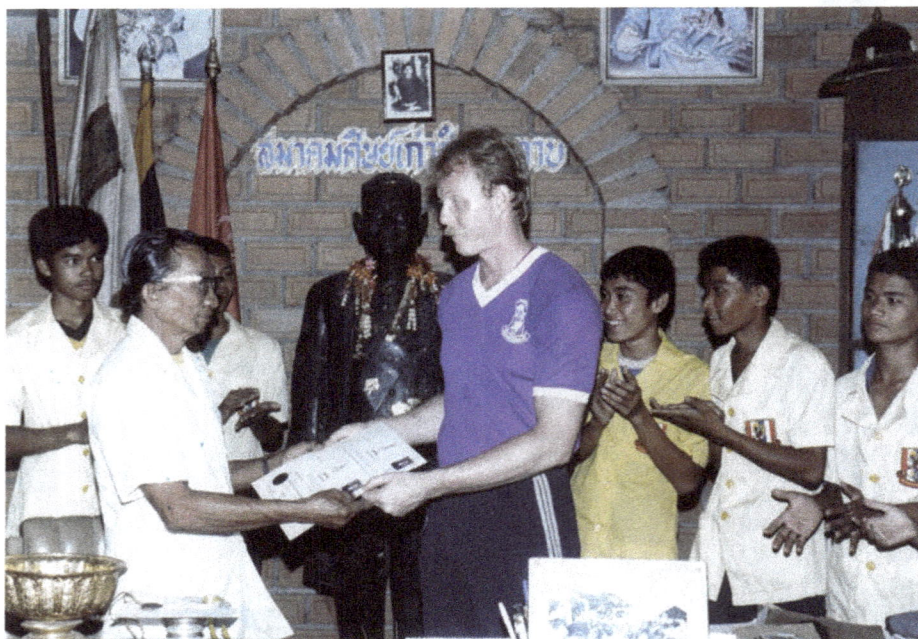

He then asked me "How many ways do you know how to break a bone?" I was floored! When I thought about it, I literally knew hundreds if not thousands of ways to: break and arm". In fact, very quickly, I realized it was a trick question for someone like myself who had been training in martial arts since age eleven. Someone, who at that moment was both a Kruu in Buddhai Sawan Krabi Krabong and holder of more than one Black Belt rank (Tang So Do Mu Duk Kwan, American Karate, Go Buddo Jiu-Jitsu Sensei Lloyd Garrard, GM Sensei Joe Corley, GM Bill Wallace, GM Jeff Smith, Sensei Phillip

Ballergeron- Seishin Kai Jiu-Jitsu/ American Jiu-Jitsu Union) in more than one different discipline, a certified Guro in Filipino Kali, Arnis de Mano, Escrima, Pekiti Tirsia Kali by G.M. Tuhon Leo T. Gaje Jr./ Guro Tom Bisio and Indonesian Penjak Silat Pendekar Suyadi (Eddie) Jaffri as well as trained and certified in Lee June Fan (Jeet Kune Do) by GM Danny Inosanto (1981 Big Springs, Texas USA)…

I knew how to break bones. After a few moments of consideration, I gave up and started my answer to Phaa Kruu that I could not answer the question as it was like "How many stars are in the sky". It was unknowable as it was so easy to break arms (or anything for that matter), that you could even trick or maneuver people into breaking their own arms like it was their idea! I said, "I can't answer". He smiled at me with a big smile. Nodding his head, he opened the draw of his desk and withdrew an envelope and handed it to me.

As I looked at the envelope he said "Kruu Antony, you don't need to practice fighting anymore. When you know as many ways as possible to fix a broken arm, then you will be the Ajahn".

The day after this, Phaa Kruu and I left the Buddhai Sawan compound early in the morning and took the long bus from Nongkam into Bangkok, first to "Sanam Luang"… the Elephant Parade ground near the Grand Palace, where we then walked past the Grand Palace to Section five of Ayurved Vidyalai behind Wat Po (Wat Chetuphon). He took me deep in the monk's quarter until we were at the personal residence of Phaa Khru Men (Uppacort). With a brief introduction to one of Phaa Khru Uppacort's aides he left there with the envelope.

Eventually, I was invited into Kruu Men's chambers where this quite elderly monk was reclining in a cool chamber on his bed (Thai style chaise). He asked why I was there, and I gave him the letter from Phaa Kruu. He mentioned that he had been a brother monk with Phaa Kruu Samaii when they had been quite young before the war. He then spoke to his aids and gave them instructions on what to do with me! I was then escorted to new quarters for me, which became my home for a time as I studied traditional Thai Medicine, Traditional Thai Ayurveda and the "Ryksaa Thang Nuad Phaen Boran Thai '' under the guidance of Ajahn Moh Boonsorn Kitnyam, Director of the School of Traditional Thai Medicine located on the grounds of Wat Po at that time.

From those days to the present, I have been dedicated to the traditional Thai culture, martial arts and Thai medicine- healing arts, eventually achieving many relevant degrees, certifications, accolades and awards in Thai Medicine and related. I have also maintained my love and practice of Buddhai Sawan Martial Arts. I continue to teach and share both in my schools today.

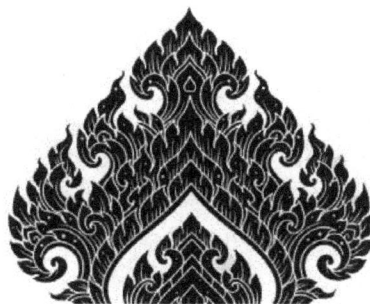

I give all credit where credit is due. Being part of the Buddhai Sawan School and tradition has brought nothing but good to my life and work as was Phaa Kruu's original vision. I credit the formal awards I have received from the Royal Thai Governments and various ministries also to GM Phaa Kruu Samaii and without his reputation and support I never would have been considered.

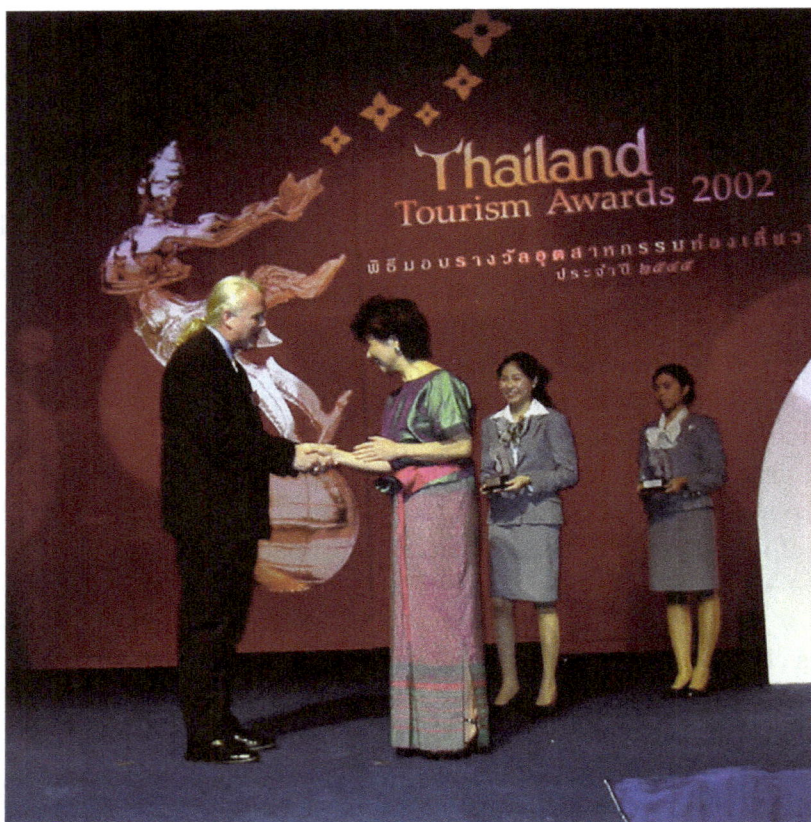

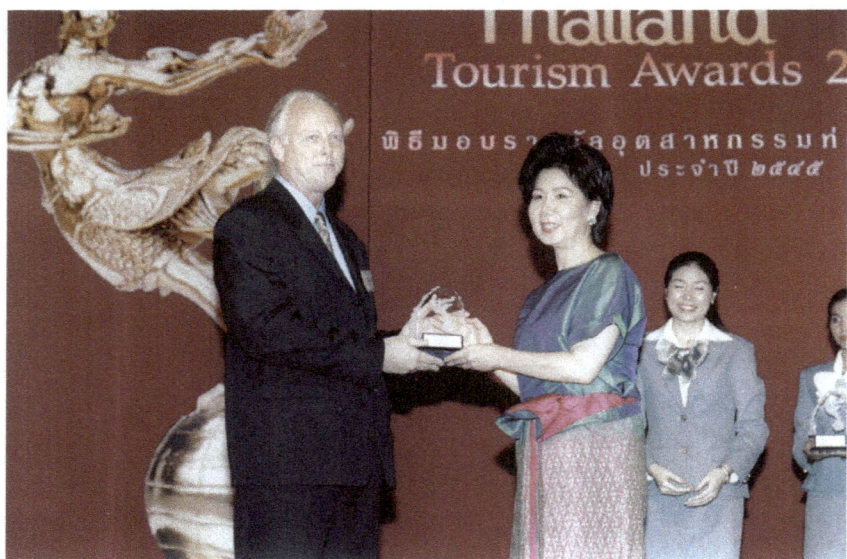

Ajahn Dr. Anthony B. James receives the "Friends Of Thailand", "Ghinari" Award 2002 September 27th., 2002, Queen Sirkit Convention Center, Bangkok, Thailand

Thai *Reussi Dottan* Hand Yoga

Every practice day at Buddhai Sawan for myself and the other students and teachers, dressed out in uniform, to begin with Reussi Dottan (Reishi Yoga) asana practice for posture, and conditioning for Spirit, Mind and Body. These morning group exercises gave us the stamina, flexibility and endurance to be able to get through the rigorous training to follow. There was some time early to do your own favorite "warmups", followed by the directed flows leading up to the postures and strength and flexibility training while using weapons of every kind. I also know that this daily practice strengthened and hardened us to prevent injury.

See the bottom of this section for information on how to become formally certified in this traditional Thai Yoga Therapy modality!

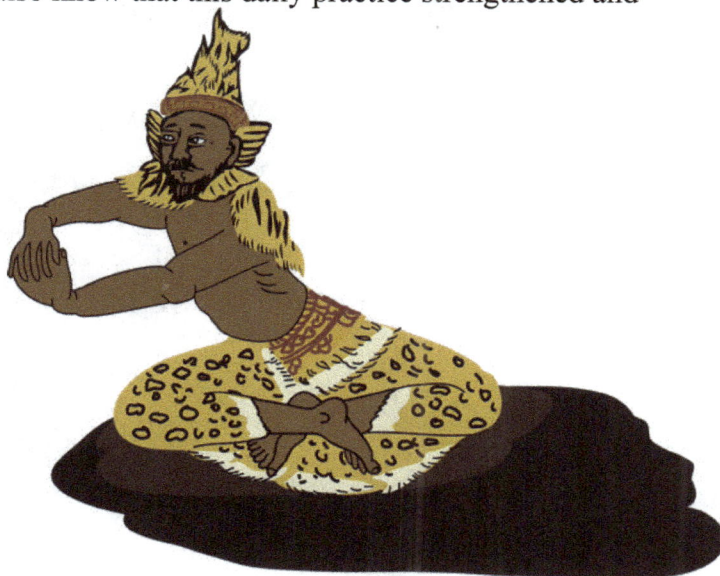

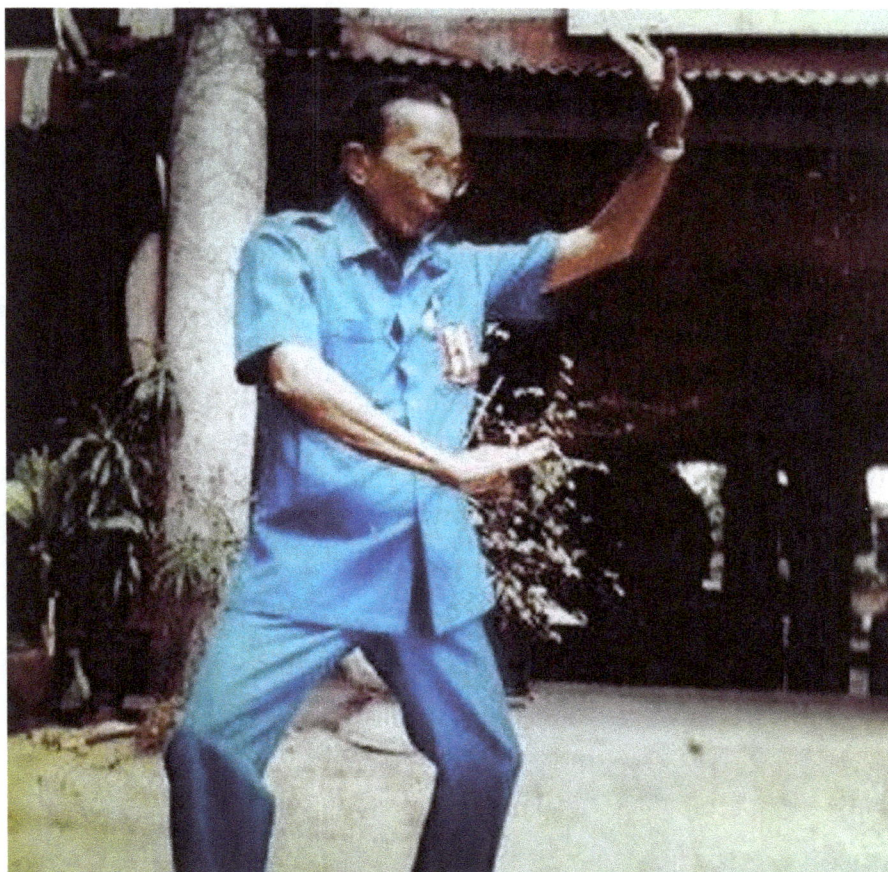

GM Phaa Kruu Samaii Mesamarn demonstrating Thai Traditional Classical Dance postures from the Ramayana mythology and their applications to Krabi Krabong and Reishi Yoga (Reussi Dottan) at Buddhai Sawan Institute, Nongkam, Thailand.

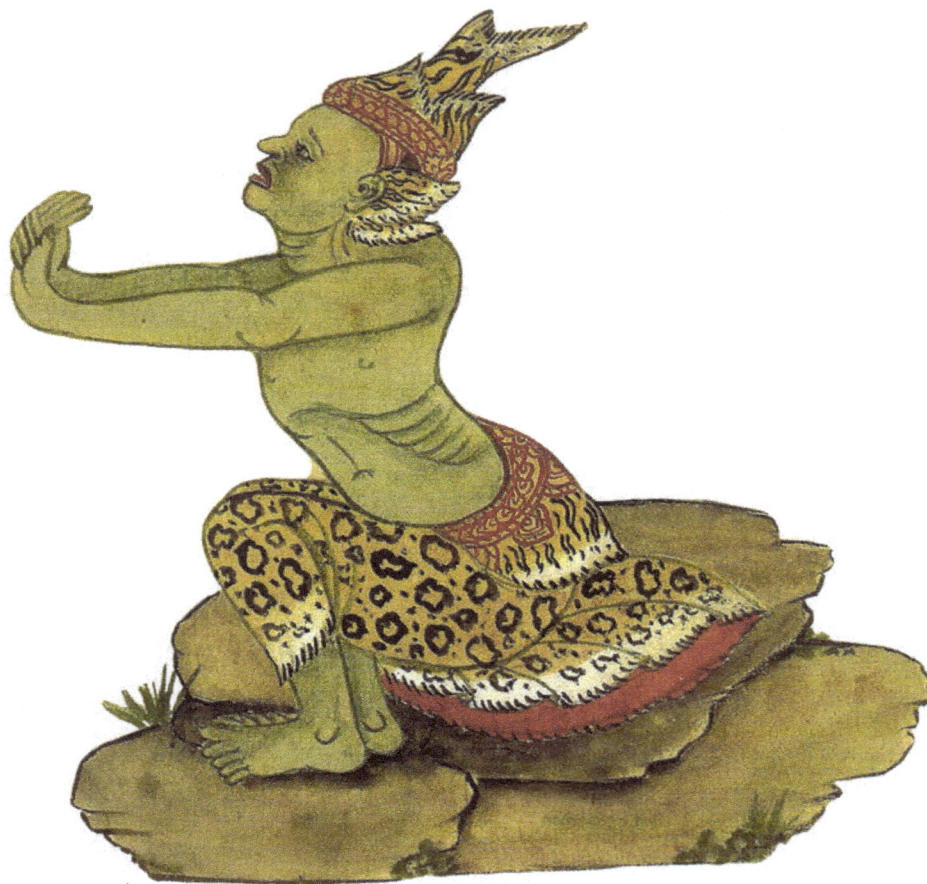

One of the key "*Thai Reussi Dotton*", Thai Yoga Hand Positions to prevent injury and strengthen the hands and arms for Buddhai Sawan Krabi Krabong sword training.

Begin learning the first form of the Buddhai Sawan style Thai Reishi Hand Yoga Vinyasa. Traditional Thai Reishi Hand Yoga is a derivative ancient work consisting of 108 Yoga Asana or postures which are primarily although not exclusively done with the hands and arms. The postures focus on the Microcosmic orbit of the body's energy and Chakras 4 and 5. All of the arms and hand meridians and PranaNadi are energized and balanced.

This work may correct and balance the harmful effects of injury, trauma and repetitive stress causing deterioration of the hands, arms and joints including wrist, elbow and shoulder. These Hand Yoga Postures and flow were traditionally used by the "Warriors' ' of ancient Thailand to strengthen and protect their arms and hands from the rigors of training and fighting with Swords ("Dap Deo") and other traditional weapons of combat.

If they can protect battle hardened warriors, they can protect the therapist and healer! Of course, if you practice Martial Arts of any kind this amazing set of conditioning hand yoga postures can reduce injury and give you more strength as well!

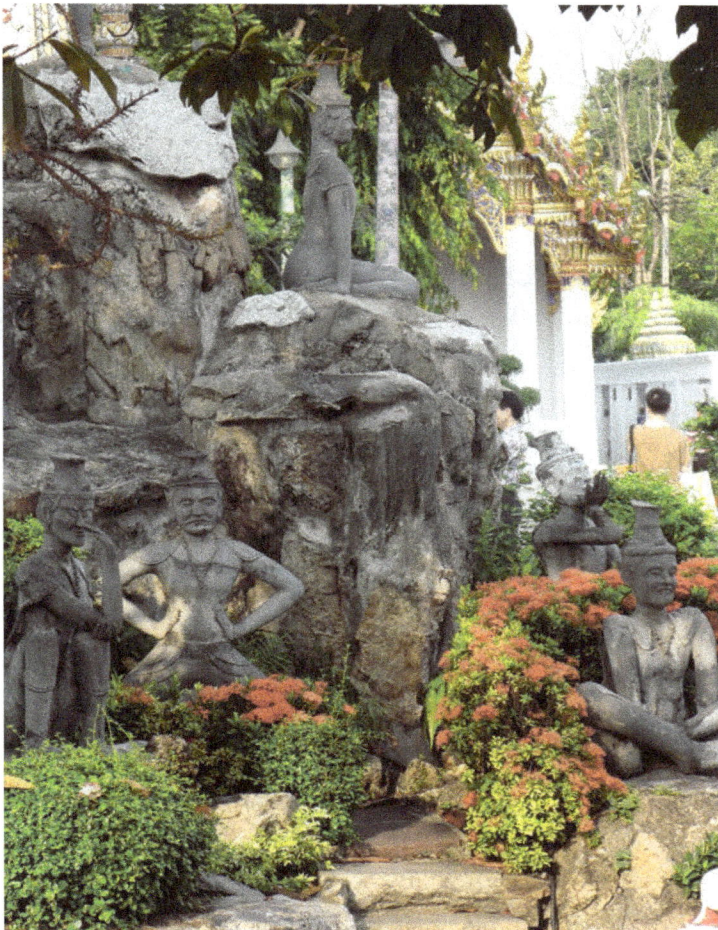

The famous Thai Yoga Reishi Garden located at Wat Po, adjacent to the Royal Palace, Bangkok, Thailand.

Circulation of breath, Prana and Chi is enhanced as well as all other forms of ManoVaha PranaNadi such as blood, lymph and interstitial fluids. Reduces and or eliminates harmful swelling and edema in the extremities.

Thai Reishi yoga is a complete system of energy balancing and wellness enabling techniques opening the hands to be the perfect expressions for compassion and loving kindness.

Those individuals suffering from hand, arm and shoulder conditions such as Rotator Cuff, Carpal Tunnel Syndrome, Tennis Elbow, Arthritis and Frozen Shoulder will be especially benefited. Arm and Hand pain can be virtually eliminated and or greatly reduced in a short time.

Learn "Amazing Thai Yoga Therapy for the Hands" By Ajahn Dr. Anthony B. James!
Visit BeardedMedia.Com New comprehensive textbook!

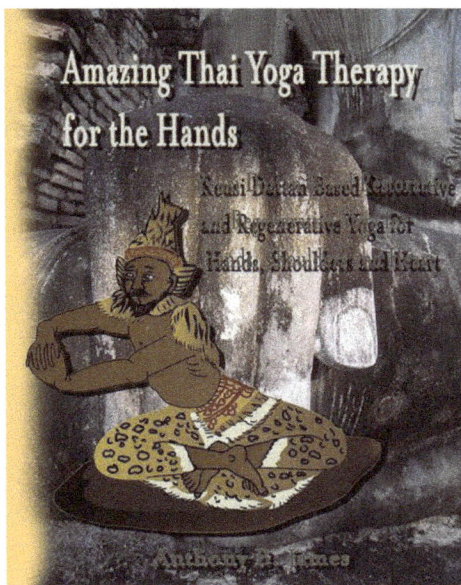

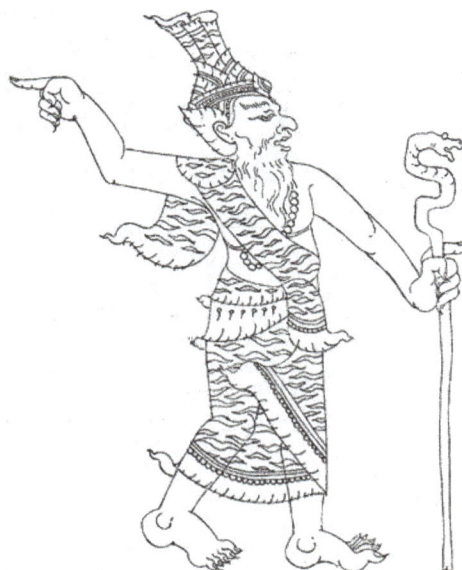

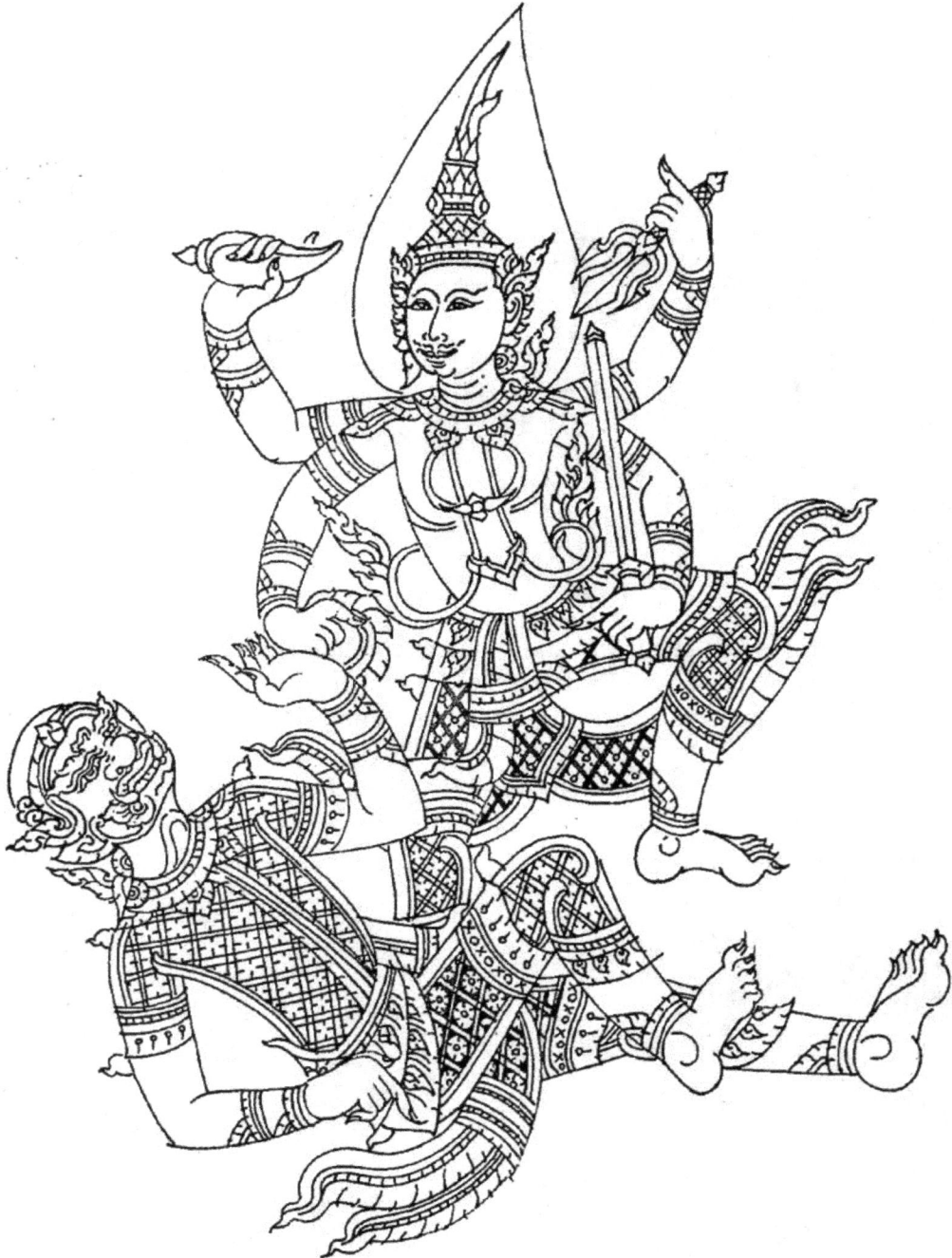

The Thai Krabi Krabong Tradition Continues

The 20th Century Buddhai Sawan school was formally recognized for this work in 1957. The school and Phaa Kruu Samaii as Dean were formally registered with the Royal Thai Ministry of Education. The former Thai King **Bhumibol Adulyadej** (*Nai Luang* or *Phra Chao Yu Hua* (ในหลวง or พระเจ้าอยู่หัว) personally presented the school with a "Victory" flag as a token of his patronage. This support or "patronage" of the Thai Royal family of the Buddhai Sawan school and teachings continues. For example, in 2006, when I was invited by the King to present Thai Traditional Medicine via live broadcast to 163 vocational schools. I was representing Buddhai Sawan, Anantasuk and Wat Po Association of Thai Traditional Medical Schools because of my affiliation as a teacher from the Buddhai Sawan tradition.

Today, there is not just one system of Krabi Krabong. Previously I mentioned Ajahn Arimeta of Chiangmai and the period of collaboration. Some of the other systems are located within the public school system at all levels from elementary to collegiate. They are more or less organized as physical education. Think, instead of football… Krabi Krabong!

Others of these schools are hard core. They emphasize traditional combative as well as spiritual discipline as their practice, mission and focus. While others are really just sport, competition focused such as in pro Muay Thai.

There is even a group for schools and teachers working together to bring Krabi Krabong (Thai Fencing) into the SEA Games and the Olympics for international competition as a combative and indigenous artistic entry or category. Consider the example, often cited, of Korean traditional Martial Arts in developing Tae Kwon Do as a sport based on an integration of Tang Soo Do, Mu Duk Kwan, Hap Kido, Jee Do Kwan, Hwa Rang Do into a non-lethal contact sport, eventually being accepted as an Olympic sport.

The Prya Phichai School of Bare Knuckle Muay Thai and Krabi Krabong is a direct descendant to the famous master of Krabi Krabong who defended his home with swords in both hands. Although mortally wounded in this battle, he gained the deep admiration of all Thai people familiar with his story of courage and action.

The Sukrat school, founded by Ajahn Thanlor follows the Mon cultures interpretation and practices with a comprehensive curriculum of the traditional Mon martial arts.

The Atema (Atrema) school traces their roots to the methods as taught by King Narasuan (Black Prince).

The Lanna Schools and systems of Krabi Krabong including but not limited to the school founded by Ajahn Arimeta, continue the unique regional heritage of martial arts passed down through the families of the Lanna or Northern Thai Kingdom.

Samnak Sri Ayutthaya Chiang Mai Fencing Club under Kru Kung

One well known and respected Mae Tang, Chiangmai school passing on the teaching of Ajahn Poo and other teachers and masters is the Muay Thai Sangha School managed by Ajahn Pedro Solana. Ajahn Solano's path is similar to that of my own as he also trained in the Traditional Thai Medicine arts in the

Wat Po Association style and that of Mama Lek Chaiya "*Jap Sen Nuad*" or Herbal Nerve Touch Massage as Ajahn Mama Lek used to call her system before she passed.

To find examples of the legacy of Ajahn Nak, previously referenced, simply go and watch the physical education programs at any Thai Public school! There you will see two unique Thai athletic sports being practiced by all the children… Takraw and Krabi Krabong.

Surviving schools that still to this day influence Krabi Krabong practice are to be found in the neighboring countries of Myanmar (Burma), Laos, Campuchia (Cambodia) and Malaysia. For example, Campochia had the Khymer and Mon cultural traditions which survived the atrocities of the Vietnam and Post Vietnam War (Pol Pot regime- Killing Fields)

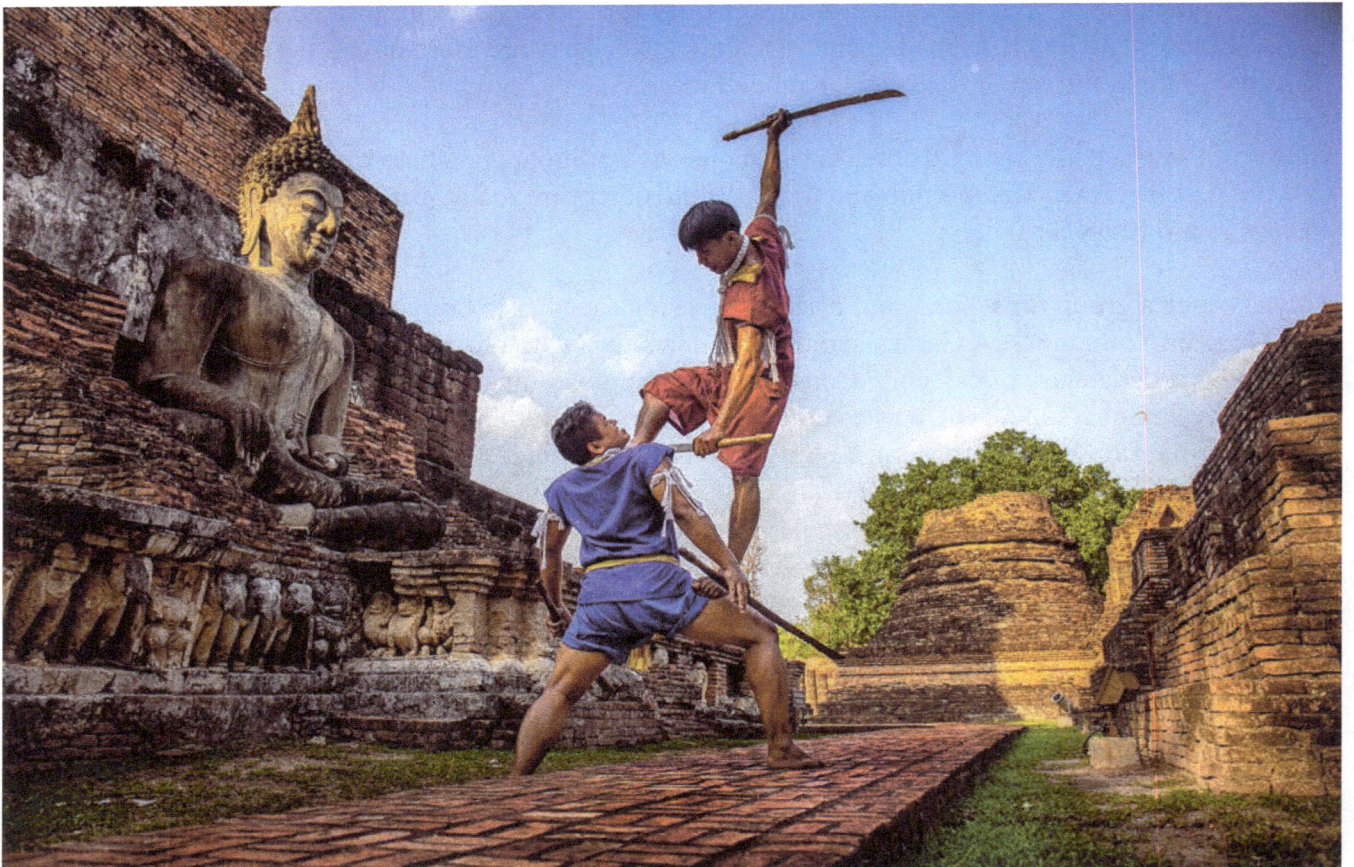

Naresuan Bin Daap Song Myyr Deo (Naresuan Flying Double Sword)

Women's Contribution to Krabi Krabong

No book would be considered anywhere near complete without some reference to the influence of women, teachers, Kruu, Ajahn's and Warriors in our tradition. Although they may not have been given their due credit for their contributions they were there. They were active and without them likely the Thai Martials arts schools and traditions are likely to not have survived, not survived intact as we find them today. Of course, we need more information and research into the roles and contributions of the "Woman Wariors of Krabi Krabong, Muay Boran".

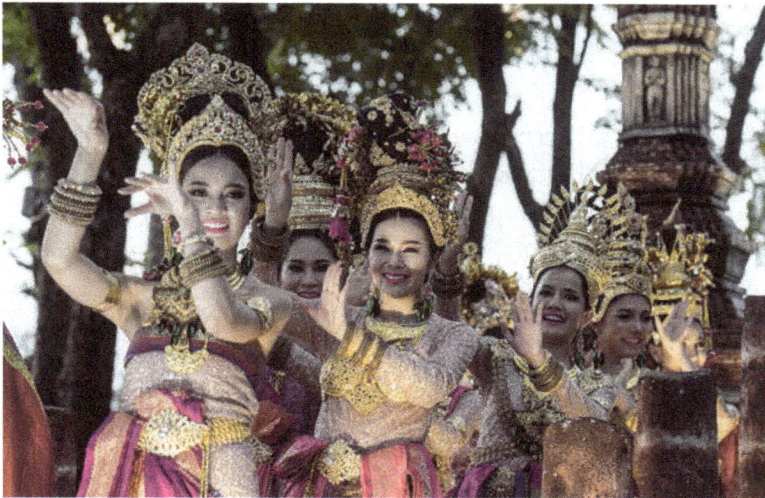

Thai women inn traditional dress with elegance and beauty during Thai Festival: "*Loi Krathong*" in Old Capital city of Sukhotai, Thailand. Having traditions of grace and beauty does not take away from their fierce and honorable character and their warrior spirit. History shows that Thai women are often a force to be reckoned with.

Queen *Si Suriyothai Mahathewi* (Crowned Queen of *Maha Chakrapat* 1548) of Ayudthaya, wife of King *Maha Chakrapat* (15th king of Ayudthaya Kingdom) entered the active battlefield and fought alongside her husband, dressed out in full fighting armor, on the top of a fully dressed out War Elephant with her daughter acting as her second. Apparently, she gave a good accounting of herself and delayed the attack on her husband long enough to enable him to get to safety. She died in battle, trying to save her fallen husband.

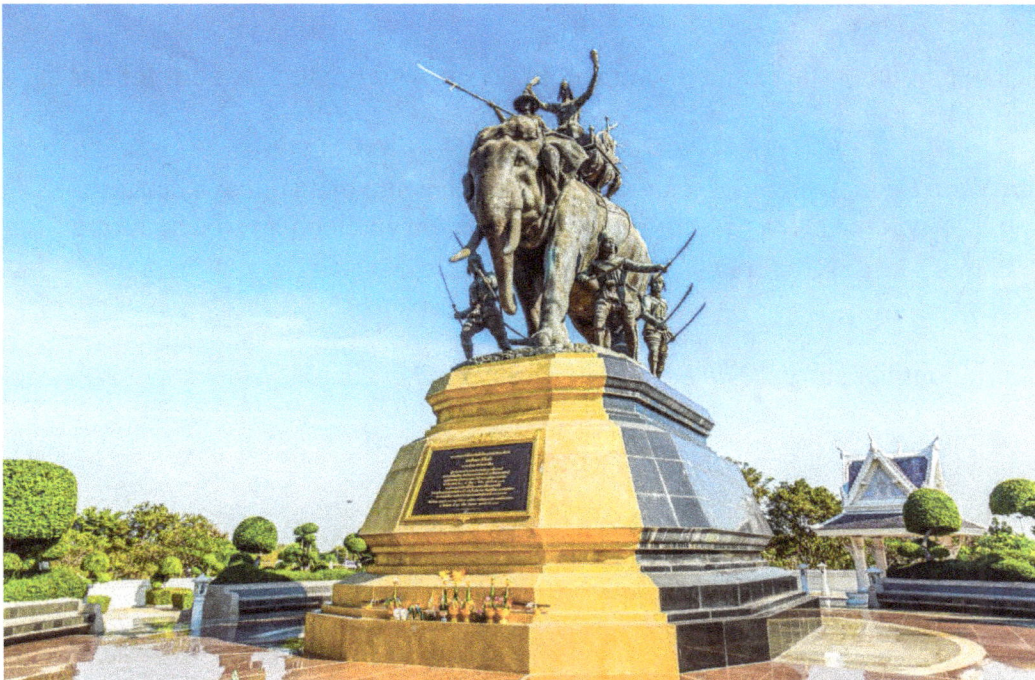

In Buddhai Sawan school of Krabi Krabong, we have always trained with the long weapons. The "Krabong", i.e., *Plong, Haw Kwan* etc. I have included some images of these traditional weapons later in the book. When I say long? I mean long enough to stand on the back of an elephant and attack either other elephants' occupants, horseman/ cavalry or infantry- foot soldiers. These weapons are immense. Some of the pole arms are nine feet in length, thick handled hardwood with forged steel blades of different configurations.

I have ridden elephants many times over an almost 40 year period of time. I have ridden these elephants, with the Mahout- Elephant handler, sitting on the tail or head. We have traversed every imaginable type of terrain from village paths to mountainous terrain with steep angle of climb, to swimming across or fording rivers from bank to bank.

The elephant is the ultimate transport four-wheel drive, all-terrain vehicle. Many times, it was all I could do to stay on the elephant! Sometimes having to lay back completely flat while the elephant was at a steep angle or completely forward hanging on for dear life. Often having to dodge brush and tree limbs and deal with the tendency for the elephant to side bar and attempt to eat at every opportunity. This is in full control, usually single file, happy elephant.

I could not imagine actually standing up in a basket with a rack of spears and polearms, Swords and Bow and Arrow… fighting. And while fighting the Mahout on the back of the elephant guiding and steering it to fight and get the best angle to do the most damage. The elephants themselves… Now called "War Elephants" were also dressed out and armored. Not to mention that elephants roar when excited? The lead officer, the Queen… would have been yelling commands to her aid (daughter) and her Mahout or driver… while fighting! To say she was well trained before this. That would be an understatement… to fight on the back of a "War Elephant" is the highest level of training. (http://www.mekongsustaina-bletourism.com/en/contents/238?ckattempt=1)

Every year the Buddhai Sawan clans attend and participate in the annual festival and remembrance re-enactments of these famous battles in Ayudthaya, including that of Queen Suriyotai in Surin, Thailand.

See "Page 55". There is a magnificent statue and monument in downtown Ayudthaya, built for her in Ayudthaya.

This statue is on Makham Yong Field, which is a historically significant site of Ayutthaya because, according to the chronicle, it is where Queen Si Suriyothai was killed on an elephant's back during a battle in A.D. 1449. (https://go.ayutthaya.go.th/en/tourist-attraction/no-temple-touring/monu-ment-of-queen-si-suriyothai/)

There is also a movie made about her story; "*The Legend of Suriyothai*" available.

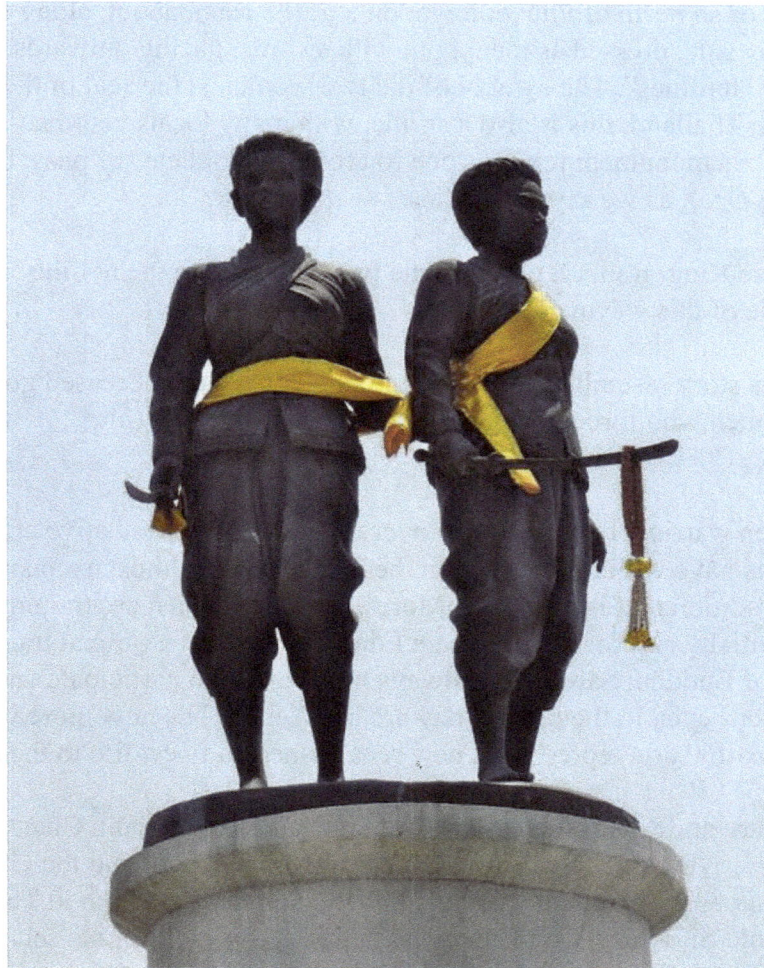

The Thao Sisters of 1785 banded together the women of Phuket Island into a formidable fighting force to militarily resist a Burmese invasion army. "Banded Together" means they organized training and practice, weapons and the fighting strategies to use them to repel the invaders.

Thai historians document that the Burmese King sent one of nine armies to invade the island of Phuket. Unfortunately, for the Burmese, the governor of the island had recently died, leaving the island without formal leadership. Stepping up and taking the initiative, the wife of the governor, "*Than Phu Ying Chan*" and her sister "*Mook*" assembled a mixed group of militias and resisted (fought) the Burmese invader army using guerilla tactics, including dressing women in military uniforms to delude the Burmese into believing that they faced reinforcements. After a month of conflict, the Burmese army withdrew, the date given for this is March 13, 1785.

They trained their army, cadre of women daily until the fighting began and according to Phuket history, after a month-long siege, the Burmese gave up and left… leaving the island free. These women are honored today with a beautiful statue in Phuket City… "In memory of their achievement in 1967 a sizeable monument to the two women was erected in Phuket province. This was a prominent event, with the King of Thailand in attendance. Every year, in March, a celebration is held in honor of their triumph.

The statues are 13kms or so north of Phuket town, on a traffic roundabout, along a major highway. The two ladies stand side by side, dressed as men, both with swords, gazing outwards. Locally, the statues are referred to as "The Heroines". The symbol of the two women is the seal of the province of Phuket. As with most statues in Thailand, this is also a shrine, with many locals visiting the site. I will point out, however, that to reach the monument requires one to cross several lanes of busy Thai traffic, so take care: "*Jog Dee*" (*Chok Dee*), as we say in Thailand, — good luck.

In gratitude the Siamese King, Rama I, elevated the two women into the nobility granting them the names listed on the title of this waymark.

Interesting enough, this story resembles that of Yamo, the wife of the deceased governor of Korat, who also led a group of women who forced the invading Lao to withdraw." (https://www.waymarking.com/waymarks/WMAVMK_Thao_Thep_Kasattri_and_Thao_Sri_SoontornPhuket_Thailand)

The honoring of women warriors does not carry over to the modern combative arts of *Muay Thai* and *Muay Boran*. These arts have with rare exception, been held in the almost exclusive male domain. However, this is one tradition that is changing. More and more women are training in both *Muay Thai* and in *Muay Boran*. Initially and for several years I did not ever see a woman training or fighting in *Muay Thai*… outside of Buddhai Sawan! We always had women to participate and train and many of the public demonstrations even to the present day are by women. The now more widespread inclusion of women in traditional martial arts represents a new renaissance and new life to these traditional arts.

I give credit to Thai Khru and Ajahn such as GM Ajahn Chai Sirute (Ajahn Chai: World Thai Boxing Association: https://thaiboxing.com/) & Khru Somchai, Fairtex school and the USMTA (US Muay Thai Association) for their support of women students, fighters and teachers both in Thailand and in the US. I also give credit to my old Sijo-Guro GM Danny Inosanto here as well for his school's support of women training in Kali, Jeet Kune Do, Muay Thai and yes, in Krabi Krabong as well. (Inosanto Academy: (https://inosanto.com/))

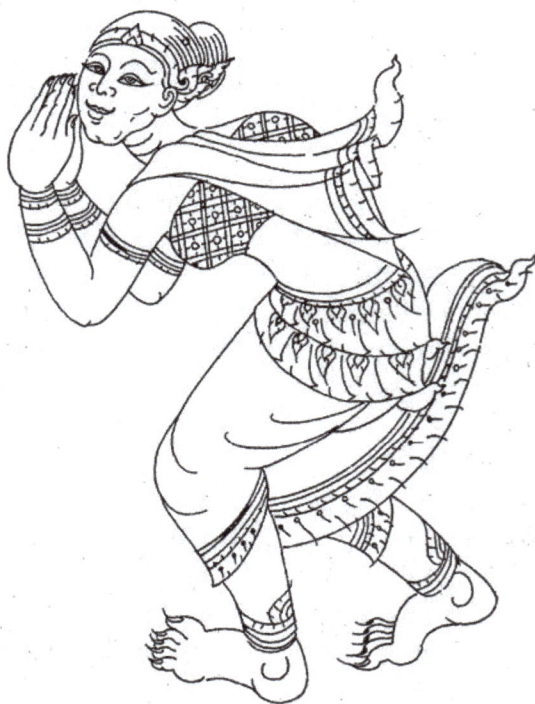

The Buddhai Sawan "Cutting The Head" Ceremony

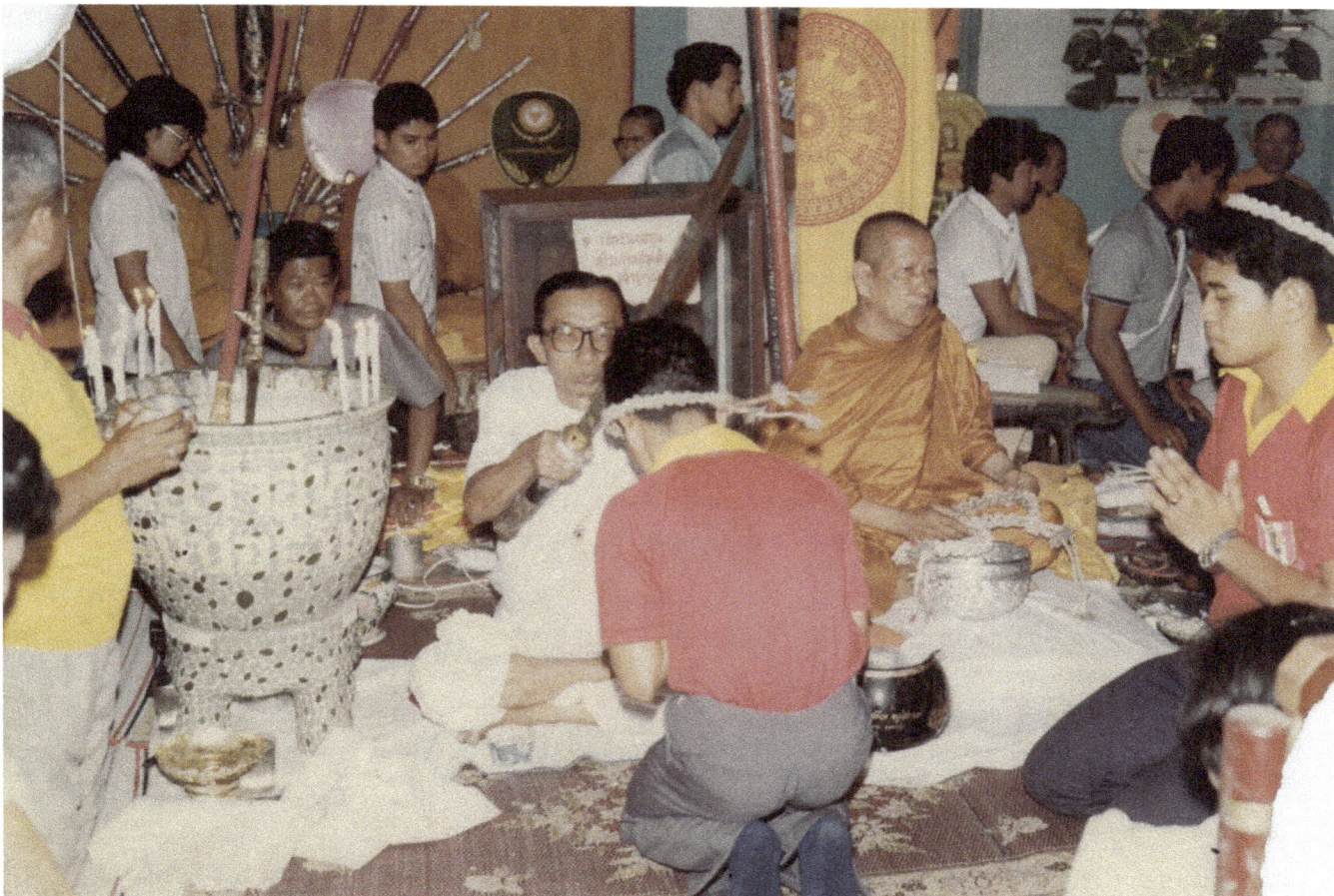

GM Phaa Kruu Samaii Performs the Puja with apprentice

Before the "Cutting the Head" ceremony, as a pre-condition to receiving the masters blessing, the student undergoes personal preparation.

There are two things the new or prospective students must learn and memorize before being inducted as a "*nakrian*" or student officially or formally in GM Phaa Kruu's Buddhai Sawan Institute and also required as a further affirmation for all Kruu or BS teachers.

The Five Precepts of Buddhai Sawan *"Sin Haa"*

(To establish a moral foundation for life and practice.) The first five are required to keep being a student. However, the final five are encouraged if the student is also on the path for Sāmaṇeras (śrāmaṇera), (and or sāmaṇerīs – the equivalent term for girls) i.e., those who choose to follow the **bhikkhu** ascetic path (towards becoming an ordained monk).

1. **Refrain from killing living things.**
2. **Refrain from stealing.**
3. **Refrain from unchastity (sensuality, sexuality, lust).**
4. **Refrain from lying.**
5. **Refrain from taking intoxicants.**
6. **Refrain from taking food at inappropriate times (after noon).**
7. **Refrain from singing, dancing, playing music or attending entertainment programs (performances).**
8. **Refrain from wearing perfume, cosmetics and garland (decorative accessories).**
9. **Refrain from sitting on highchairs and sleeping on luxurious, soft beds.**
10. **Refrain from accepting money.**

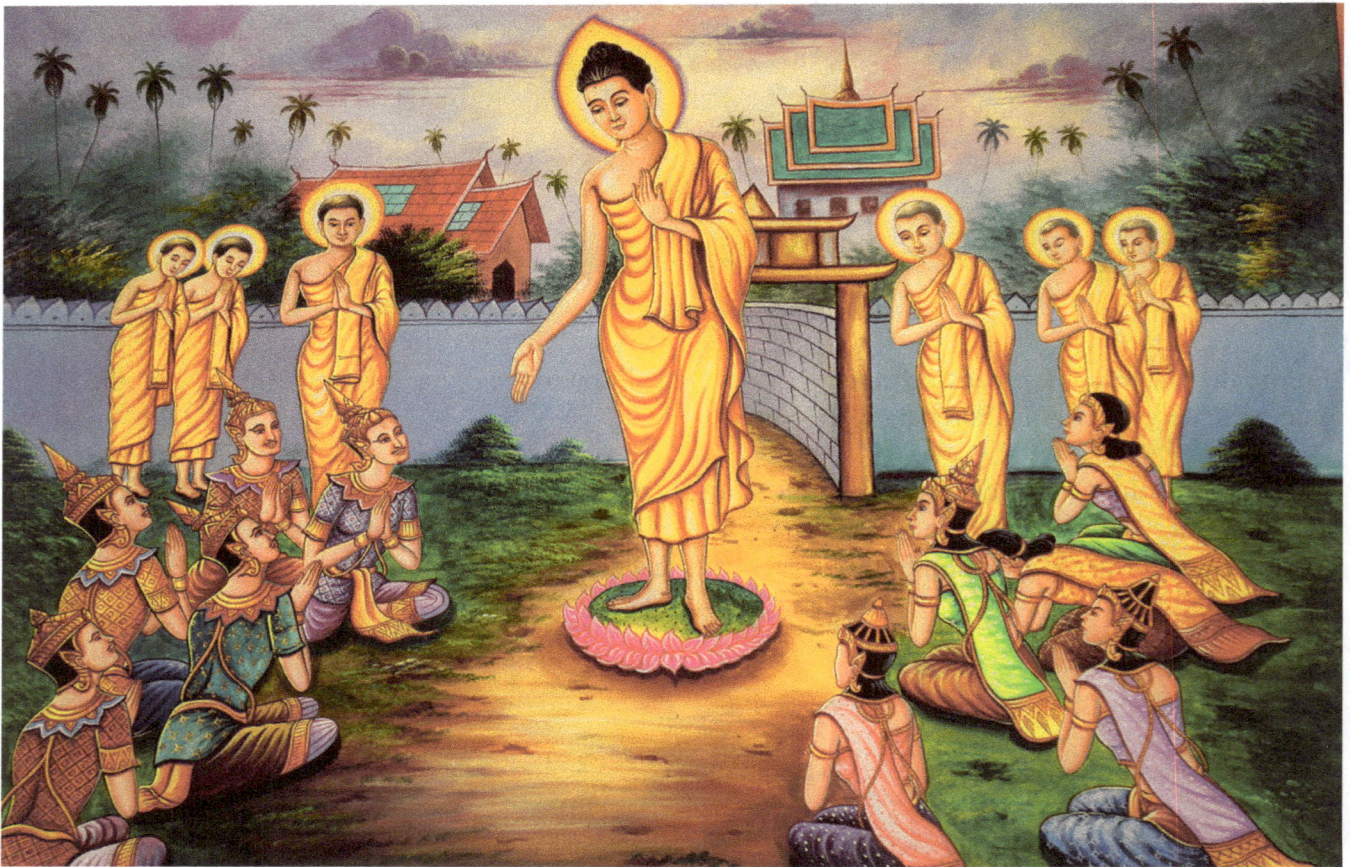

Buddhist art painting, Wat Nong Khee, Wapipatum, Mahasarakam

The Buddhai Sawan Student Oath (A vow to preserve the heritage)

We have come to honor the teacher and solemnly promise to be honest disciples.

We will respect you and have complete trust in you, father teacher.

We will treasure all traditions, rules and everything we will learn from you.

We will make your style and technique our own.

*We will never think, say or do anything to harm the school or our friends
and fellow members of our community.*

*We will swear that our words are honest and to be kept forever.
Earth, Heaven and the four directions are our witness.*

We beseech you to always protect us with the strength of our bodies, our words and our soul.

*Thus, we beseech you to teach us everything you know to protect us from failure, to protect us from
danger and to bless us with love and happiness forever.*

New students first make an application in writing. Once accepted either as a group or single individual
the process is the same.

An offering is made to the Buddha. GM, Phaa Kruu Samaii brings the offering to the main altar.

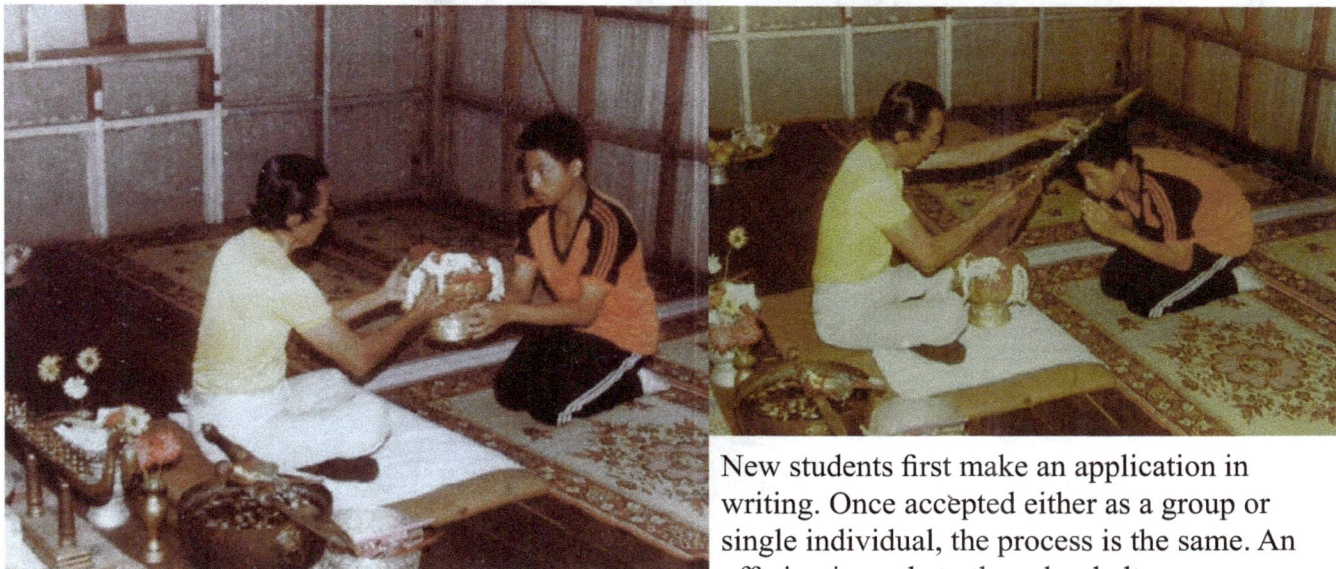

New students first make an application in writing. Once accepted either as a group or single individual, the process is the same. An offering is made to the school altar.

GM, Phaa Kruu always loved to preside over the kid's classes personally.

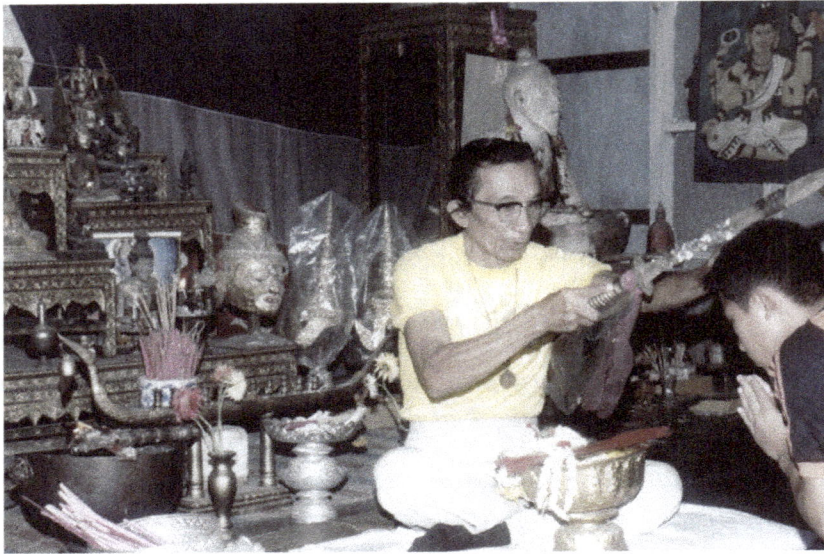

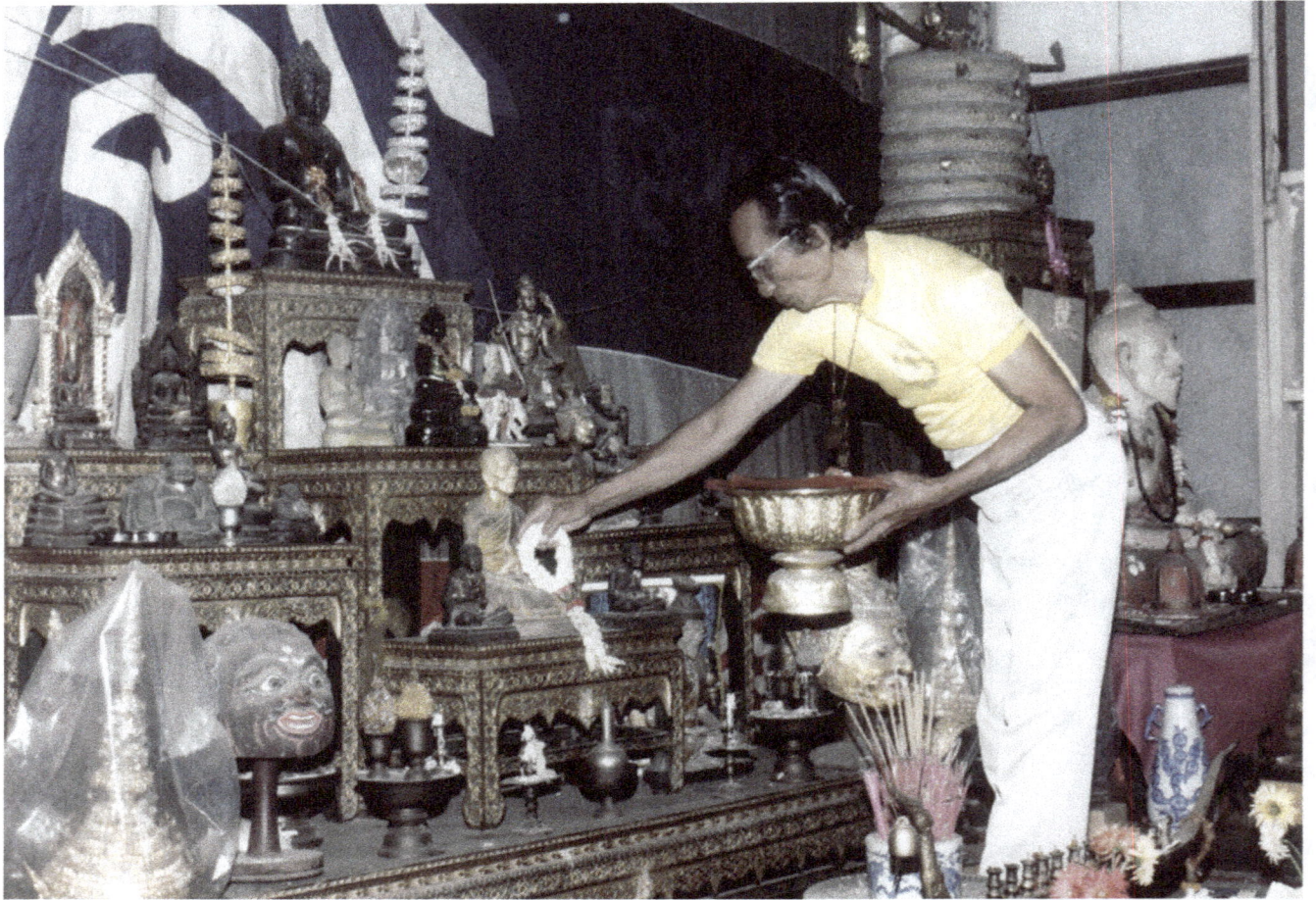

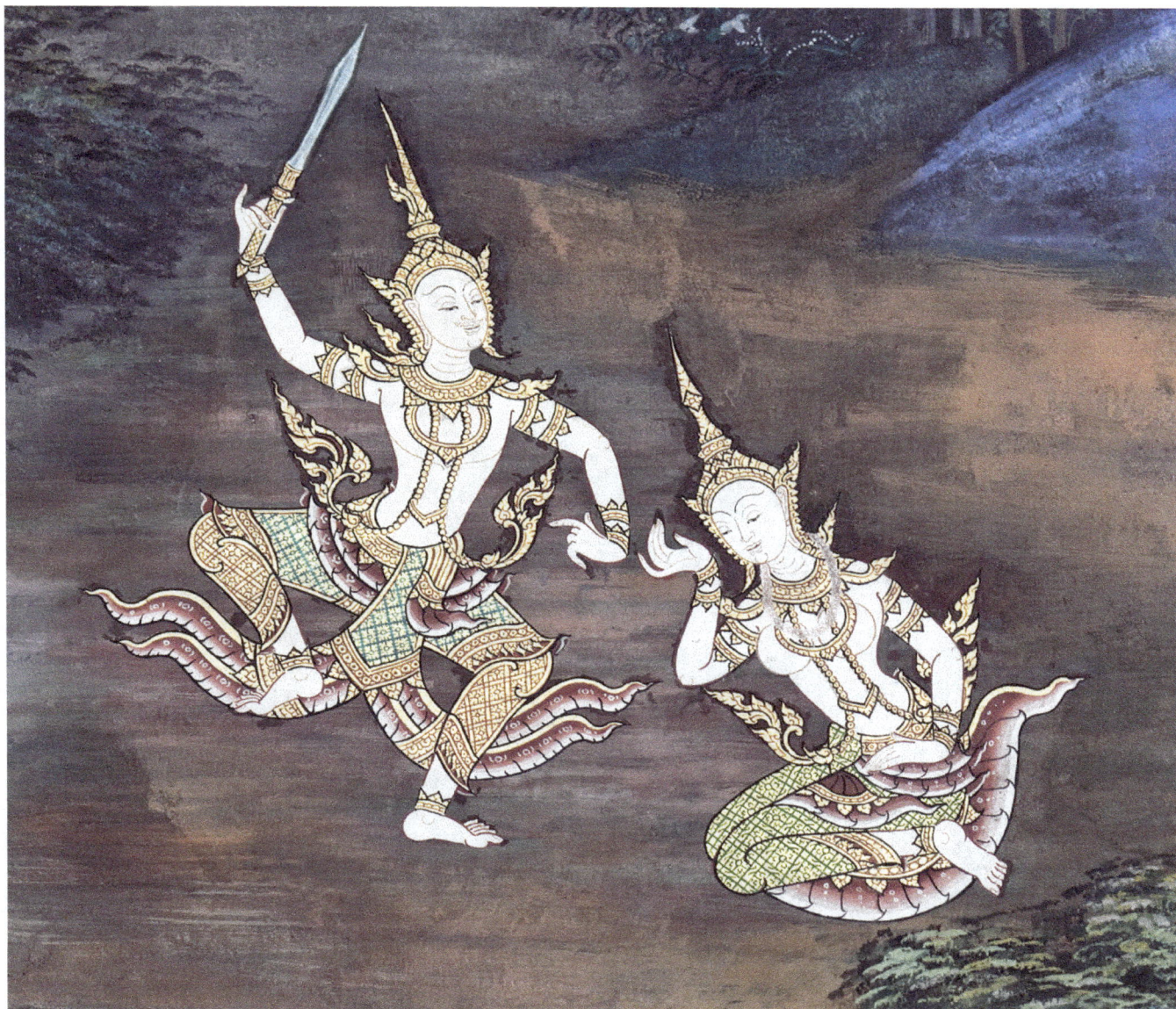

Rama with Sword Dancing, Panel from Ramayana Edic, Wat Phra Khaew, Royal Chapel, Bangkok, Thailand

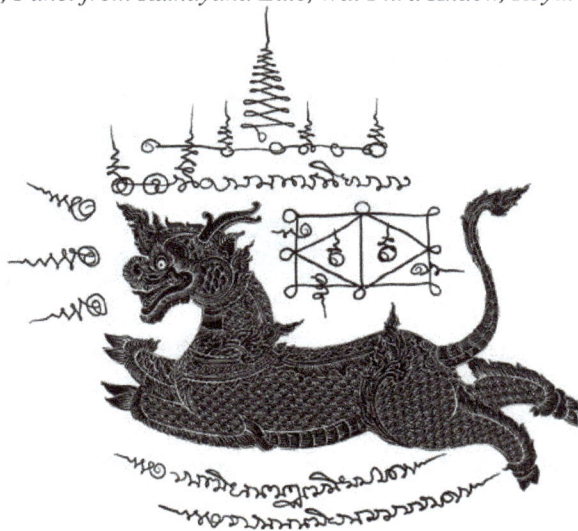

Large group induction and blessing ceremonies have always been a part of Buddhai Sawan life.

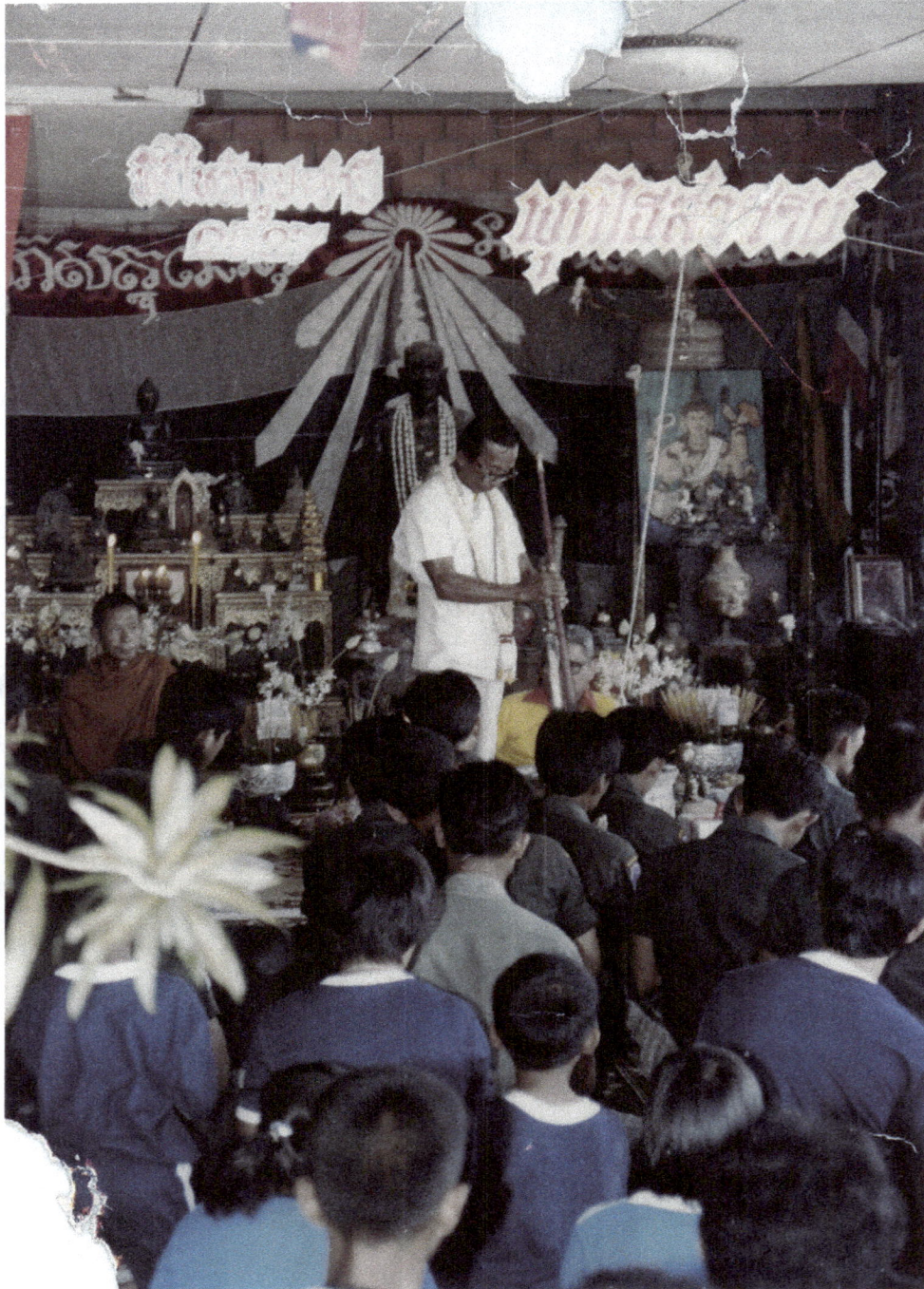

GM Phaa Kruu Samaii Mesamarn accepts a large group of Thai Special Forces/ Elite Border Patrol Servicemen into Buddhai Sawan Krabi Krabong community. At this time, Buddhai Sawan Krabi Krabong was being taught and practiced formally in the Thai Military forces. Many quite well known officers and Generals are former graduates of the Buddhai Sawan Krabi Krabong training.

The Tiger Sword Of Thailand
"The Ancient Art of Siamese Sword Fighting: The Science of Fighting with Eight Arms!"

Attacks seem to come from every angle with lightning speed, impossible to counter, impossible to follow. You're hardly able to interfere with, much less able to stop, more than a mere percentage of blows. You counterattack immediately only to find .... emptiness. Although, not for long. Pain suddenly explodes across your back as you whirl, only to find a wall of flashing steel. You're good, and you manage to thrust into that morass of whirling death just in time to realize that one of your legs has been crushed; crushed by a kick which seemed to have materialized from nowhere, and you're going down.

Those flashing blades never stopped, they never deviated from their inevitable progress. It's as if your opponent had eight arms!

Nightmare or dark fantasy? Neither. You've just encountered the Tiger Double Sword of the Temple Buddhai Swan of Ayudhya, Thailand--also known as the "*Krabi Krabong Budddhai Swan,*" or "long and short weapons of the Buddha's heaven".

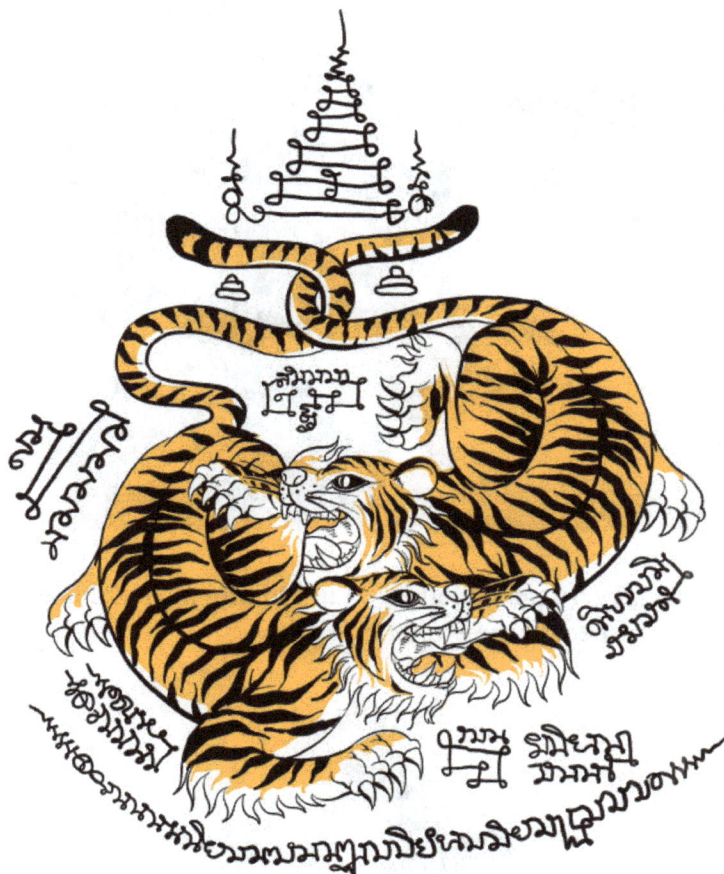

Buddhai Sawan Sri Ayudhya in Nongkam/ Thonburi (Chonburi)

The original home of Buddhai Sawan Krabi Krabong Sword Fighting Institute and Center for Revival Culture

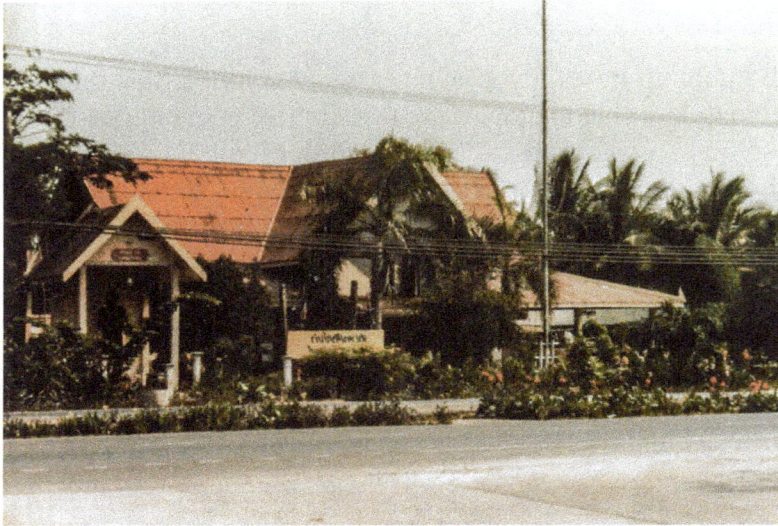

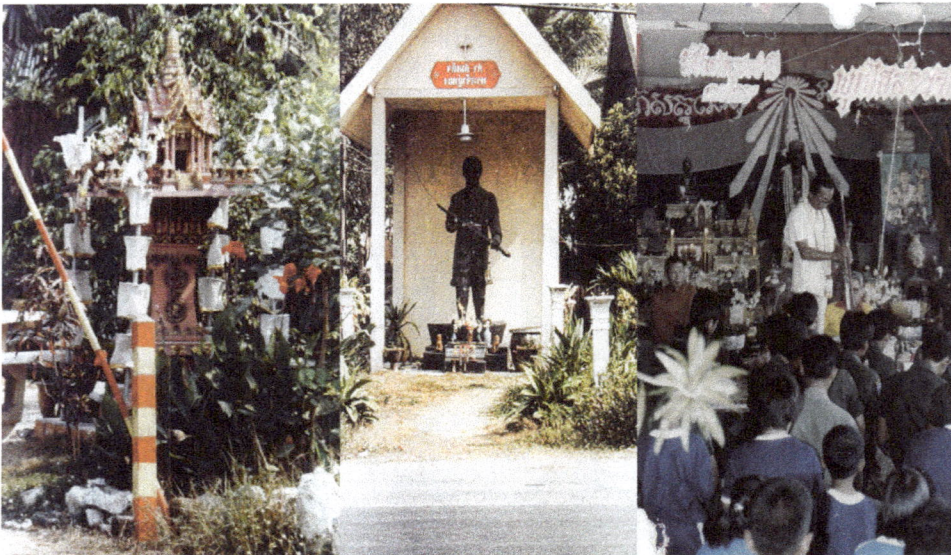

Following tradition, every day, every person engaged in training at Buddhai Swan Institute in Nongkam, Thailand was required to pay respect to three alters:

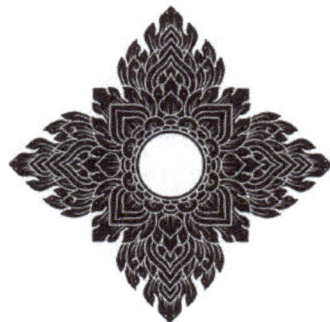

An Ancient Heritage

Allegedly, the Temple, *"Wat Buddhai Sawan,"* was the first meaningful structure erected when the first Thai kingdom was established in *Ayudhya* or northern Thailand. This temple, erected by the Buddha's disciples as a center for understanding and culture was to become the home and the training ground for the Krabi Krabong Fighting Arts. It remained so until around 1943. The school was relocated at that time to a new location in the Nongkam (Phetkasem Road – Hwy.), Thonburi/Bangkok area.

Many Thai historians attribute Thailand's 700 years of independence to the fighting skills of the kings, princes, and warriors trained in Krabi Krabong. Because of this, no Thai cultural exhibition is complete without a reference or demonstration of the Tiger Double Sword.

The strength of the Tiger Double Sword is found in the school's emphasis on the inner or the spiritual growth of the individual student. The Buddhist values of humility, compassion, and respect are prerequisites for training and are continually reinforced. The monks taught Krabi Krabong as a way of life for the warrior. This way of life fulfilled the path of Right Action, one of the eightfold pathways to perfection, according to the Buddha.

The sword is not only an efficient way to part an enemy from his life, but more importantly, it is a tool used to separate that which is nonessential from that which is productive and of value in the student himself. This cutting away or casting off of the negative or unclean aspects of the personality is first emphasized in the initiation ceremony of the Buddhai Swan where the Father/Teacher uses a sword to cut the head of the new student, thus symbolizing the setting aside of the old for the new.

The sword expresses the internal qualities, strengths, and weaknesses of the person who wields it. Hence, the spiritual and emotional development of the student is emphasized early in the training. Most prospective students think that all there is to fighting effectively with the sword is to pick one up and swing it in some particular fashion. This, however, is not true. To use the sword effectively, there must be a melding of the mind, the body, and the spirit.

The sword is an extension of the hand which is an extension of the mind; the sword is an extension of the mind. If the mind, heart, soul, or the spirit of the warrior is weak, no matter how correct the methodology used, there will be flaws. The impure person is not a spiritual warrior. However, if the heart is true this will be reflected in the blade—the blade having a veritable mind of its own will find its mark a most regardless of the technique used.

Ajahn, Kruu Anthony B. James, teacher of the Buddhai Swan Sword Fighting system located at The Thai Yoga Center in Brooksville, Florida, compares the "Tiger Sword" technique to the tiger in nature. It is unquestionably powerful, capable of subtlety and deception.

The Tiger attacks with such speed and ferocity that it literally overwhelms its prey, yet the tiger is quite capable of waiting calmly for its prey to come into range of its own accord. Before the Tigers attack, there is a "springiness," an alertness in the stance. Tiger's hunting tactics are sometimes described as being "stealthy".

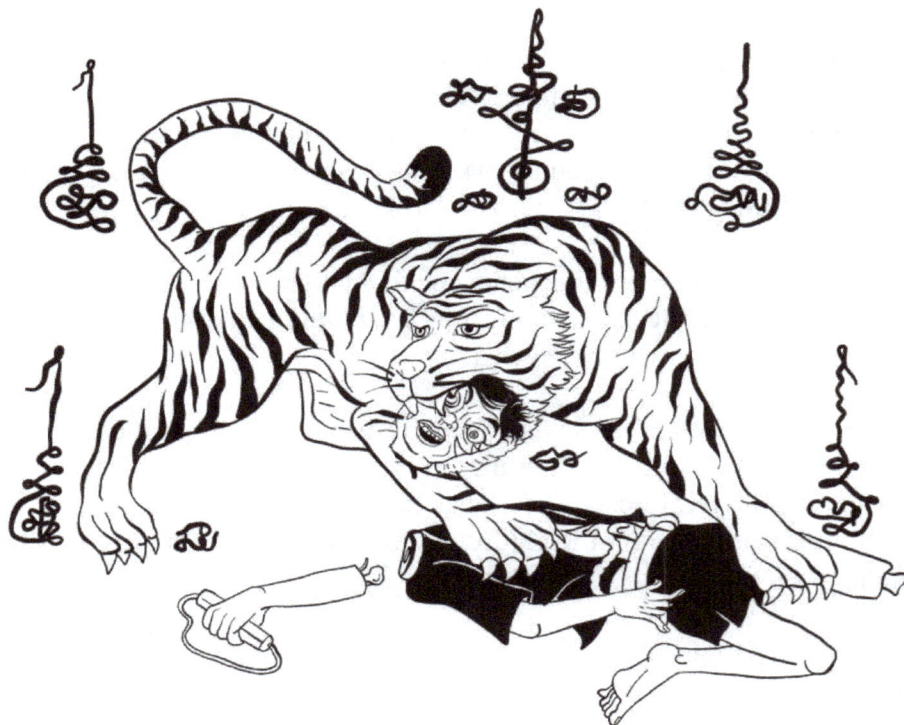

Once an attack has begun it continues with full force until completed. All parts of the body are brought into the attack as weapons. It is as if attacks are coming from all directions at the same time.

Elbows, knees, shins, and forearms are routinely incorporated into the offensive and defensive applications. Where some systems are more or less oriented defensively, that is to say to receive an attack and to counter, the Tiger Sword emphasizes attacking explosively and aggressively.

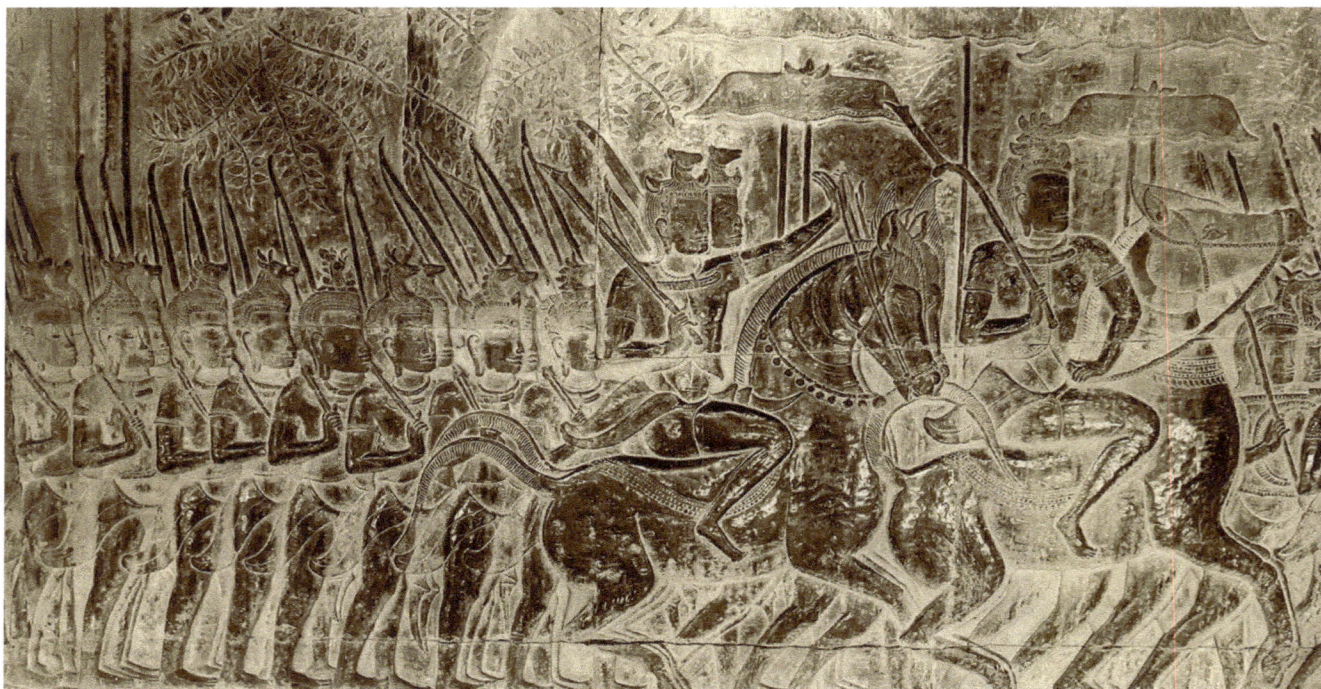

Temple illustration of Thai battle with Khymer armies

Buddhai Sawan Krabi Krabong Techniques

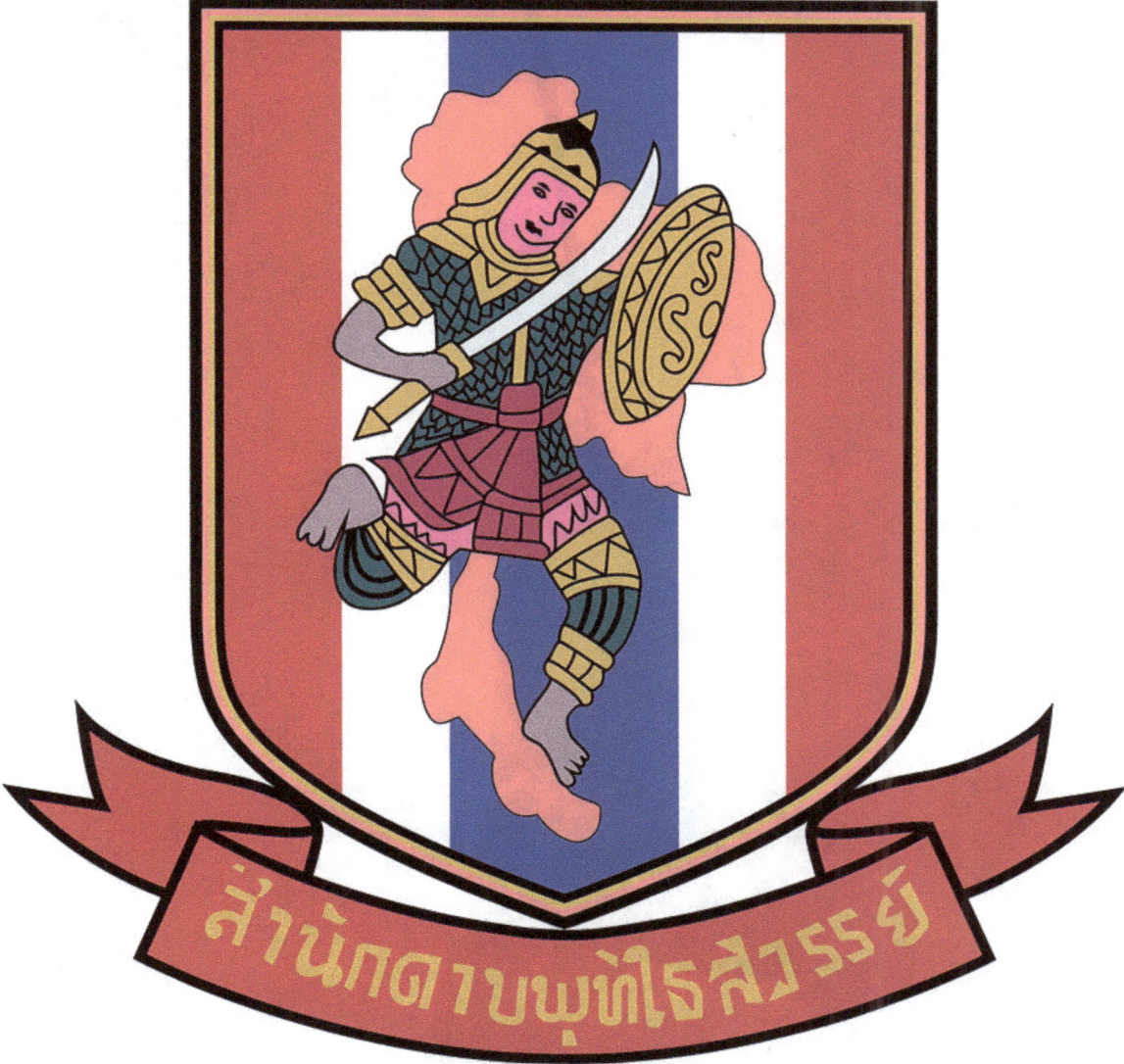

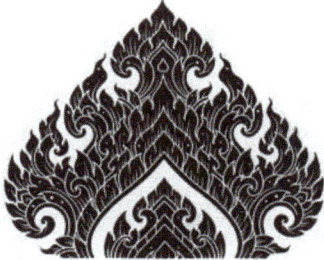

Krabi Krabong
Embodiment of the Warrior Spirit

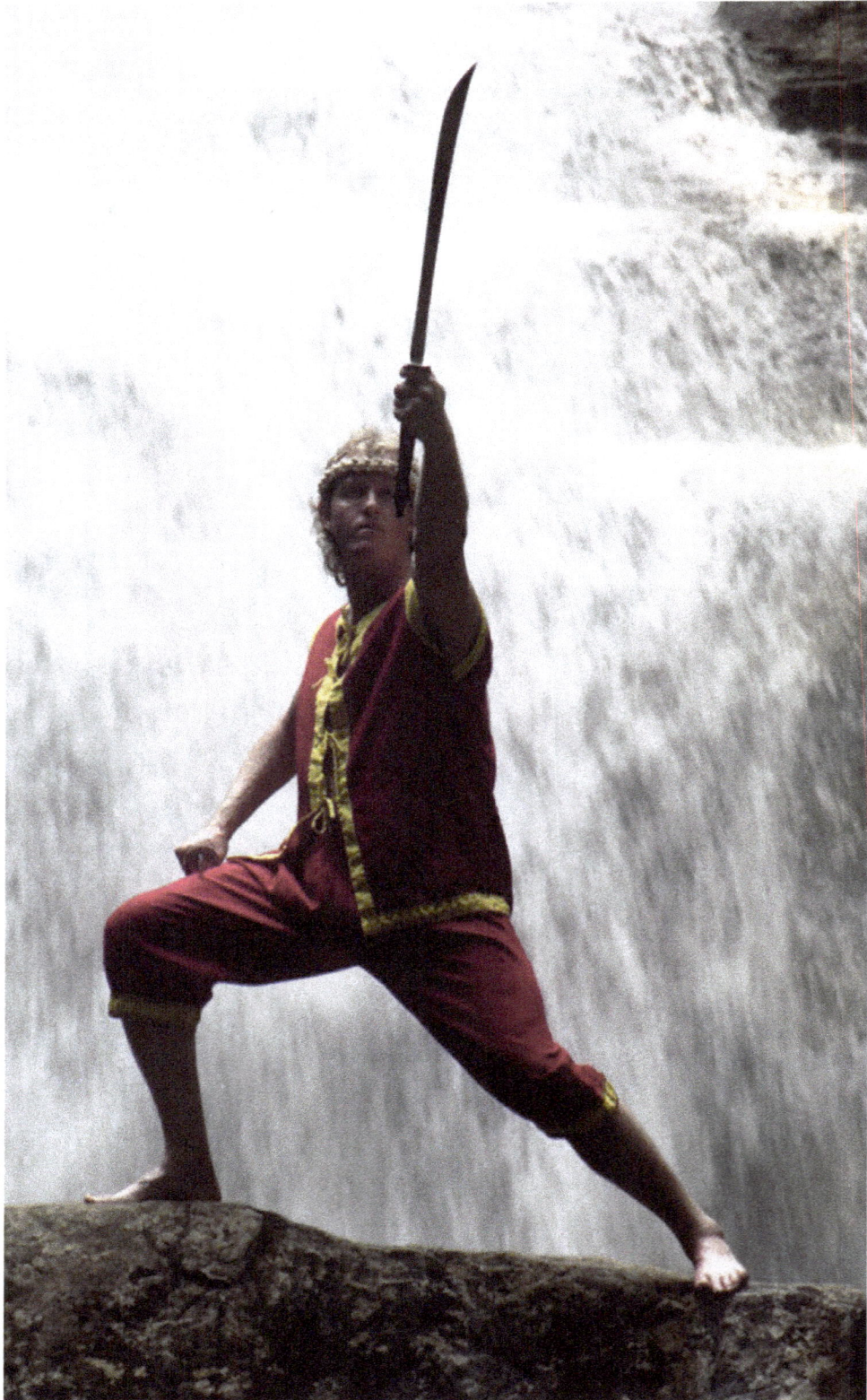

Parade Attention ("Khwām ริncı" ความสนใจ)

Traditional Military Style "Standing Attention". This is the first posture to be assumed before either kneeling to begin the "Wai Kruu" or stepping back and raising the swords into the "*Ksum*", Basic fighting stance. Attention!

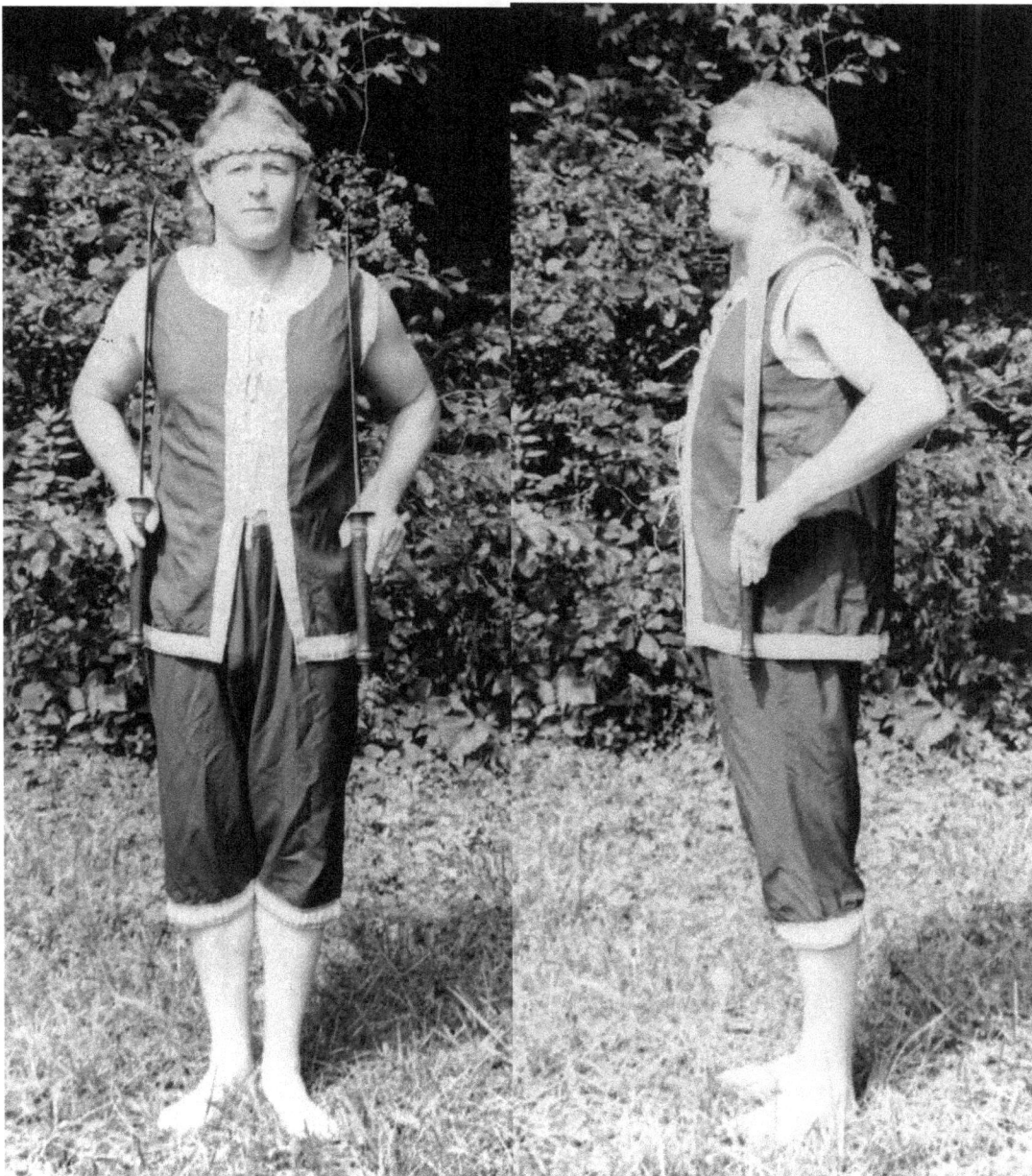

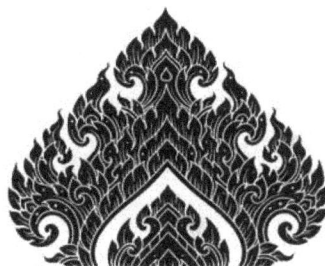

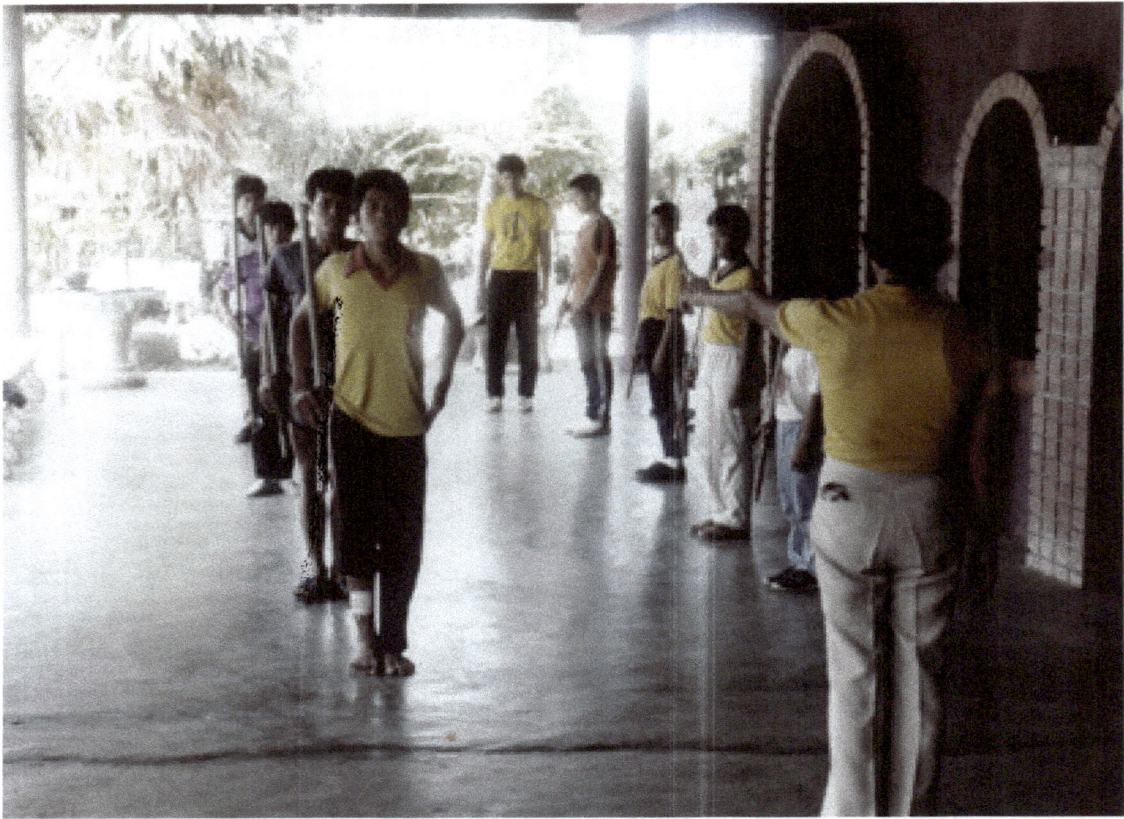

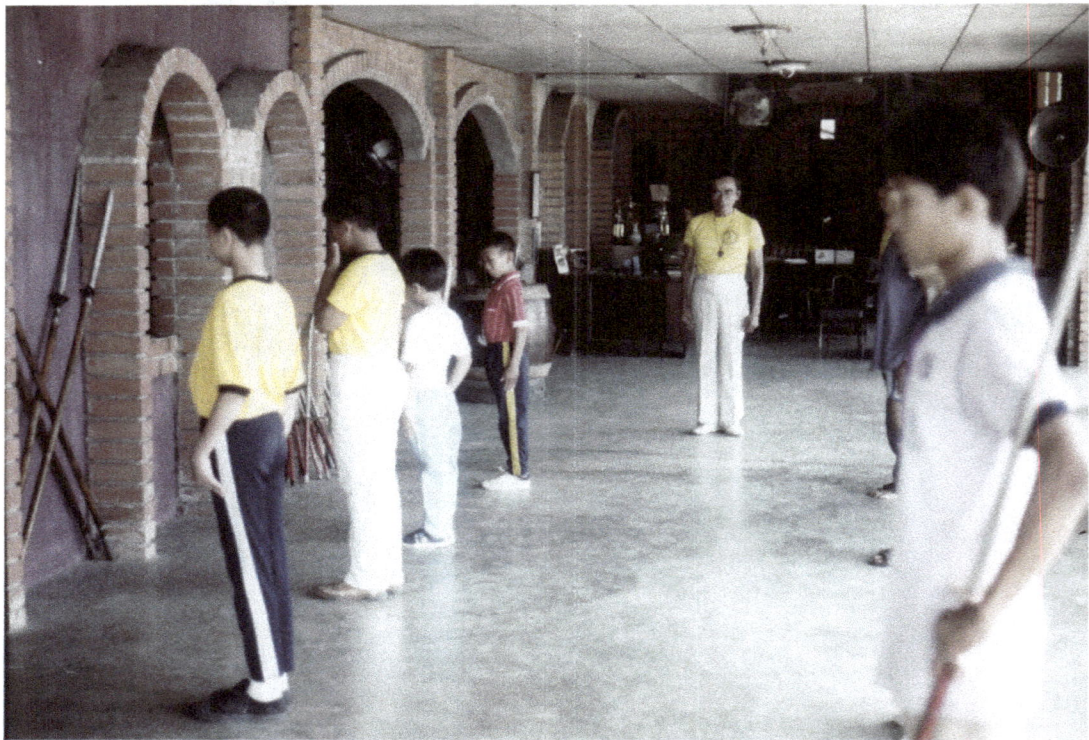

GM Phaa Kruu Samaii teaching Buddhai Sawan Parade Attention

Phaa Khruu Samaii would drill every step repetitively, over and over again! He obviously believed in repetition. He also stated that repetition was a means to an end. By driving the simplest technique deep into what we call "muscle memory" we are then free to react and to move with freedom and spontaneity. The Tiger does not think about what comes next or what to do next… the Tiger is patient, then pounces explosively!

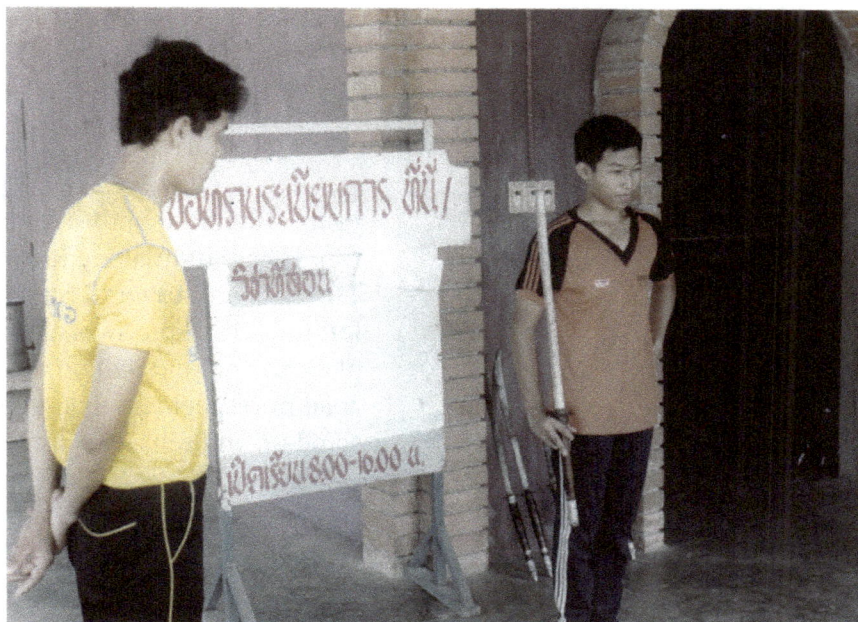

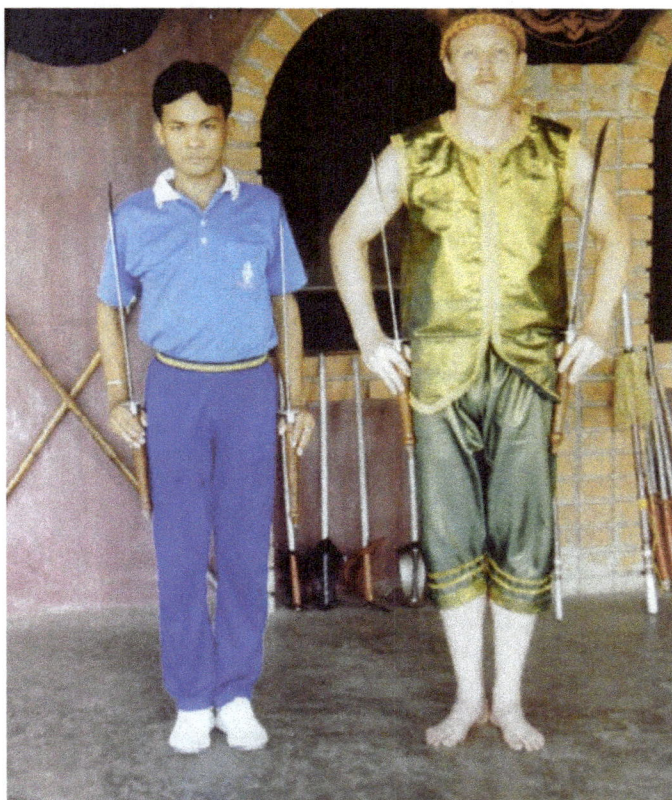

It wasn't enough to be technically correct, he wanted to see the Tiger spirit in every little detail from the way you held the swords to where your eyes were looking or focusing while you were in a stance or preparing to move. These rules and emphasis applied to all students, regardless of age, rank or skill.

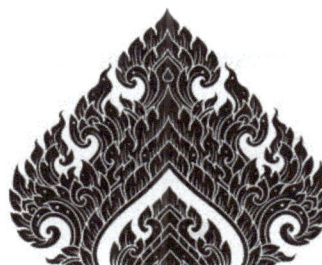

Wai Kruu

Bowing with Double Swords... *("Dap Song Myr Deo")*

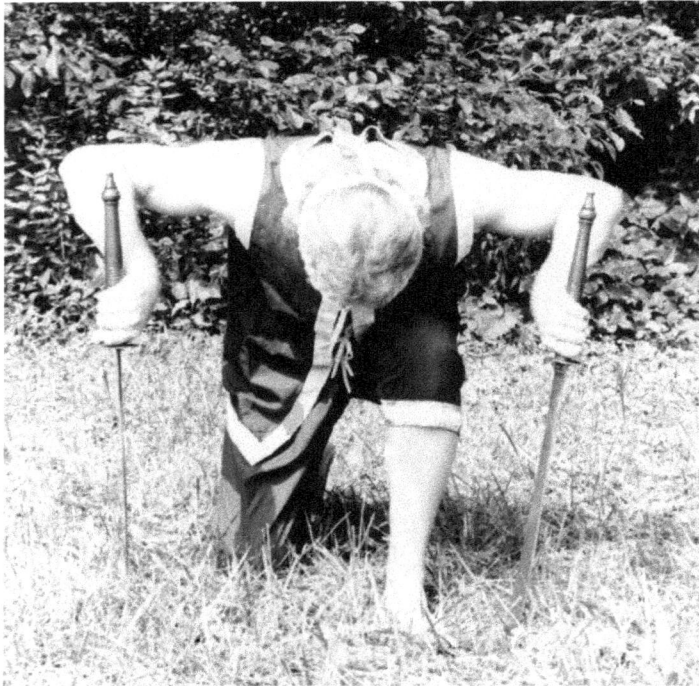

From Attention, both swords ("*Dap Song Myr Deo*") held tight along the sides of your body. The eyes are forward. Step forward with the left foot. Turn the swords over one time and place the point down on the ground. Bow the head in respect and then in one smooth motion, stand up and return back to attention.

"*Wai Khru*" is an exotic Thai language phrase literally meaning "to salute the teacher" or "pay homage to the teacher." The phase is also used as a reference to an exercise called "Four Directions." *Wai Kruu* is the first and most important step in learning all traditional Martial Arts of Thailand. The teaching of Wai Kruu is found in all five styles of Krabi Krabong and in all the variations of *Muay Thai*. It is so predominant that any illustration of Thai Arts without a representation of it cannot be considered as accurate.

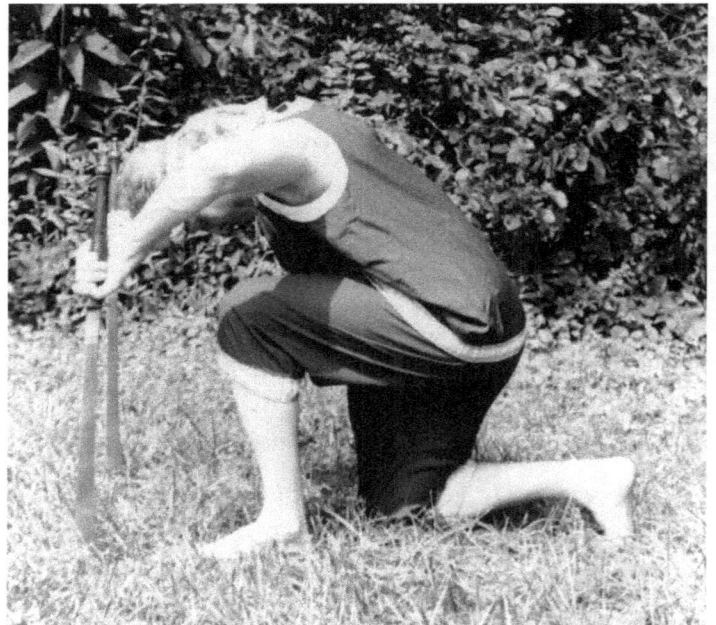

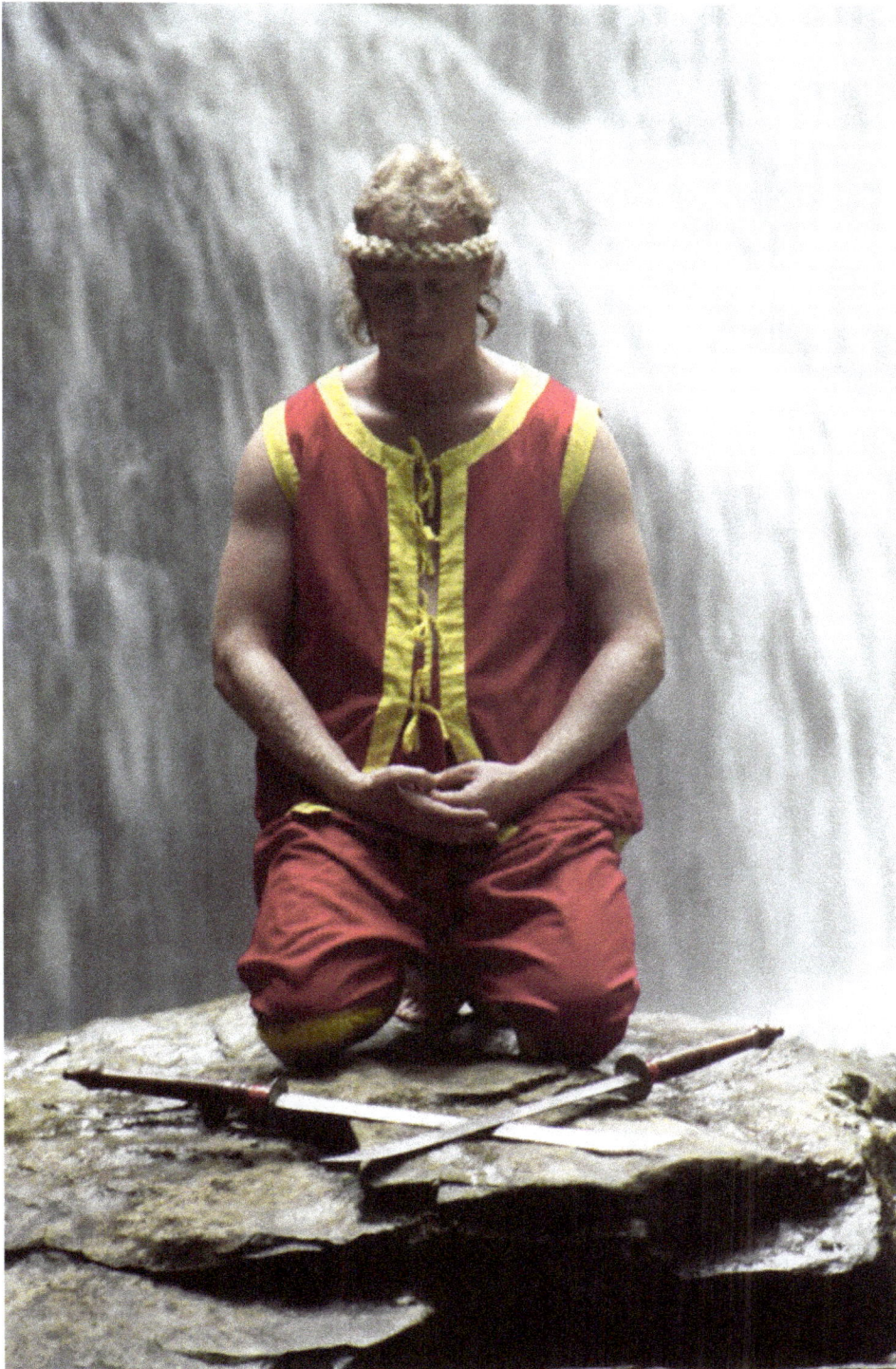

The *Wai Kruu* is where the warrior takes on the spirit of the warrior; where the student acknowledges his teacher and pays respect to him. If the warrior is a practicing Buddhist, it is where he comes to the Buddha and pays respect and solicits favor and protection. The *Wai Kruu* is part of a magic ceremony where the warrior is made invincible to harm and spiritually empowered to do well what he needs to do.

The *Wai Kruu* is an aid to concentration and visualization. As you go through it, images are brought to mind; pictures of what is to come. You may see the evil or unwanted thing before you and you ward it away with a hand motion. You symbolically carry out a series of various attacks on your opponent, visualizing their success and anticipating any counters.

As you flow, you acquire power and demonstrate your prowess to your opponent or to the spirit of your opponent.

Each and every school of Krabi Krabong and of Muay Thai has its own form of *Wai Khru*. Sometimes the *Wai Kruu* may be called a sword dance. GM, Phaa Khru Samaii called the *Wai Kruu* the *"dance to the gods."* He said that the performance of the *Wai Kruu* with a proper spirit brought favor or merit from the gods. This favor was brought into your spirit and with it came protection and insight. The particular dance signifies which particular school or style from which it originates. This is immediately obvious to the trained observer.

Bowing

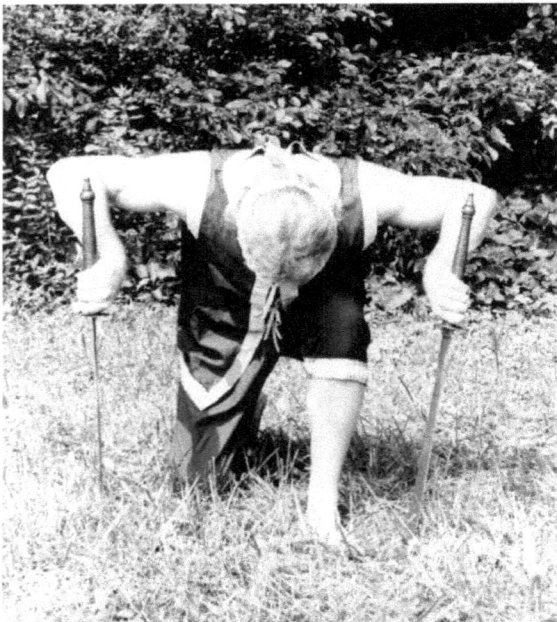

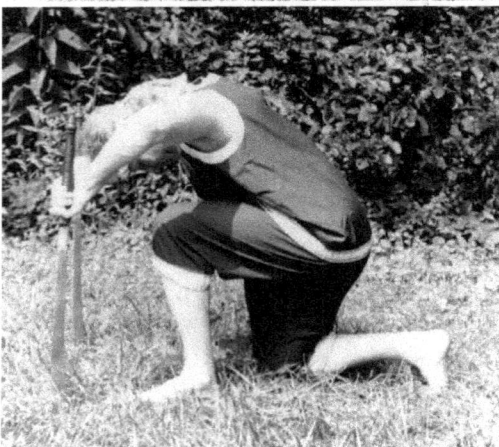

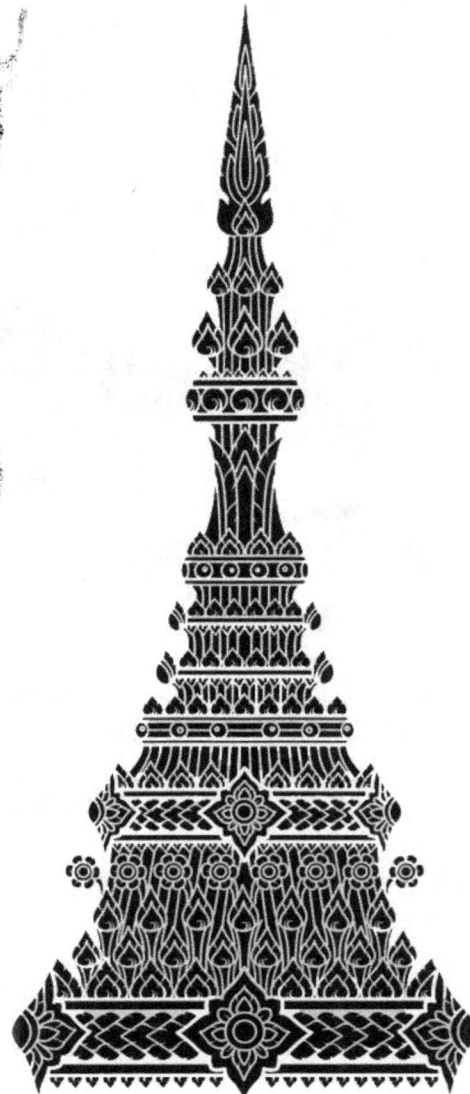

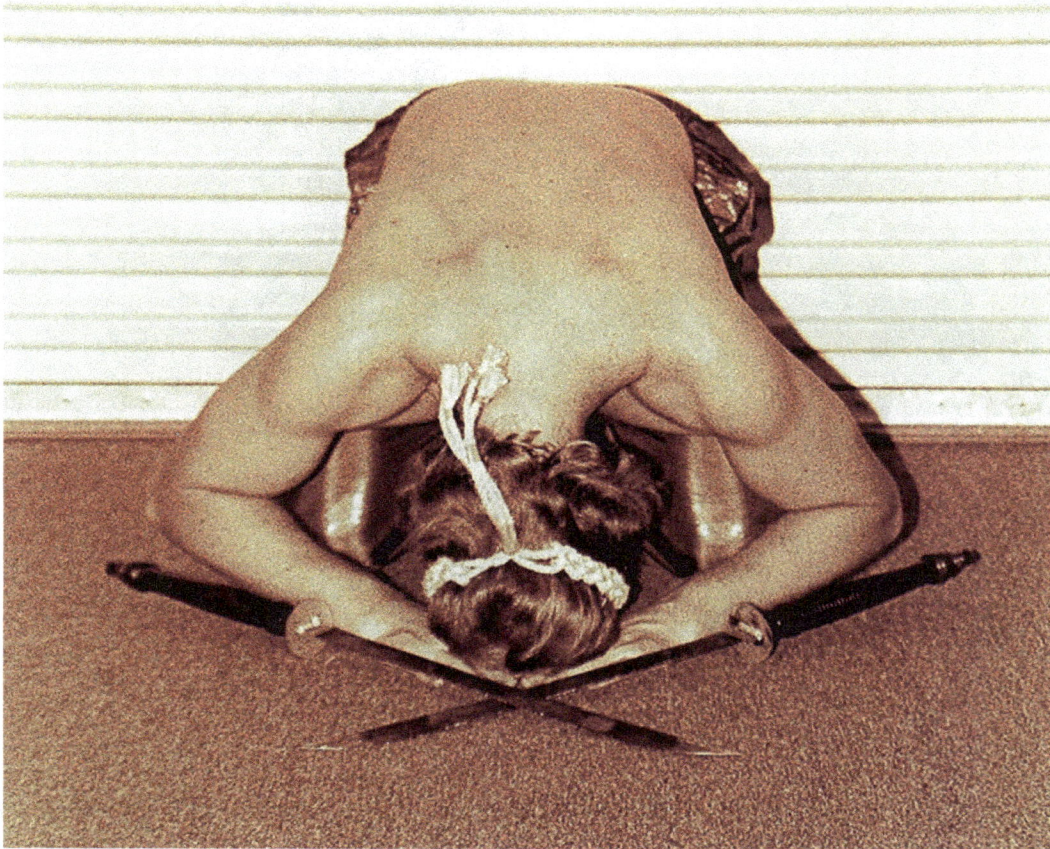

Make a triangle with your fingers and put your forehead in it! Bow three times… One: for the Buddha (Figurative and literal), Two: for the Dhamma (teachings) and Three: for the Sangha (brotherhood of men and women who follow and practice the precepts of the teachings!

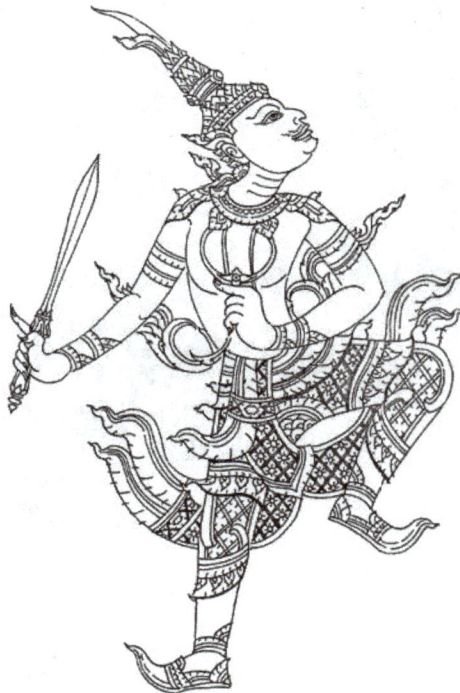

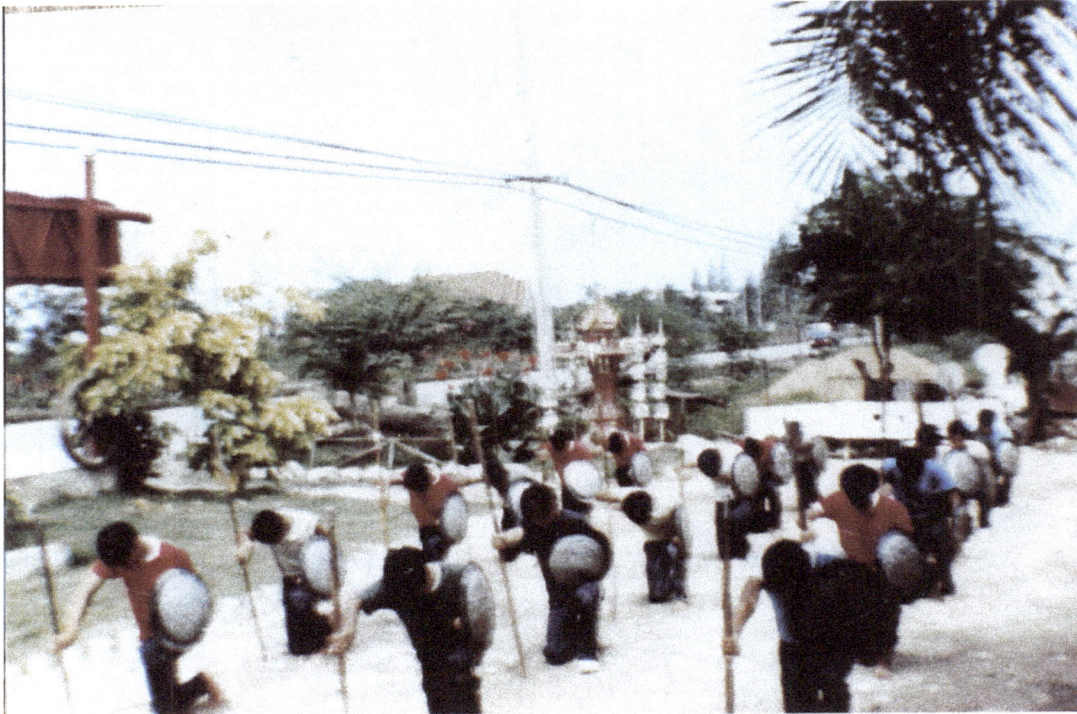

For instance, our style, that of Krabi-Krabong -Buddhai Swan style, is the "Tiger '' style - the *Wai Kruu* of royalty, allegedly first codified by the "Black Prince '' of Ayudthaya. As such, it is very grand and royal in its motions. Sweeping steps and powerful demeanor characterize this style. Conversely, in the "monkey" style, the motions are short and compact and revolve around one another; less of a dramatic form and more of an even comical aspect. Both dances would be correctly called *Wai Kruu* but are distinctly different in nature and appearance.

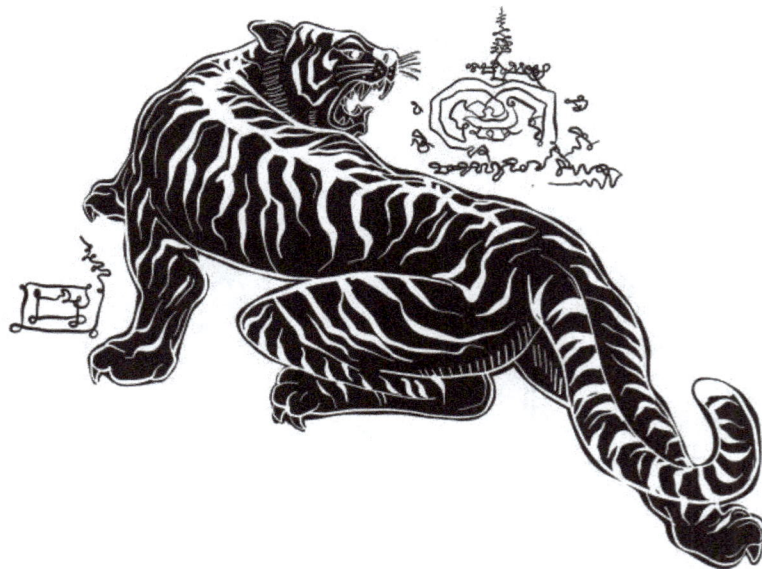

"Paying respect to three teachers"

Performed solo as well as in a group. This is the first and last teaching of Buddhai Sawan style Krabi Krabong. If you do know the "*Wai Khru*" you do not know Krabi Krabong!

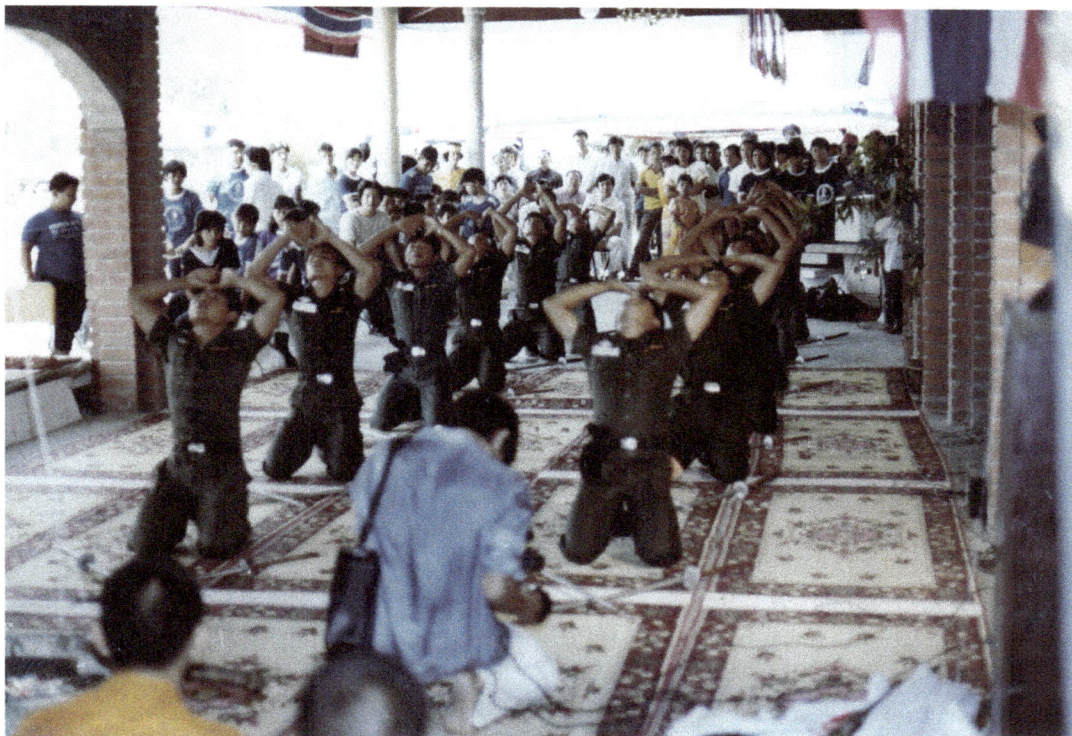

Members of the Thai Airborne, Special Warfare Operations Group (Thai Elite Border Patrol) Practice Wai Khru in the courtyard of Buddhai Swan Institute in Nongkam, Thonburi Thailand. The school after Phaa Kruu's passing was returned to old original location of *Ayudthaya* Thailand. Even members of the Thai equivalent of Green Beret's must learn and practice this sacred dance.

The *Wai Kruu* in itself is considered to be a complete preparation of the warrior for battle or the priest for prayer and meditation. It is recommended for daily practice in order to give the maximum benefit over time. The *Wai Kruu* in this regard is similar to a traditional Yoga Vinyasa or flow. It is also a similar practice as "*Kata*" or "Forms" practice of other oriental martial arts. Especially where the "*Kata*" are not only meant to be conditioning but they are mnemonic devices coding the techniques and repertoire of the given system or school. Before there were books or literature such as the one, I'm presenting here, the *Wai Kruu* was also the "catalog" passed down from one generation to the next in the form of an oral tradition.

In the *Wai Kruu*, there is a certain reservation, a certain aloofness. The eyes are focused on some distant perspective or toward the sky. This is the posture of royalty, of nobleness. It is the paying of homage, or the giving of respect, or the demonstration of understanding. Understanding that all things are connected and that nothing is done or accomplished without the blessing or the observance of God and the Buddha.

In the *Wai Kru*, the warrior bows to the Buddha three times, as three symbolizes perfection, and the Buddha stands for perfection. There is also the consideration that one is bowing or acknowledging "The

The "Buddha" (Thai Lang. "*Phoota*") is not just referring to the historical person of *Gotama Sidhartha Buddha* or *Amithaba Buddha* of Compassion... The first teacher represents metaphorically the origin of all teachers as far back as back goes. God or whatever is your concept of God, Great Spirit, Deity or Conscious Influence ("C" Influence)... connection to the Absolute, creator or origin of all things.

The "Dharma" (Thai Lang. "*Damma*" or "*Thamma*") represents the teachings derived from the Buddha as codified both by the Buddha personally, such as in the formulations of the "Eightfold Noble Path", but additionally, it includes the thousands of learned commentaries written and passed down through generations by the people who think highly or venerate these teachings... The Sangha (brotherhood)!

The "*Sangha* '' (Thai Lang. "*Sanga*") represents the flesh and blood of actual people, Men and women who both followed the teachings derived from conscious beings and their Dharma, but who additionally thought enough of these teachings and commentaries, understandings and disciplines to hold them sacred and pass them down from one generation to the next in the form and practice of an oral tradition.

The Sangha in this respect is especially important as it then becomes the tangible basis for the lineage and heritage for healing and Martial Arts such as Buddhai Sawan Krabi Krabong. This lineage passed to and recovered by GM Phaa Kruu Samaii Mesamarn and then by him, passed on to the next generation of Ajahn, and teachers both Thai and "*Farang*". We are non-ethnic, "Farang" Thai (foreigner) are the first such generation to be inducted into this ancient Warrior tradition with an especially hard task... to learn, practice, preserve and pass it on to the next. My prayer always is that we will not be the first generation to drop or fail to pass on the teachings and true values of the Buddhai Sawan Krabi Krabong to the next following generations.

Buddhai Sawan Krabi Krabong is first and foremost a cultural heritage of Thailand and The Thai People and we preserve its teachings for them. However, at the same time our teachers told us to go out to the world and teach as they were led to believe that the world needed these teachings, and it was to be the duty and obligation of students and teachers like myself to bring it to the world.

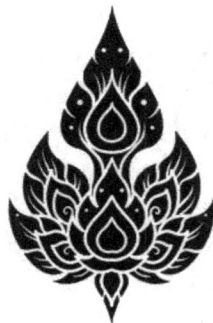

Details on Performing the "Sword Dance!"

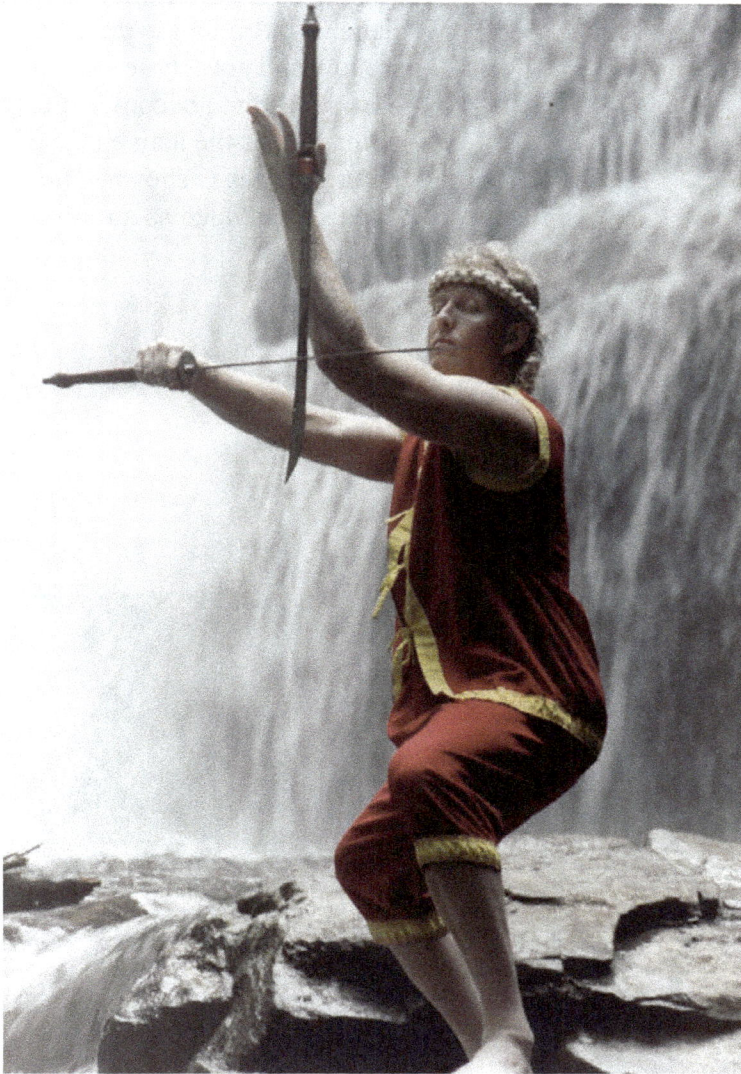

After bowing, the warrior washes his spirit, taking off the impure and unclean and putting on that which is right and proper. He takes his hands and washes his whole body and then casts the dirt or uncleanness behind him. This may be symbolic of coming to the fight without prejudice or preconceptions that act as interference to be in the moment. In a fight, one wants and needs to be present!

The warrior then salutes each of the Four Directions. The four directions are representative of "*all things*": of everything. Four directions are representative of "*Thaat Thang Sii*", the four divine elements: "*Lom Fai, Dim, Naam*", "Sanskrit Lang. *Pancha Mahabhuta*" which forms the f oundation of all that there is... Air, Fire, Water, Earth. In Thai Ayurveda, the "Sanskrit Lang. *Pancha Mahabhuta*" of Ether and Air are combined into the nature and processes of one element "*Lom*".

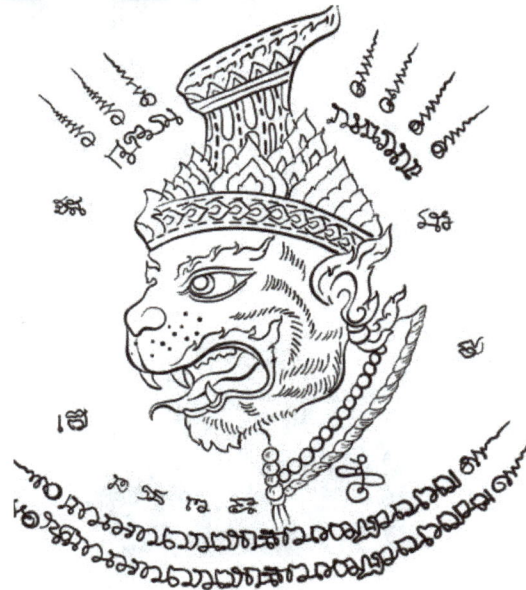

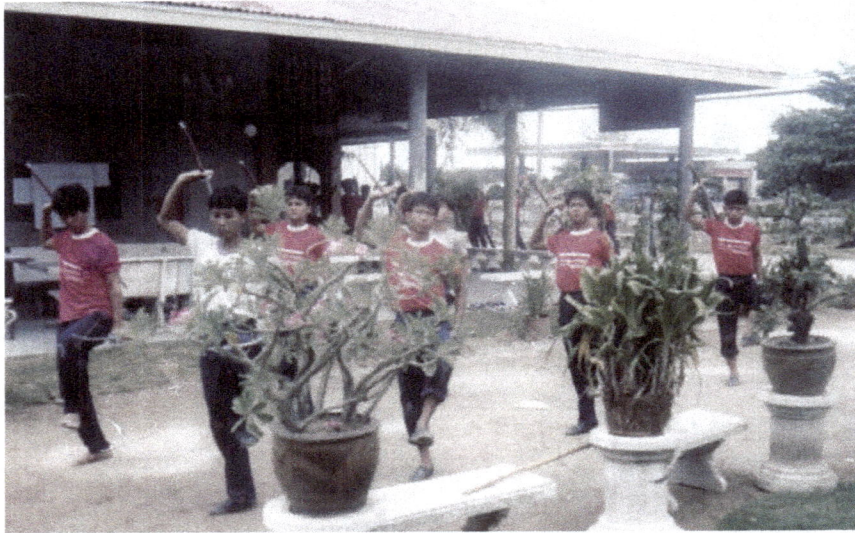

Four directions are representative of the gods. Lastly, there is dancing. At first, the dancing is slow and soberly reverent. The dance then becomes more animated, as the active part of natural forces is shown. The dance is intended as an offering to the gods.

The *Wai Kruu* of Buddhai Swan of *Ayudthaya* is a repository of information, much like the kata or forms commonly encountered from Japan to Korea. There are many nuances of eye, hand, foot, and weapon position. Each one of which is highly significant.

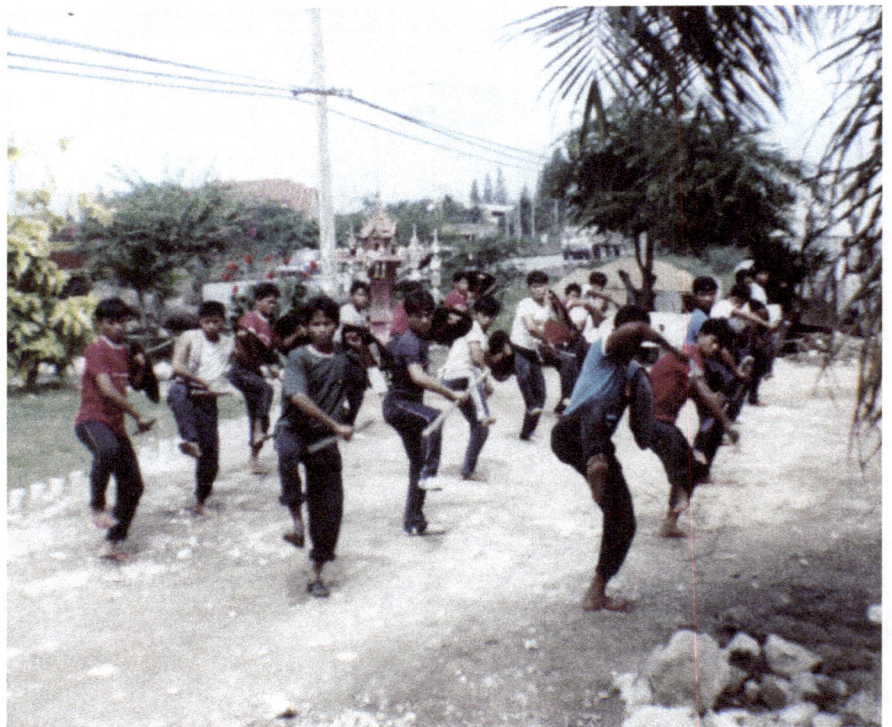

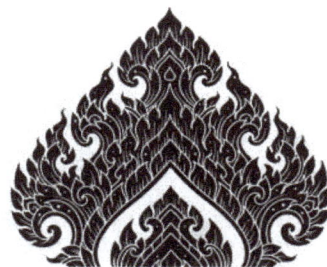

Ksum (Basic Fighting Stance)

The swords are held one in each hand, alongside the body, parallel to the arms. The elbows are positioned close into the ribs. This is called being "at attention." The feet are angled 45 degrees apart at the toes, and the eyes are straight forward. The chest is out. The shoulders are held back in a military fashion.

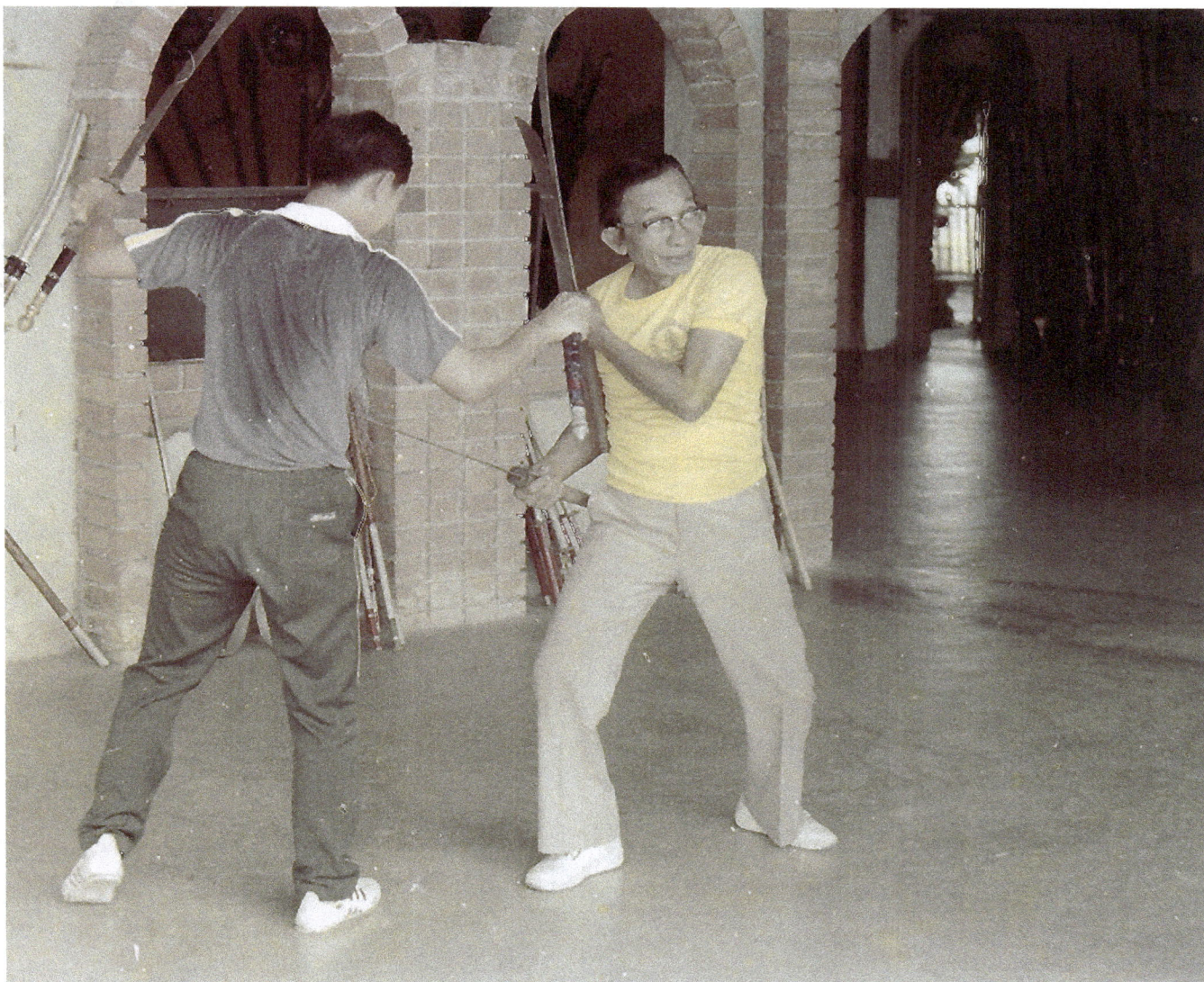

GM Phaa Kruu Samaii demonstrates a good, strong stance means adaptability and responsiveness and deadly effect to any threat or opportunity!

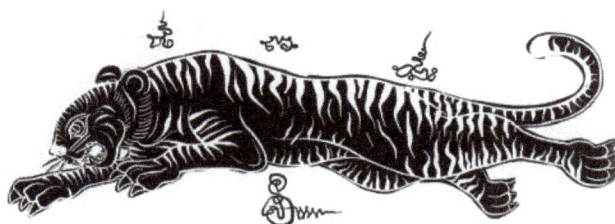

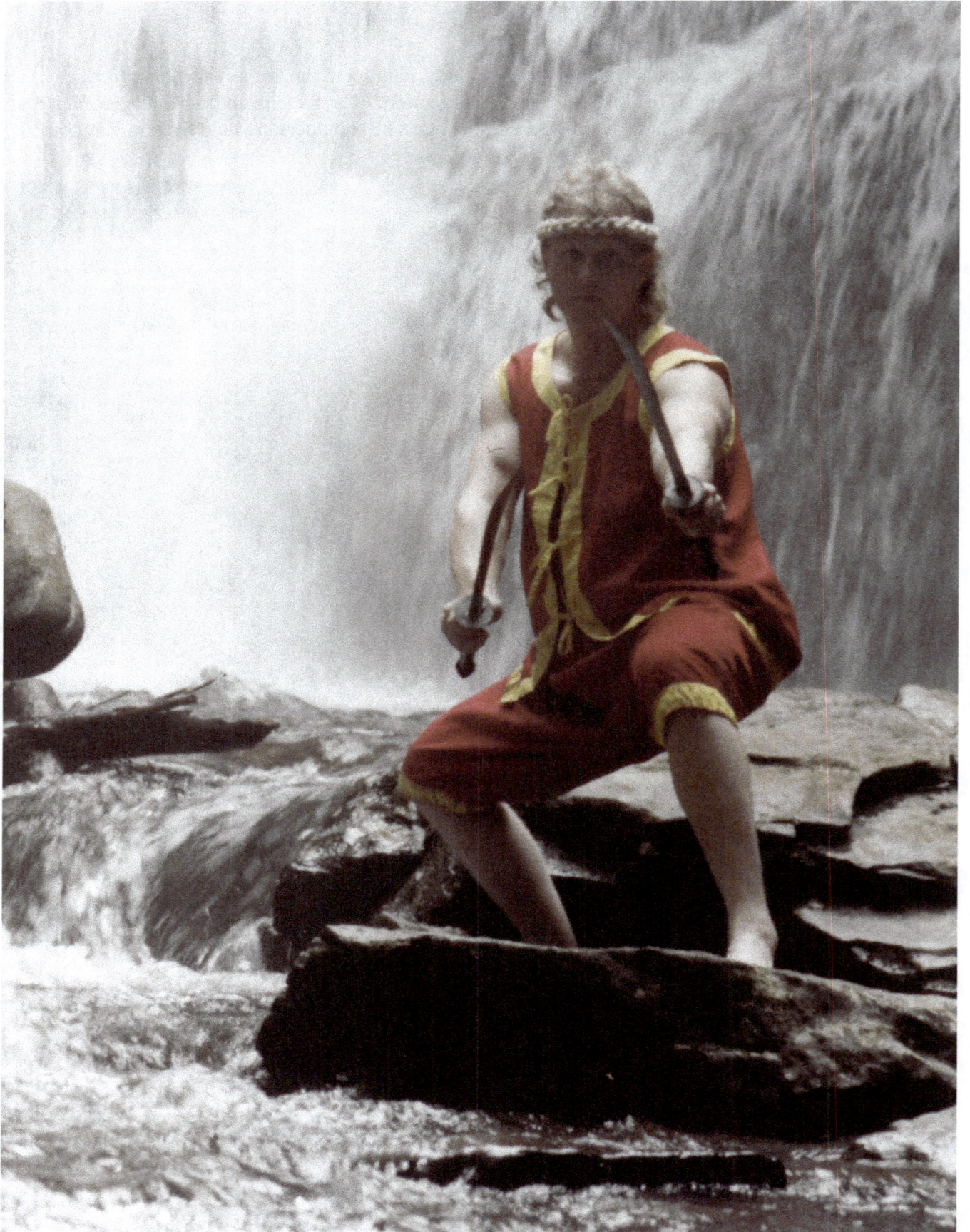

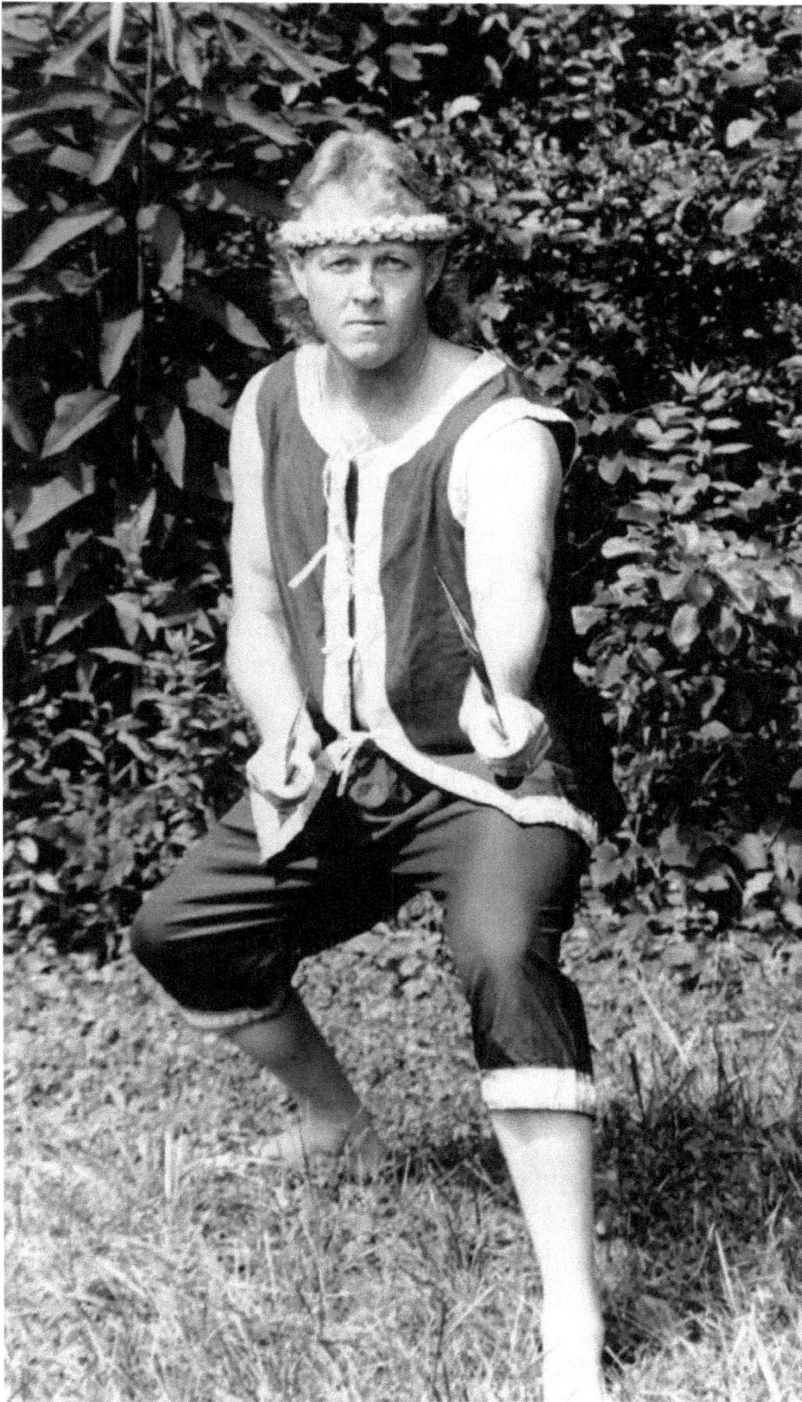
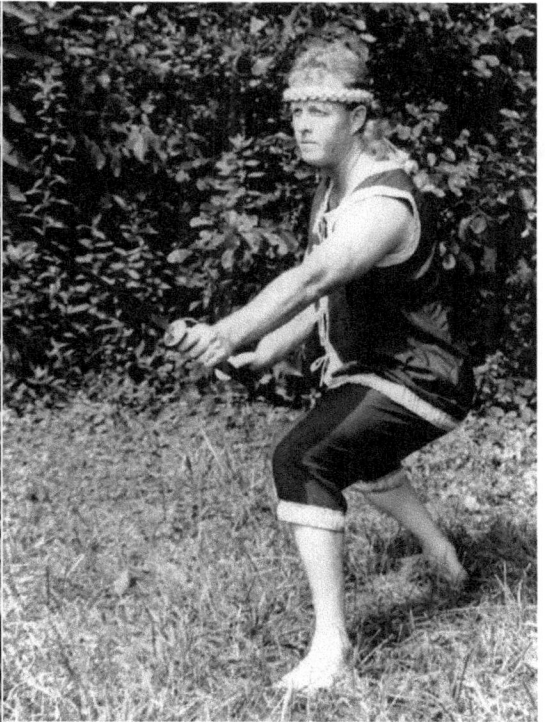
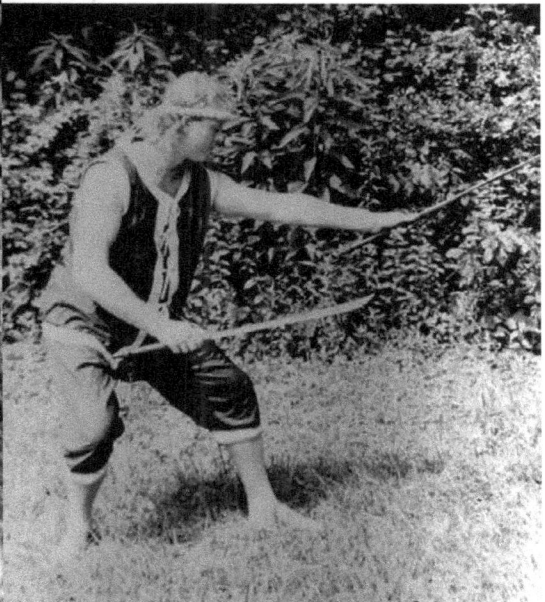
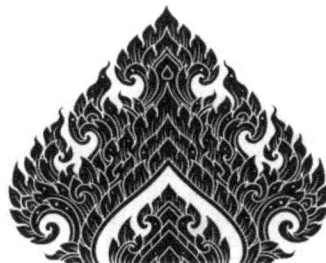

"The Tiger's Claws"

Although there are more than one hundred different striking methods with the sword, Ajahn Kruu James focuses initially on the five basic cuts from which form the foundation of the Tiger Double Sword technique. Notice that all five cuts begin with a simultaneous step.

1.   The **"Kaw"** (Neck) cut is the most common and the most powerful cut. It is an inward, downward diagonal usually aimed at the base of the trapezius and neck area. Most cuts in Krabi Krabong are made with a driving and then a drawing motion. Contact is initially made fairly close to the sword guard and as the sword moves into and through the target area, is withdrawn. This allows the narrow leaf shaped Thai blade to cut most efficiently. As the blade reaches waist height it is chambered with a snap to the outside of the hip. This is done with a downward turn of the wrist in order for the long handle to clear the body. In preparation for a following cut, the opposite hand is raised to a high position at the same time.

2.   The **"Aeo"** (Elbow) cut is an inward horizontal cut at the height of the elbow. It is generally intended to strike the side or the mid-level area of the torso. This cut is withdrawn as the blade approaches the centerline or the mid-point of the opponent's torso. Again, it is returned to the outside of the hip.

3.   The **"Ka"** (Knee) cut is a rising inward diagonal to the region of the knee or groin. The strike scoops upward from low to the ground with a similar drawing motion found in the other cuts. Chopping or hacking motions of all kinds are frowned upon in the Tiger style of Krabi Krabong. They do not allow maximum utilization of the blades cutting or, more accurately, slicing action. Even a very sharp blade will slow down and wedge tight in the body as a result of friction against the sides of the blade. By incorporating a drawing or slicing type of movement, a new edge surface is constantly being brought into contact with the target's surface allowing deeper and more penetrating cuts.

4.   The **"Hua"** (Head) cut is a descending vertical strike to split the opponent. It is timed with the step so that the body's weight is in the sword at contact. When done correctly it is not uncommon to shatter the opponent's sword if he attempts to block it.

5.   The **"Trong"** (Straight ahead- Thrust) cut is actually a direct thrust to any viable target area. The pommel of the sword and the tip of the blade are lined up with the target and thrust forward with a lunge into and through the area and then withdrawn sharply along the line of entry.

In the *Tiger* style, Double Sword style (weapon in each of both hands), of Krabi Krabong, the entire man is considered a weapon at all times, and even though there are ten different weapon systems the fists, elbows, knees, and shins are fully utilized. All parts of the sword are incorporated into attack and defense from the tip to the pommel.

At any time, an opponent may expect to be hit, tripped, or kicked bearing the brunt of an unorthodox attack.

Any technique or movement which will expedite the fight, to injure or otherwise intimidate or interfere with the progress of the opponent, is considered a viable tool. "Whatever is necessary" is the rule. "Whatever is practical" properly defines the strategy.

The warriors of the Thai Sword (*Dao/ Deo/ Dap Song Myr Deo etc.*) are creative and innovative, as well as having exceptional skills in basic technique. They are hard to surprise because from the first lesson they are exposed to the unexpected. It is made clear that to not make a right effort from the first to the last may be to die. To become confused or bewildered, or to show the result of fatigue before the battle is over, is to die. This results in a sense of commitment to even the simplest interaction.

In practice, the total person becomes involved in every strike.

Every cut, every punch, and every kick are fully expected to be the one which finishes the fight. Most techniques are designed to go through the opponent. Quite often if a cut is missed, the attacker must turn completely with it, allowing the weapon to carry him. You see instances when even though the defender successfully and correctly blocked an attack he was still knocked to the ground. Steel swords shatter, sticks snap, and staffs are broken in pieces. The Thai warrior feels that this is the way to develop the mind, body, and spirit. If this is how you practice, what can your opponent expect?

However, the most important aspect of BS Krabi Krabong practice is the showing of respect! The Buddhai Sawan concept of "*Wai Khru*" is both a literal and a metaphorical honoring practice of paying respect Thai style! It is also a Yoga like Vinyasa or "Form" as Karateka say, which acts as a catalog of techniques and sequences actually used individually in practice and combat. It is also a catalog of concepts such as the "Animal Styles" such as "Tiger, Elephant, Monkey, Snake and or Boar style. It is the practice of cultivation of discipline and fierceness and the steely demeanor of a warrior.

Kaw

Cutting neck

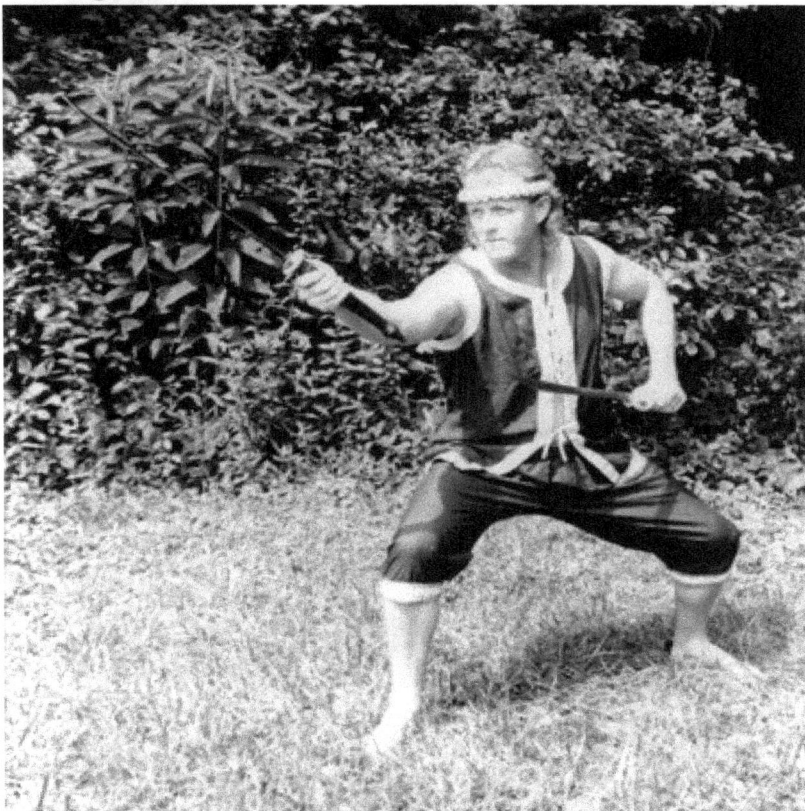

Aeo

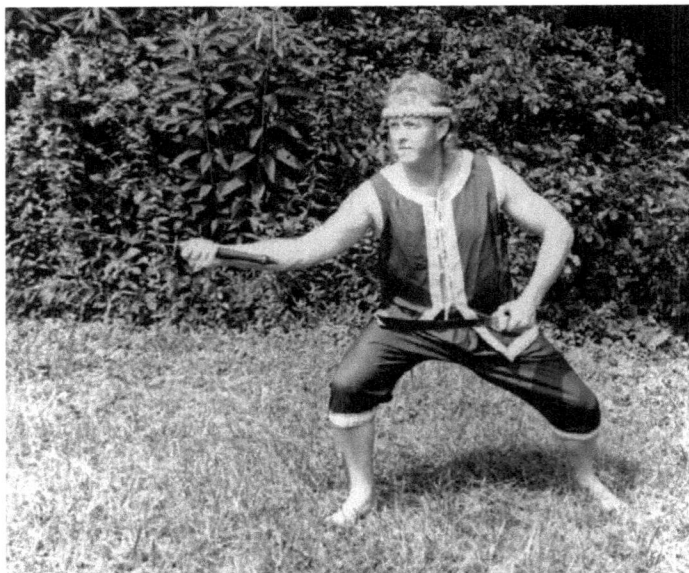

Cutting Elbow

The stance and footwork is the same for both cuts. Only the target changes. In Krabi Krabong basic training consistency of application from a simple basic structure is everything. To adapt for a change in the height of a particular target, bend the knees a little more or less. The idea is to keep the actual cutting motion itself in the power range as much as possible.

Ka

Cutting the knee

The footwork is again the same for Ka and Hua, (knee and head).

For the knee attack, deepen the stance. It is important to NOT lean over, or to bend forward to cut a low target.

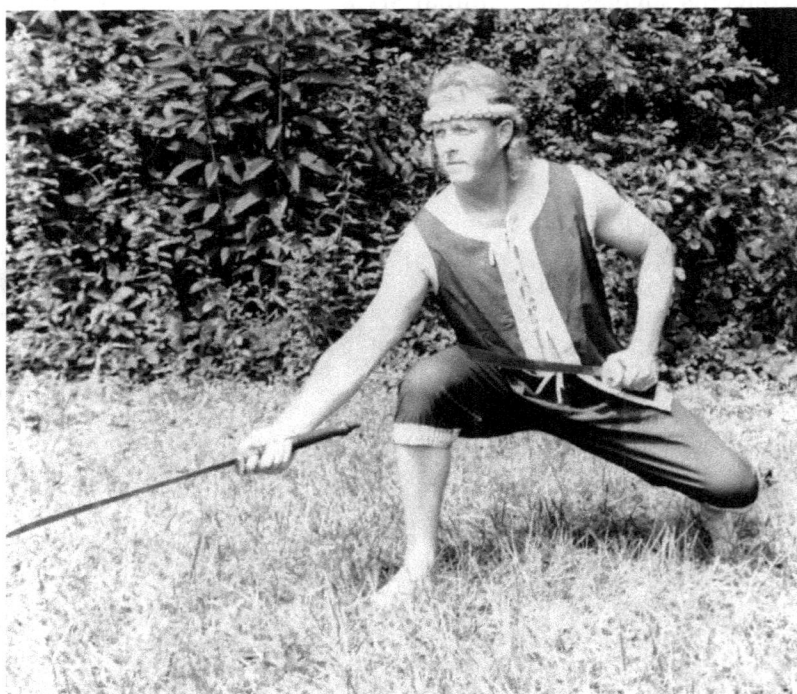

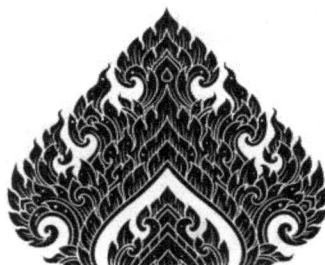

Hua

Cutting the Head

A powerful stroke capable of literally cutting an opponent in half! You rise straight up to bring the sword over for the head cut. This strike looks like the "*Kaw*" or neck cut. The only difference is that the angle is straight forward and down. Remember all of the basic cuts are made with a drawing in motion. This involves more of the blade.

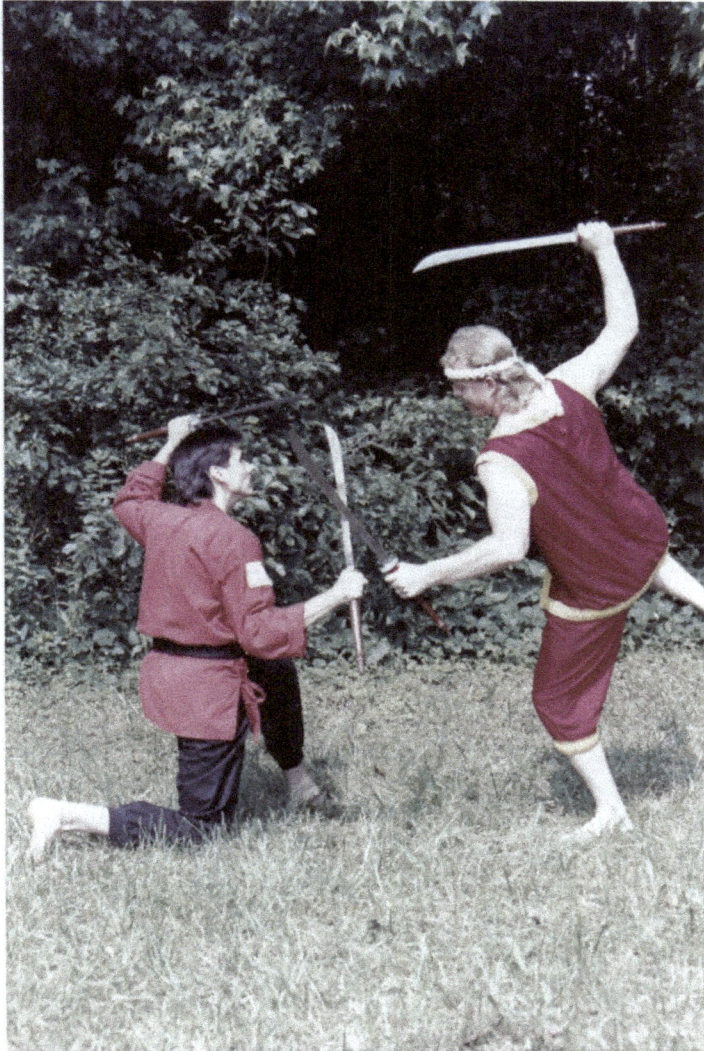

There is no "chopping" or "hacking" movement in Krabi Krabong. The drawing and pulling into the cut are a "slicing" motion. By allowing the sharp edge of the sword to do the work you economize energy and have less wasted motion. This becomes vital when fighting multiple opponents.

It starts high and pushes forward and drops into the top of the head with the dropping weight and leverage of your whole body behind it.

Even so, the finish is to recover the sword directly back to chamber without dropping the point of the sword any more than necessary to be effective. Phaa Kruu was always critical of over compensating or dropping the blade downward as this indicated a slower recovery to guard and or an opportunity to get hit with a counter strike while your blade was not pointing at the opponent.

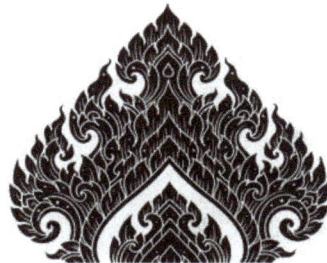

Trong

'Straight Ahead Cut'

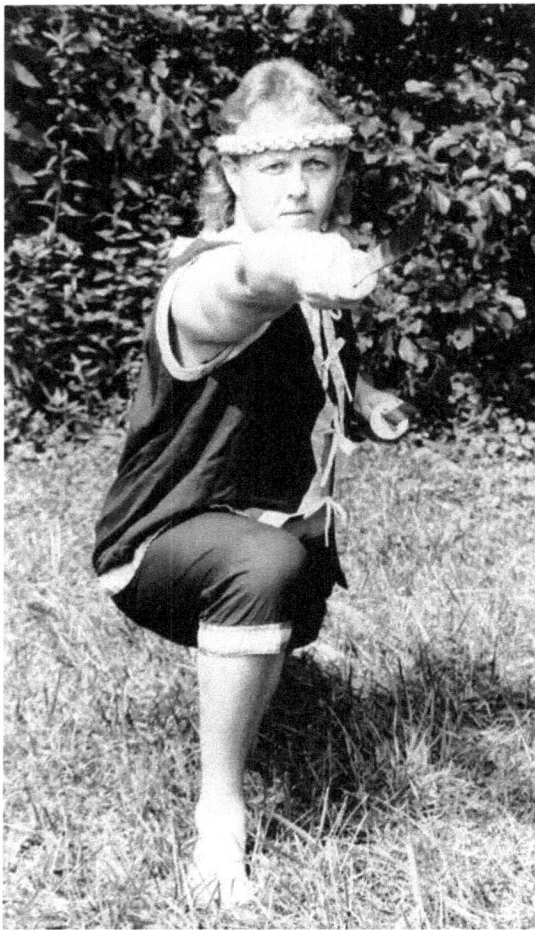

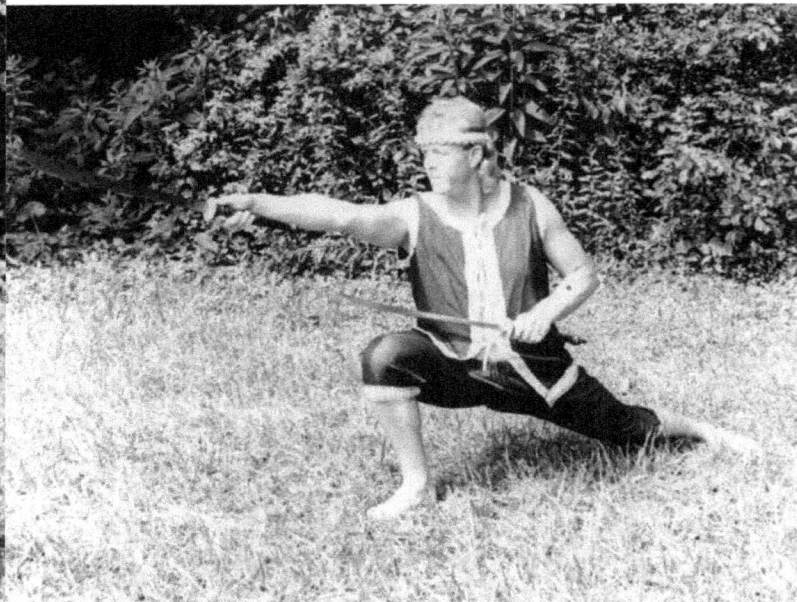

The sword is thrust forward, with a powerful lunge, as if punching. This "*Trong*" is performed quick, fast… blinding fast, if possible, to surprise the opponent. The guarding hand is ready to follow through or defend as necessary. The entire weight of the warrior is positioned behind the straight thrust. With a sharp weapon this technique is designed to pierce both the armor and body of the opponent. There is commitment to go "through" any barriers or resistance.

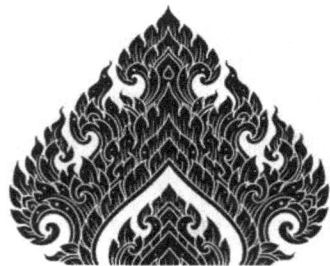

Block and Cut

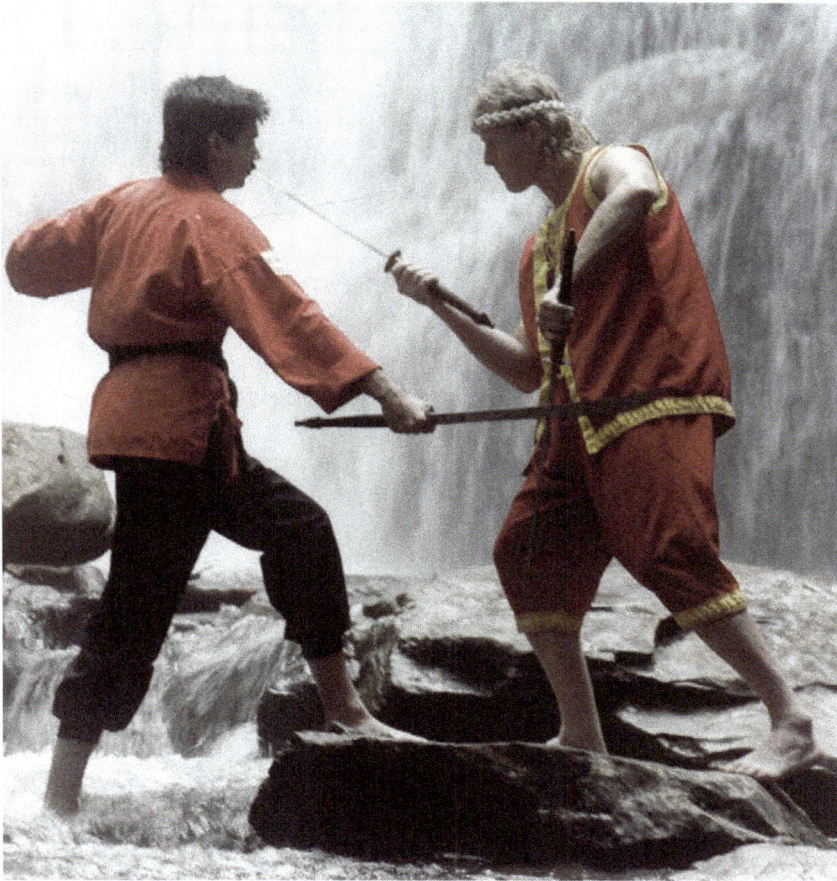

With two swords you are never idle and combination attacking and defensive motions at the same time are the norm. You may block with the blade. However, it is just as common to guard or block using the extended handle as well. It is no accident that the Thai "*Deo*" has such a long handle!

Stomping, kicking, sweeping, tripping, knees etc. are all commonly used when fighting with two blades. In practice you never want to just block, always hit while blocking at the same time is the practice.

Middle Outside block/ deflection with "Kaw" neck cut

The concept of "Block & Cut" has I believe unlimited or infinite variations possible. Consider the blocking sword can be over the head, high, middle, low or very low position with the blade either pointed up or downward. The tip of the blade can be pointed at the opponant or slightly turned out or inward... in more of a classic European "Parry". Deflecting a bit versus stopping the incoming blow.

Add to that the possible attacking and or counter attacking motion possibilities of the "live" sword... either to use cutting edge, back blade, point, cutting forward or backward, thrusting, spinning, twisting etc.? Circumstance, opportunity, strength, skill, timing and some luck are the only limitations.

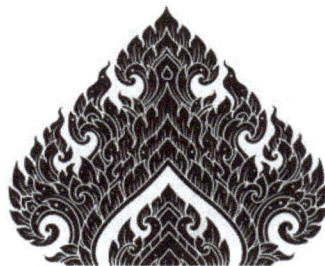

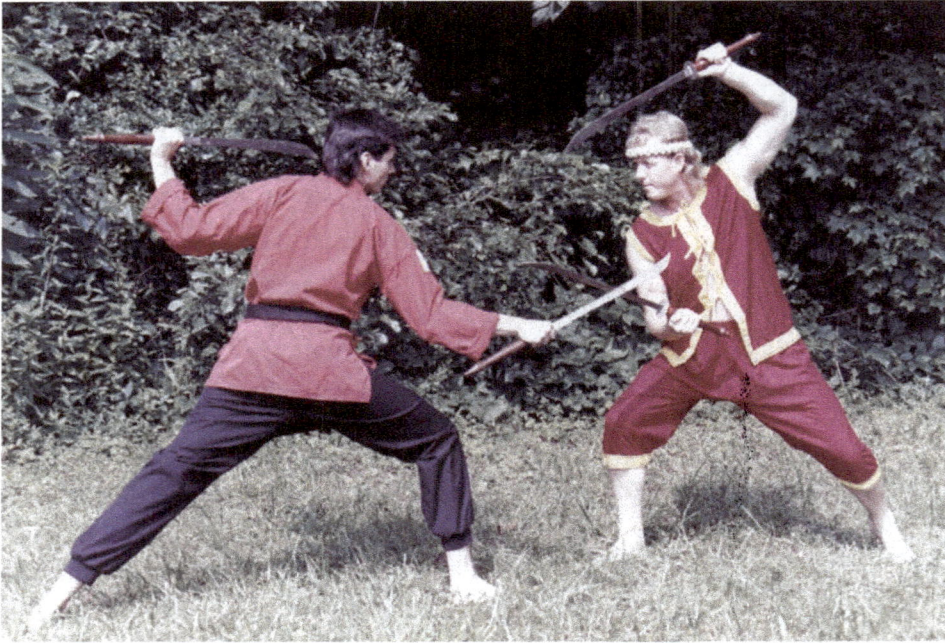

Middle Inside block/ deflection with Kaw or Hua cut

Below: Phaa Kruu demonstrates Block and Cut with Inside parry/ deflection coupled with middle thrust to belly.

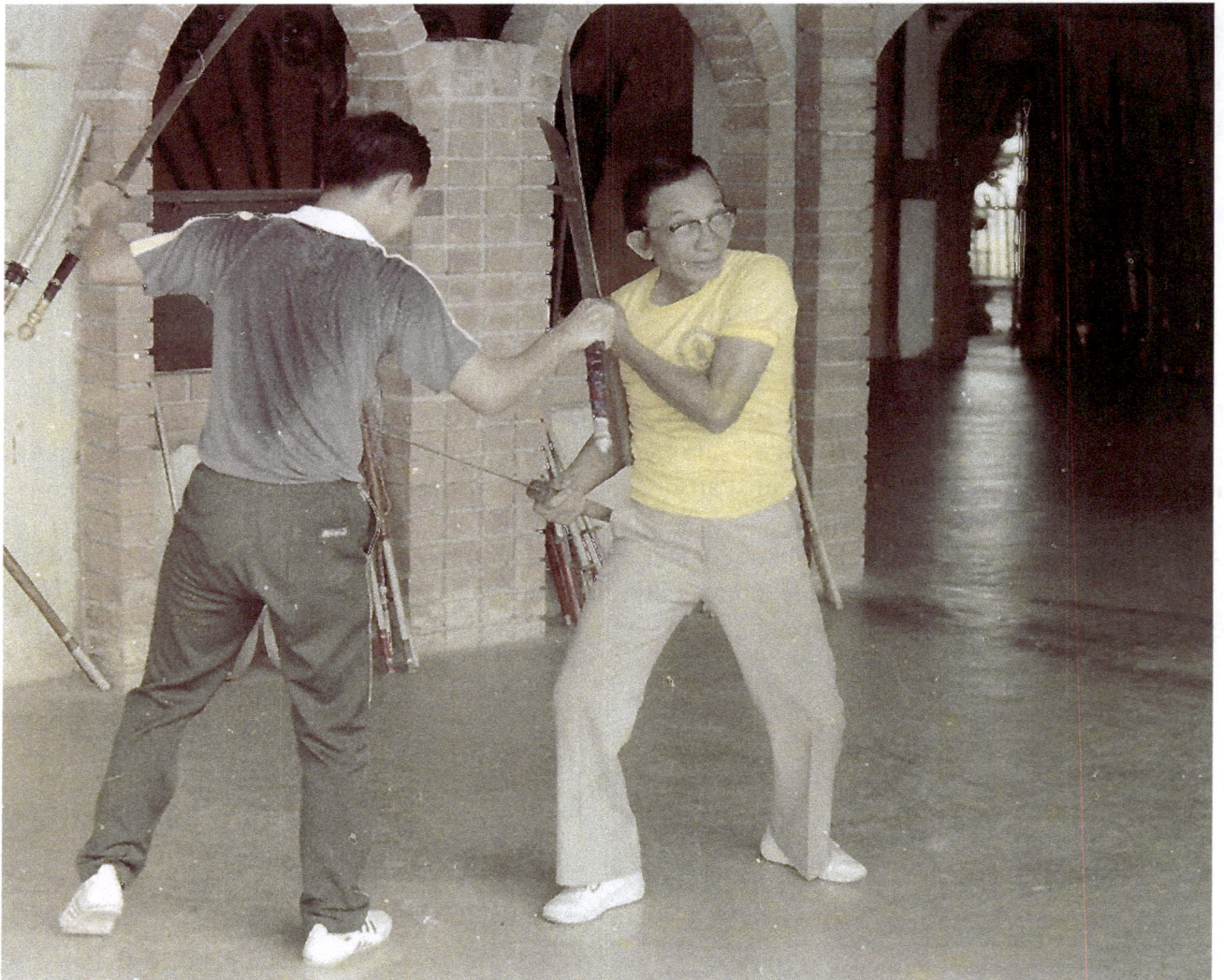

Gripping The Sword

Usually when attacking the sword is applied with a snapping motion. The proper gripping method should allow for flexibility and for correctly applying force.

The weapon is held firmly with the first two fingers.

The bottom two fingers are touching but are relaxed. They are only tightened when actually about to strike. The thumb is extended along the handle to a point just behind the guard while not actually pressing against the guard in a modified Saber grip. This position allows you to apply some springiness to the blade action. (On occasion, the sword may be gripped in a reverse fashion, but this is not really favorable due to the force with which most attacks arrive).
This grip method is beneficial for several reasons. It allows you to point the tip of the sword at the opponent with less stress to the wrist.

This hand position increases thrusting power and control. The thumb position enhances the incorporation of twisting and drawing motions which originate at the wrist. On the defensive side, it provides a triangular-like support to the blade to keep it from collapsing upon impact, acting like a spring or shock absorber.

However, you hold your weapon, however and whatever type of stance you have either chosen or been placed in by chance, your total objective is to cut the opponent; to cut your opponent well and with feeling. Whether your first motion or movement toward making the initial contact with your opponent is to block or parry, you should continue that movement and hit him strongly. If you hit him first, so be it. If he strikes first and you parry you still must cut him. In real-life combat, there can be no sense of testing as any motion or tactical procedure which does not finish or at least disable your opponent is an opportunity for him to finish you.

Boxer's spar--that is, trade out and exchange contact of various levels--by mutual contract. This testing and probing continue until a mistake is made, an opening is presented, or fatigue affects one fighter. The objective is to score points or maybe knock out the opponent. I am not talking about this type of contest. In a boxing match, the loser often walks away or "comes to" later. In real-life combat, this is seldom true--usually to lose is synonymous with death.

There can be no such thing as a wasted moment or wasted motion; in fact, any contact with the opponent where you have not been productive and damaged his capability physically, emotionally, or structurally is a missed opportunity.

Don't fight your opponent's weapon or weapons, cut him! In other words, the object is not to make his weapon ring but rather to make him sing.

No one type of attack or defense will automatically guarantee having this ability. That is, to always hit or cut the opponent. It is not so much a technique as it is of a certain kind of attitude.

This attitude which should always be present becomes manifested through the application of various techniques during combat. There are two variations:

1) The same weapon which initiates the attack continues to make the cut

2) Multiple weapon attacks simultaneously or staggered in such a fashion as to allow one to cut at all times or at any time.

When not attacking or defending, the proper grip allows you to relax the hand, thus, conserving strength in the hand. There are, however, two other methods of holding the swords.

A)   **Closed Fist:** This is recommended when using the handles for blocking.

B)   **Reverse Grip:** It is the opposite of the saber grip and is used by the skillful when some deception is called for.

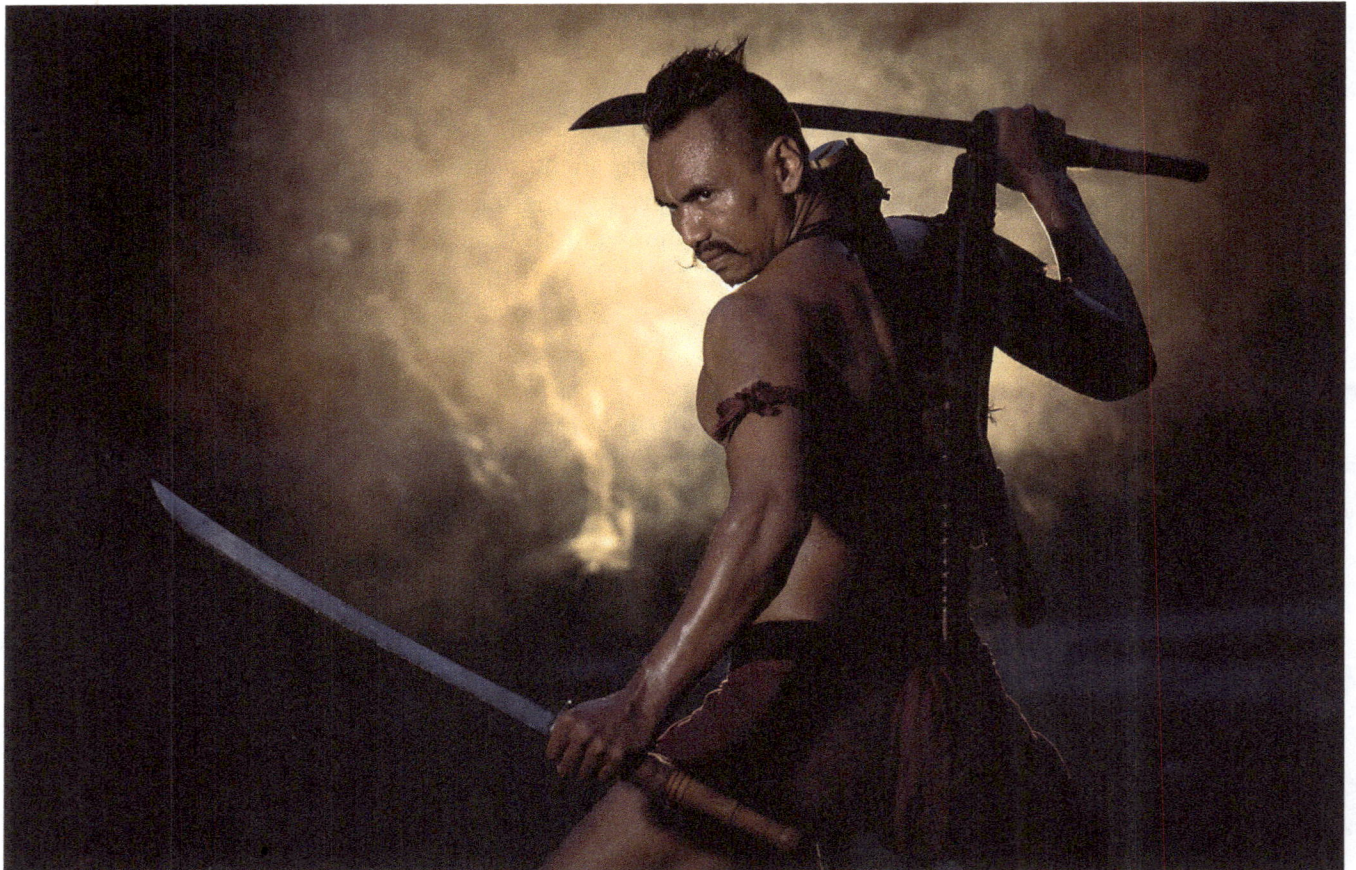

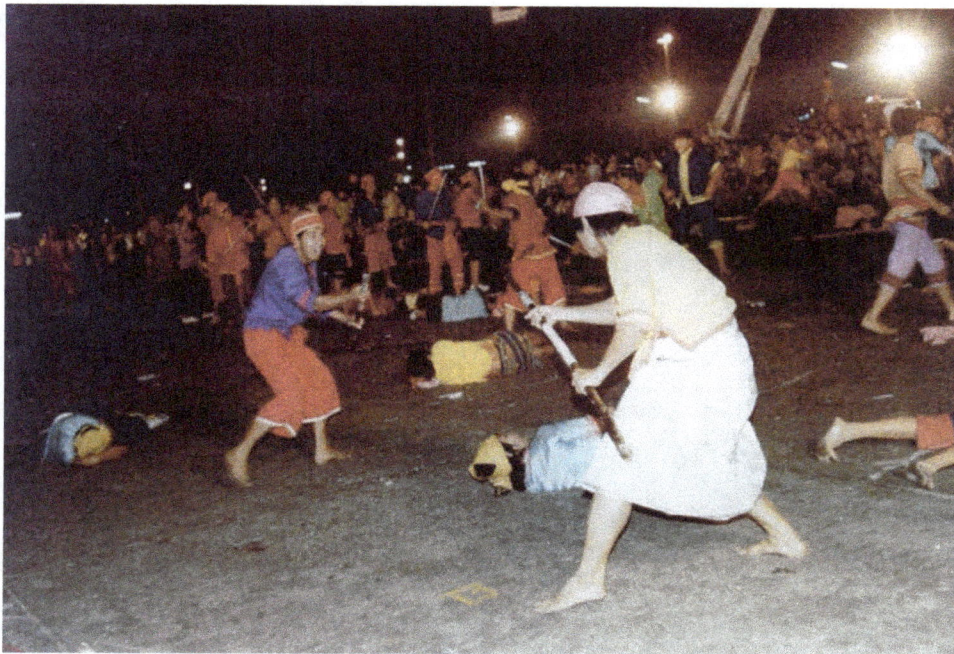

Two on One

Multiple Attacker Method (Two or More!)

Reenactment of famous melee battle between the Thai and The Burmese Armies at the Annual Surin Elephant Round Up, Surin Thailand 1983.

Now imagine thousands of warriors from both armies going at it all at the same time and you begin to see the utility of training for multiple attackers!

Buddhai Sawan Krabi Krabong participates at Annual Annual Surin Elephant Round Up, Surin Thailand 1983. GM Phaa Kruu Samaii leads the parade holding of him being honored by the king. Please note Ajahn, Kruu Alfonso Tamez in first row behind Phaa and Maa Kruu.

Lets give credit where credit is due! This humble and fierce man opened the door for so many of us! Originally from Monterray, Mexico, Ajahn Tamez was the first non-ethnic Thai to graduate as a Kruu under Phaa Kruu in the Buddhai Sawan Krabi Krabong tradition and is the person who personally introduced me to Buddhai Sawan.

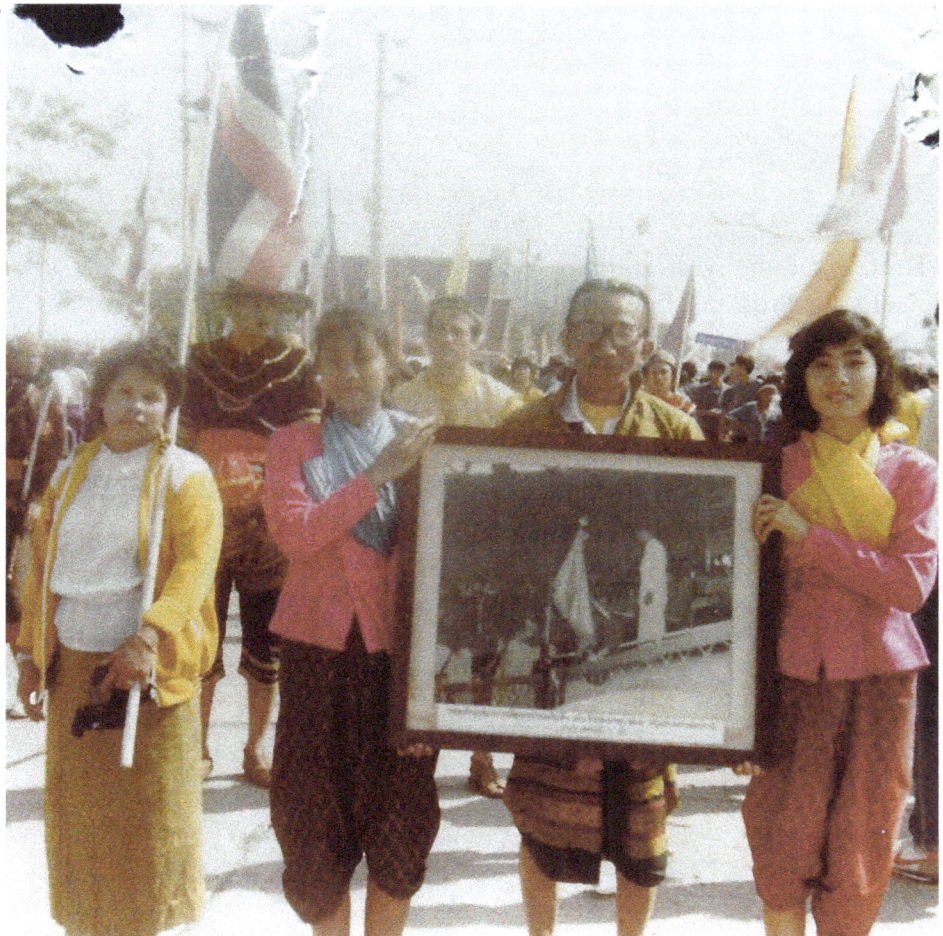

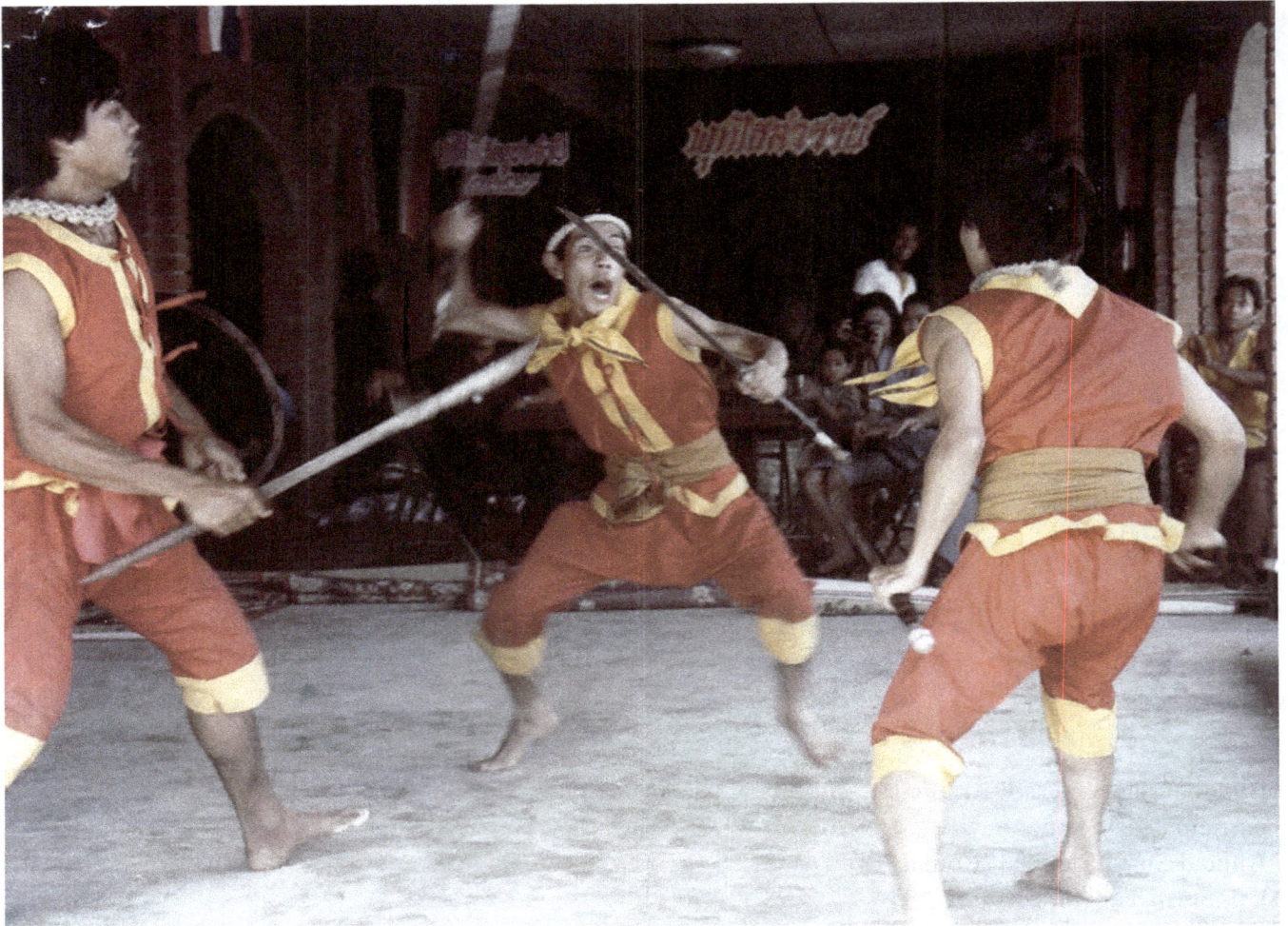

Buddhai Sawan Khru- Teacher Certification Requires fighting multiple attackers simultaneously

Krabi Krabong was originally intended for warfare of large groups or armies. The basic methods are well suited for multiple attacker types of situations. When fighting with a sword in each hand it is imperative to maintain a good grip and control.

"Two on One" practice becomes the basis for "Five on One". "Five on One" is a metaphor and practical training for Melee or group combat with an unknown number of assailants such as in a battle with dozens, hundreds or perhaps thousands of combatants all going at it at the same time!

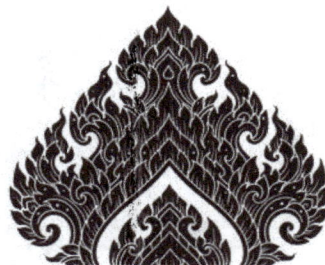

Sword Fighting Combinations

"The opponent who cannot stand cannot fight."

Please Note! *Even though for simplicity's sake I list these double sword/ weapon striking combinations as always leading with the "Right Hand- Mūxḵhwā", They are meant to be practiced with either side leading. This is to avoid always favoring or attacking from one side. Also know that every combo can also be done with ANY other weapon or combination of weapons. This includes adding Shields and Mai Sok to the mix!*

Additional Note: Every strike has a corresponding block, parry and counter strike! Every strike has a footwork to avoid the attack, slip the attack, get inside the attack or otherwise change the range of the attack or distance between the fighters. As is common ion other martial arts such as Filipino Kali, Pekiti Tersia, Arnis de Mano, Escrima, Lastra Maharlika, Canete, Serrada etc. there are six different fighting ranges which may favor one weapon or tactice over another.

Usually when training and or "drilling", we keep to one range to build the muscle memory. However, as Ajahn Tamez once told me... *"Mix it up! In real life there is no range... there is only hit or be hit!"*.

Repetitive drills build muscle memory, coordination and as they are isokenetic and isotonic "load bearing" exercise, they also build strength, increase joint and connective tissue extensibility and accessible range of motion. Because of the load bearing attributes based on the weight of the weapons and the "lifting" of them there is also hypotrophy with increase in lean muscle mass and increase in bone density. Think of how a baseball pitchers arm can have up to 50% greater bone density than the non throwingn arm! Perform the drills at speed and see the cardi- aerobic effect.

Eight Strikes: *(Advance forward or backward with each strike in pattern)*
1.   Right Neck - Ḵhwā Kaw (Right side: pronounced "Kwa")
2.   Left Neck - Ŝāy Kaw (Left side: pronounced "Sai")
3.   Right Elbow - Ḵhwā Ao Sok
4.   Left Elbow - Ŝāy Ao Sok   (simple= Ao),(advancing with each attack)
5.   Right Knee - Ḵhwā Kaow (simple= Ka)
6.   Left Knee - Ŝāy Kaow
7.   Right Head - Ḵhwā Hua (Ḥąwĥn̂ā)
8.   Left Head - Ŝāy Hua (Ḥąwĥn̂ā)

Seven Strikes: (Advance forward or backward with each strike in pattern)
1.   Right Neck - Ḵhwā Kaw
2.   Left Neck - Ŝāy Kaw
3.   Right Head - Ḵhwā Hua
4.   Left Elbow - Ŝāy Ao
5.   Right Elbow - Ḵhwā Ao
6.   Left Elbow - Ŝāy Ao
7.   Right Head - Ḵhwā Hua (Instead of stepping forward or through with the right leg, step out, to the right side, 90 degrees, and pivot as you bring the sword with an upward thrust toward the neck.)

Three Strikes: (Advance forward or backward with each strike in pattern)
1. Neck (right side) - *K̄hwā Kaw*
2. Neck (left side) - *Ŝāy Kaw*
3. Head (center) - *Hua*

On the defensive side, on count #3, make a long sidestep under the attacking arm to avoid the descending blow, then spin around to make a counter cut to the head (high target). Then begin 3 Double Sword Sweeps "Dap Deo Fan Sapai Long".

Nine Strikes:
1. Right Forehand Neck - *K̄hwā Kaw*
2. Right Backhand Neck (to the left side) - *Ŝāy Kaw*
3. Left Forehand Neck (to the right side) - *K̄hwā Kaw* (Follows #2 in a sweeping motion)
4. Left Backhand Neck (to the right side) - *K̄hwā Kaw*
5. Right Forehand Neck (Follows #4) - *K̄hwā Kaw*
6. Right Backhand Neck (to the left side) - *Ŝāy Kaw*
7. Left Forehand Neck (to the right side) - *K̄hwā Kaw*
8. Left Backhand Neck (to the right side) - *K̄hwā Kaw*
9. Right Forehand Head – *Sap Hua* (Chop the head) (Step out to the side with the right leg. Before continuing, there is a downward block with the left hand to negate a side cut and an inward block to counter a thrust.

Note: Between each two cuts, before the backhand movement, the guard is corrected with the tip held high and the handle down. If there was a thrust inserted, it would be deflected by the handle.

Six Strikes:
1. Right Neck - *K̄hwā Kaw* (Right side: pronounced "Kwa")
2. Left Neck - *Ŝāy Kaw* (Left side: pronounced "Sai")
3. Right Knee - *K̄hwā Kaow*
4. Left Knee - *Ŝāy Kaow*
5. Right Knee - *K̄hwā Kaow*
6. Back of Right Knee - *Kaow* (With the right hand in a figure eight motion as you do a back spinning movement away with the right leg to avoid the same attack on your own leg.)

Five Strikes: (Begins like Nine Strikes)
1. Right Neck - *K̄hwā Kaw* (Hits Right side)
2. Right Backhand Neck - *Ŝāy Kaw* (Hits Left Side)
3. Left Forehand Neck - *Ŝāy Kaw* (Hits Left Side)
4. Left Backhand Neck - *K̄hwā Kaw* (Hits Right side)
5. Neck - straight thrust with the right hand – *Thit Kaw* (Also "*Tid*")

Putting it all together

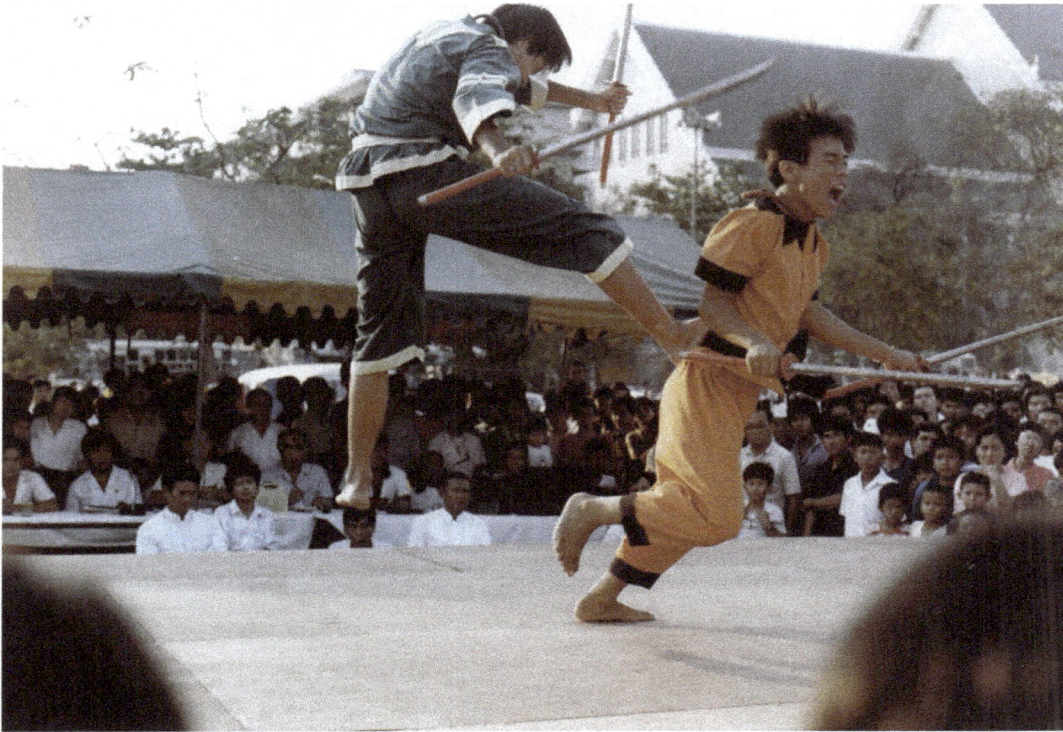

Advanced students of Buddhai Swan spar free style full contact with rattan swords. Rattan swords are favored for demonstrations as in the past steel swords would shatter and send pieces flying into the crowd.

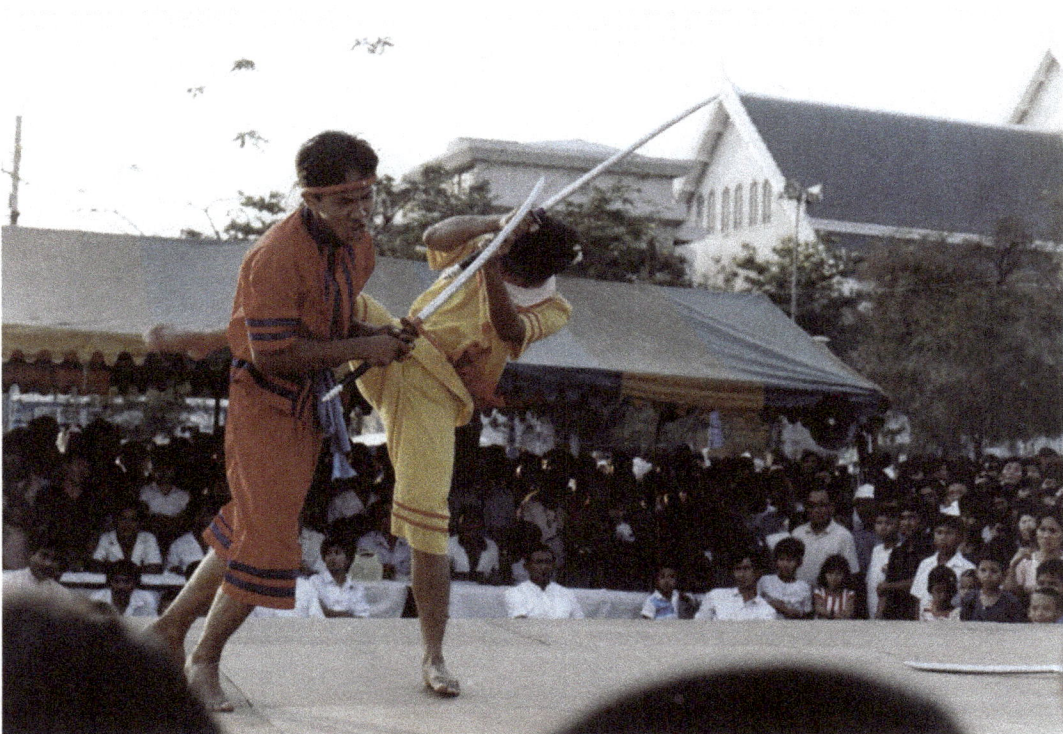

These photo's photo was taken on the King's birthday Dec. 5th, 1984, on a platform built in front of the Grand Palace. Members of the Thai Royal family are sitting in the pavilion to the back.

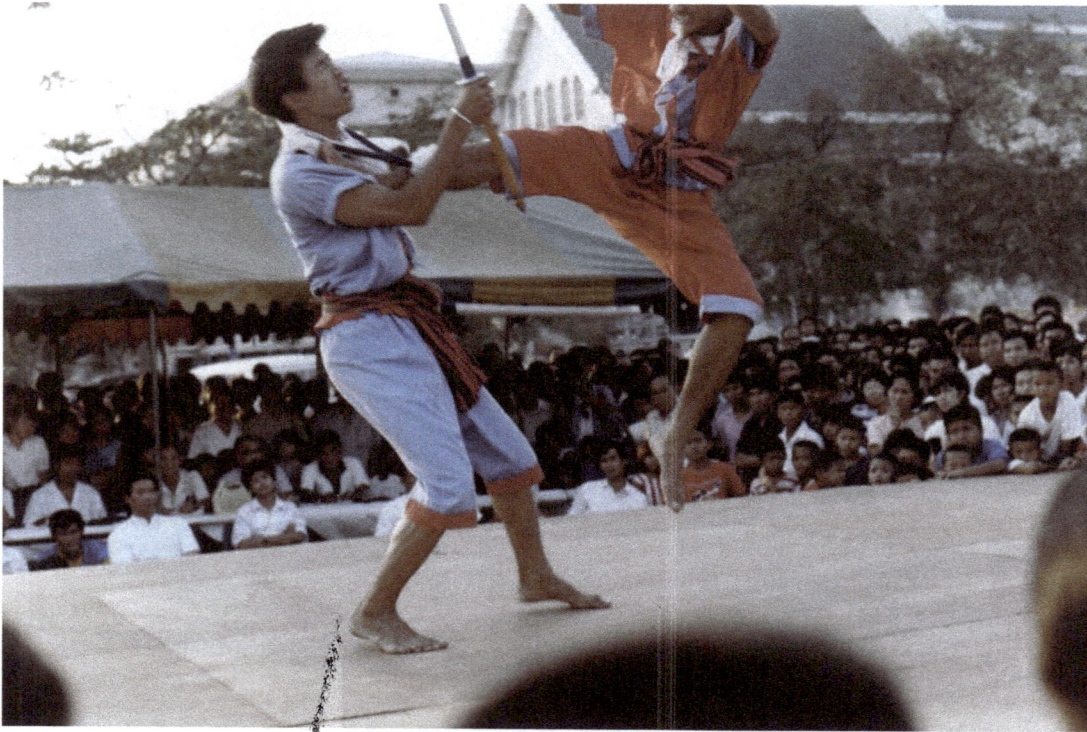

The sparring depicted above is typical of the intensity and exuberance shown by practitioners.

Energy levels are high and a great deal of pure athleticism is displayed without the slightest hindrance. The challenge, the fun and adrenaline of fighting with swords against capable opponents provides one with moments of pure unbridled joy!

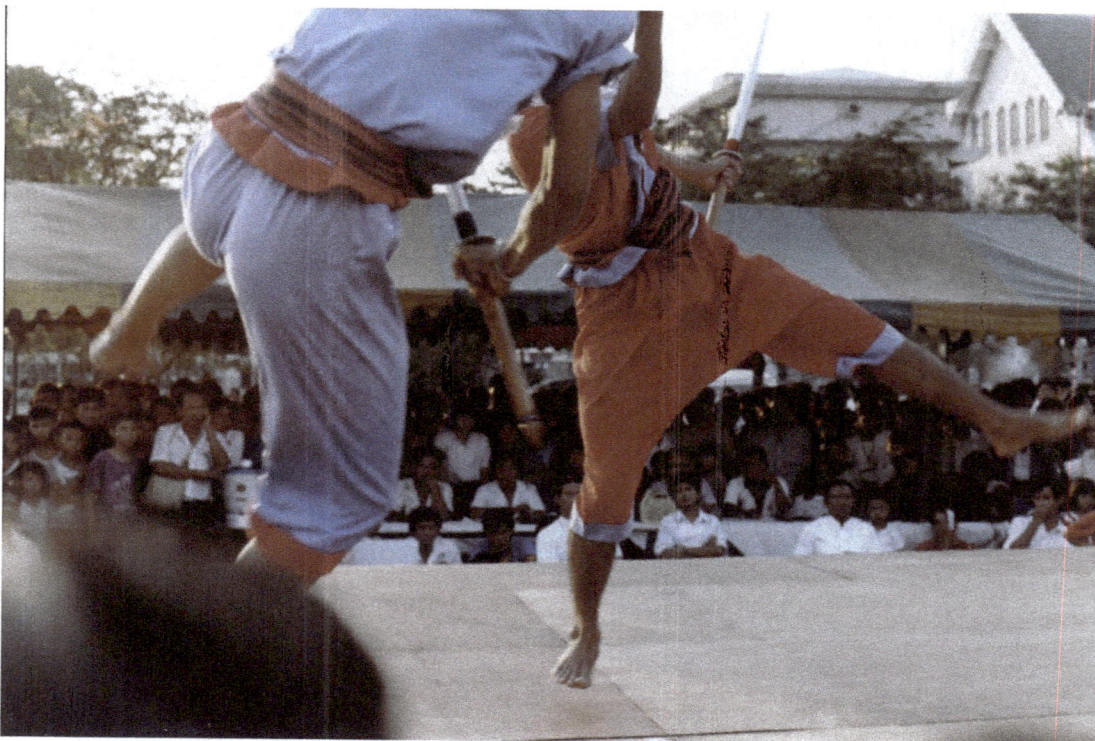

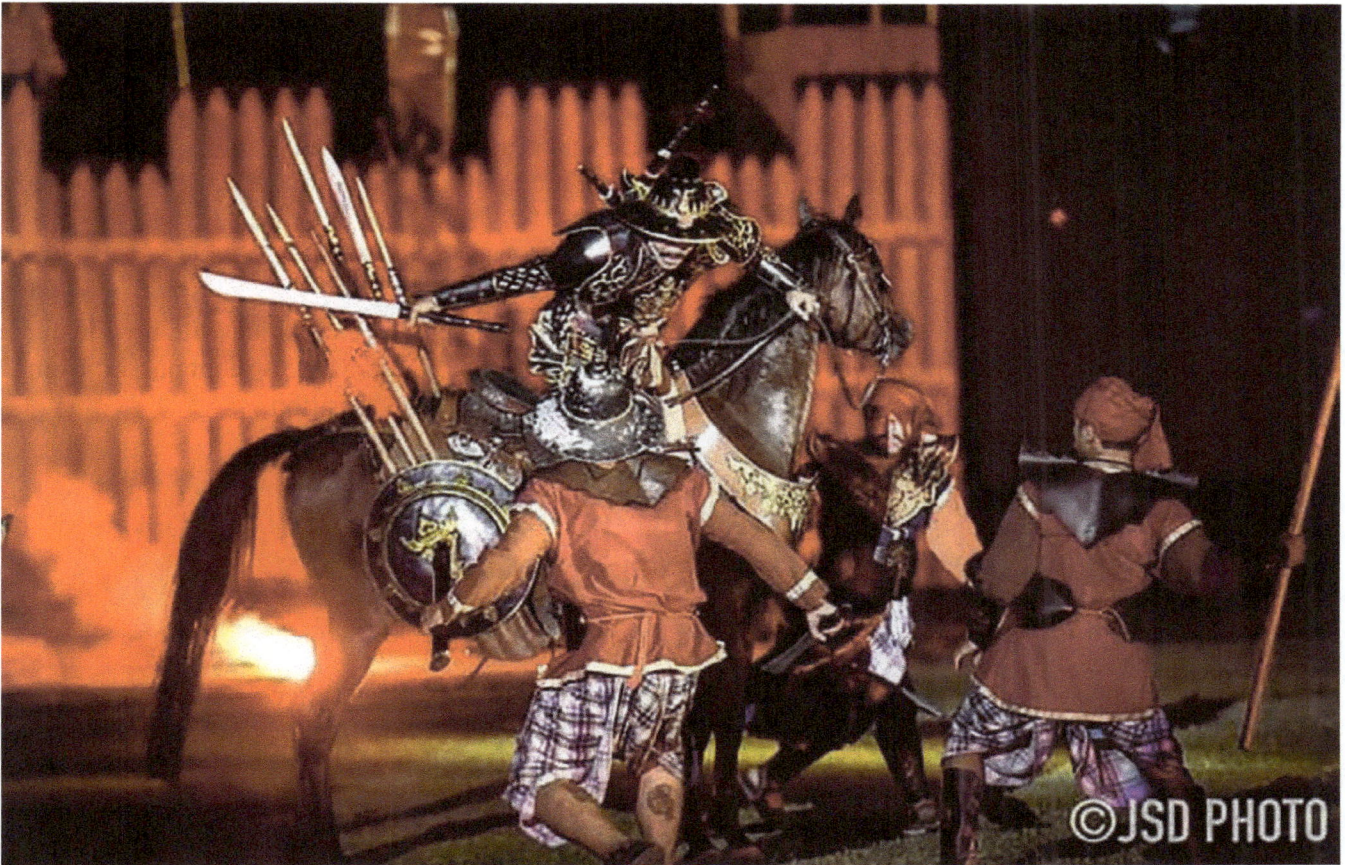

Buddhai Sawan Thailand, Reenactment of Black Prince fighting against infantry on horseback. © Courtesy of Ajahn Jira Mesamarn

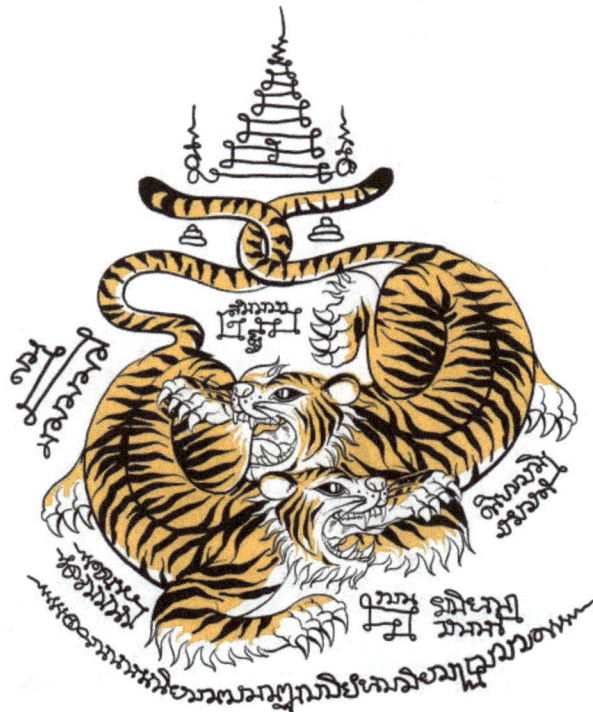

Traditional Offensive Sword Fighting Techniques

1. "*Fan Sapai Lang*" (Double Sword Sweeps)

From a high position both swords are brought downward in a crushing type of movement. Both swords are capable of cutting and the full weight of the body is behind them. Begin with the lead sword turned inward in order to snap it outward on the cut.

2. "*Puab Pang Pai*" (Lotus Shield)

Block an oncoming thrust with the lead hand. As you step and slide rearward continue with a wide circle overhead with the rear hand which cuts the opponent from the left shoulder. Make a diagonal cut from high drawing to a low position.

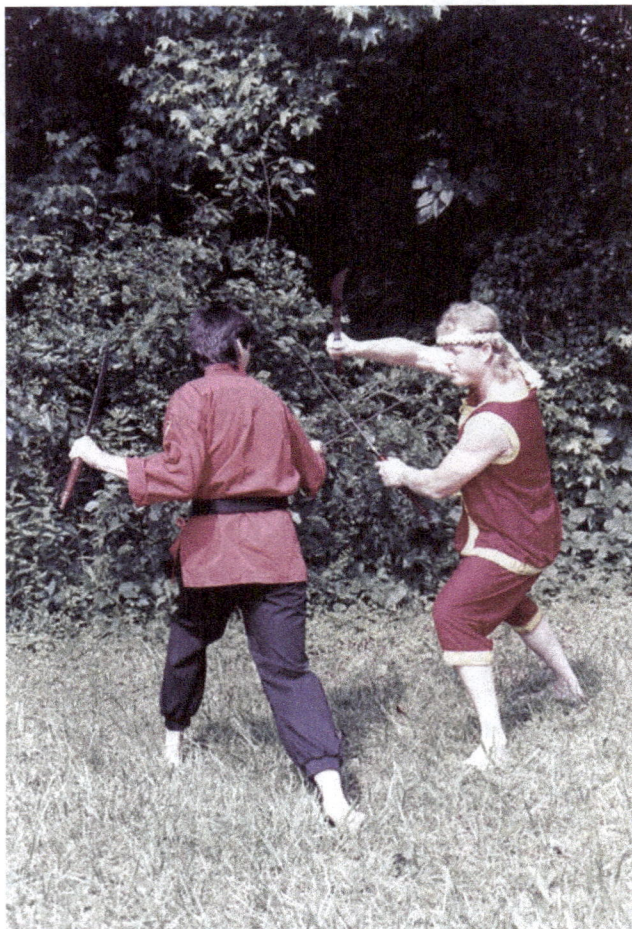

All of the traditional fighting combinations are drilled to both sides, left and right. The combinations are practiced repetitively until there is no hesitation, and they appear as second nature. They simply must be executed as if clapping their hands.

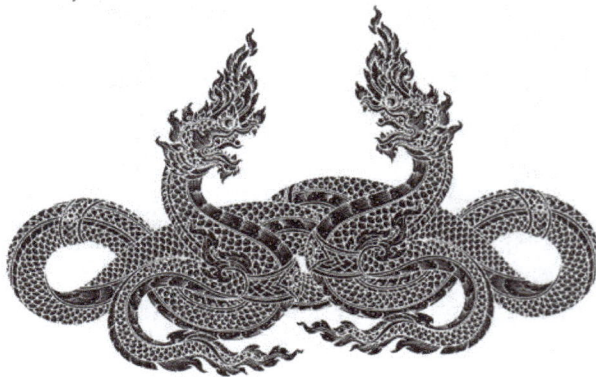

3. *"Kwang Puab"* (Cut Diagonally the Flower)

Block incoming thrusts with the lead hand as you step and slide to the rear. With the same hand, continue by cutting back with a level cut across the neck or arms of the opponent. As you block, turn the wrist inward to give more snap to the backhand cutting motion.

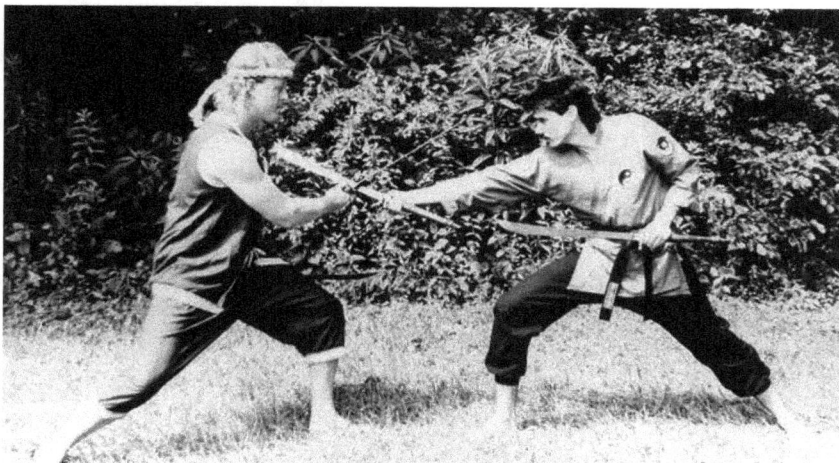

4) *"Puab Silaat Baai"* (Flower of the Leaf Blown)

Same as Kwaang Puab except that you return with a rising diagonal backhand cut upward across the midsection. Don't forget the rear hand is ready to counter-thrust at any time.

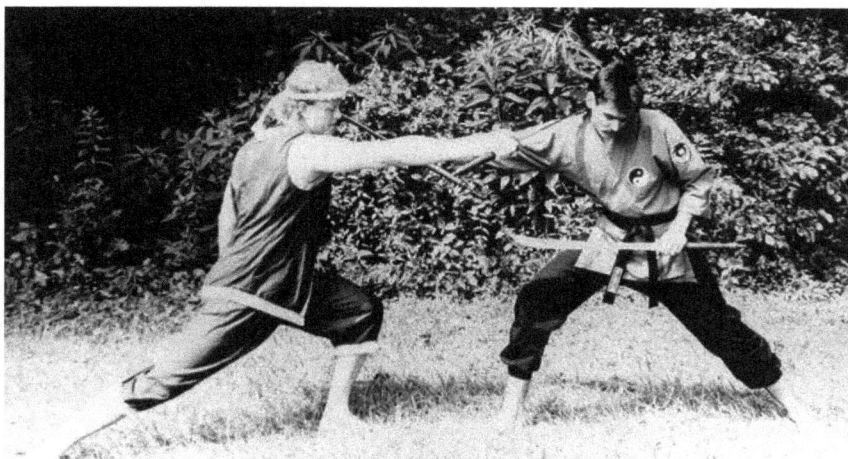

5) *"Huab Pan Lak"* (*"Kwai Pan Thum Mai"*- *"Khwāy p̄h̀ān t̂nmị̂"*, (The Buffalo Passes the Tree Coming Closer)

As the opponent lunges with his rear hand, parry downward with the front hand as you step back changing sides. Step in with the front foot as you scoop his sword upward and around toward his neck. Step through with the rear leg and brace your left sword against the back of his neck. Pull the swords away, cutting both sides. As you cut him, kick him away hard.

6) *"Nok Peek Hak"* (Bird with Broken Wing)

As the opponent thrusts or cuts toward the head, defend with a cross block pushing upward. Once the swords are high, sweep them outward and downward to then execute two crossing/rising cuts under the opponent's arms. Continue by snapping the wrists downward sharply and pulling the hands apart. This executes two simultaneous cuts across the mid-section. Follow with a kick to the opponent's body.

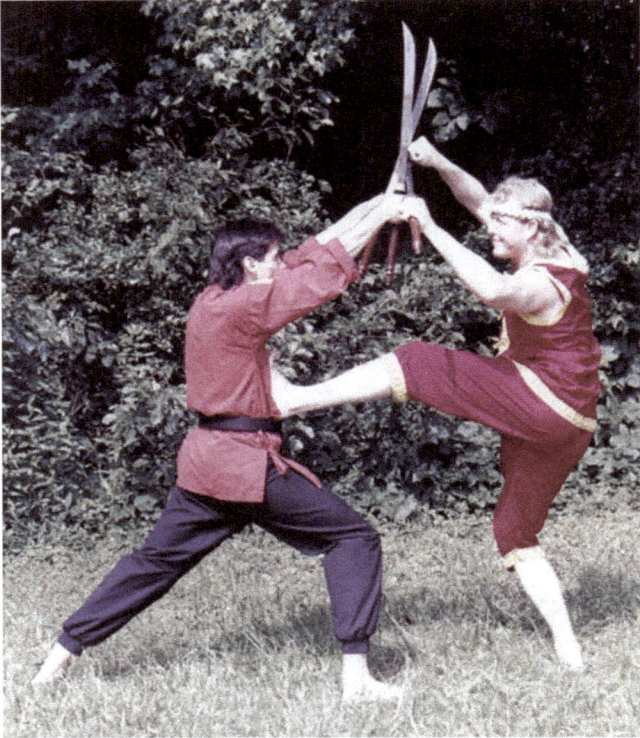

7) *"Ga Long Sai"* (*"Nok Kad Thaung"*, *"Nk kạd tĥxng"*) (Bird Bites the Stomach)

As the opponent thrusts with the lead hand, step back with the rear foot and simultaneously execute an inside sweep block with the front hand. This is followed with a thrust from the rear hand. The thrust arcs around into the target. Follow with the same attack from the opposite hand. The feet follow the hands.

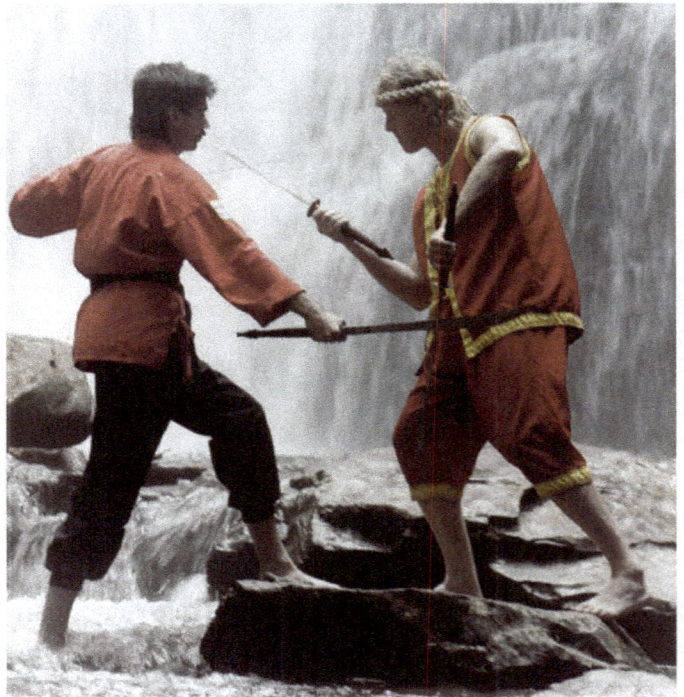

8) *"Kruan Kratop Fuan"* (Wave Flowing or Rolling)

As the opponent leads with the thrust, block with a high outside wing parry with the rear hand. At the same time, sidestep 45 degrees with the lead foot to the outside of the attacker's lead leg. Countering off the wing block, continue with a downward diagonal backhand to the back side of the attacker. As the cut is made the rear foot spins around to add torque.

9) *"Krater Tri Mai"* (Rat Runs Up the Tree)

The attacker leads with any cut and the defender receives the attack by stepping back through with the lead leg (changing sides) and meeting with his new lead leg. The defender sticks to the blade and snapping or turning the wrists cuts directly into the opponent's hand, arm, and into the body. Against a vertical head cut, the defender uses a horizontal block with the lead hand and as soon as the attacker's motion is checked, picks up the opponent's blade with his rear blade. He then cuts inward and downward with the lead hand. (Rhythm: tap, tap, cut).

10) *"Syya Tom Lai Hang"* (The Tiger)

As the attacker gives two downward cuts, the defender cross-blocks, but with only the tips crossed. This allows the tips to get between the swords, sweep the swords apart, and kick into the opening created. When the opponent thrusts to the body, the block is performed downwards and outwards.

11) *"Noong Tai Roun"* (Rats Running on the Arm)

As the attacker lunges with a thrust to the body, the defender steps back through and picks up the attacker's sword with an outside sweep or backhand. As this is done, the defender hooks the lead handle of his sword behind the handle or pommel of the opponent's weapon and strips it away from his hand. Continue with a backhand cut into the body.

12) *"Hok Kho Chang Erawan"* (Head of the Elephant)

A single sword technique. As the attacker thrusts with the backhand, the defender steps back through and blocks with both hands. The front is high on the arm of the attacker. Grab the attacker's outstretched arm with the backhand.

Drop the sword under the arm and return back over so as to hook the sword under the attacker's chin and turn it against the neck. Lever the attacker to the ground with your sword, simultaneously cutting.

13) *"Mon Kon Chon Gao"* (Little Animal Cuts the Jewel)

As the attacker leads with an attack to the head, the defender blocks with a cross block and then s tepping out with the lead leg to the side cuts the front of the knee with the backhand and then spinning cuts the back of the same knee with the lead. May also be done with no block and a well-timed sidestep.

14) *"Jara Ka Kwan Klonq"* (Crocodile Stops in River)

As the attacker lunges or thrusts, the defender steps back and parries the thrust down with a low outside wing deflection. Just after clearing the opponent's weapon, execute a quick back leg round kick to the side or back of the attacker's leg. This can sweep.

IMPORTANT NOTE! These are NOT all of the traditional techniques or combinations! Of course there are many more traditional offensive sword fightng techniques! Buddhai Sawan Krabi Krabong and it variations of both traditional and modern schools and teachers have an amazing catalog to work with. The terms for all the important tools are not entirely standardized and individual schools and their teachers hae and make popular their very own. This variety and allowance for genuine creativity is not just hallmarks of identifying characterics but part of the "secret sauce" that has aloowed our tradition and it's off shoots to survive for centuries.

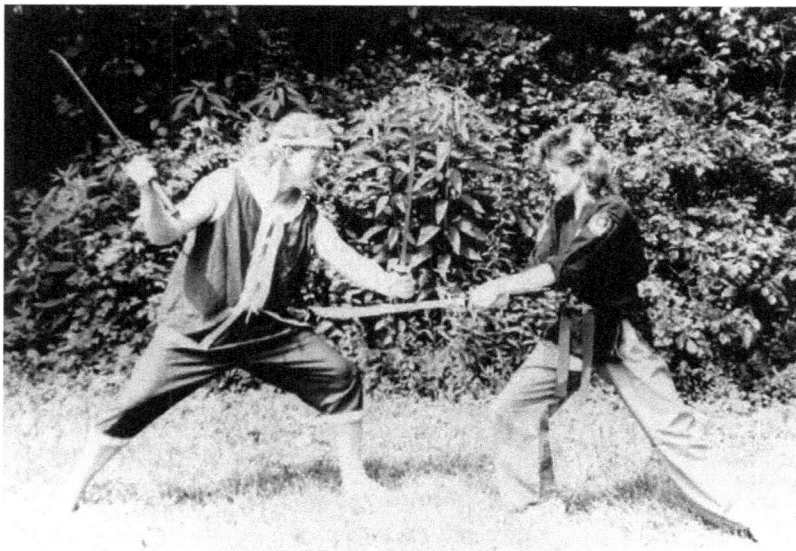

15) Inside Sweep - Back Hand Cut

As the attacker thrust with either front/ lead hand (two handed long sword), inward sweep block using the handle of the lead sword. Control the weapon away from centr line while making a big cut with the rear or back sword. This is a power cut or finnishing technique. You can literally cut the opponant in half with this technique.

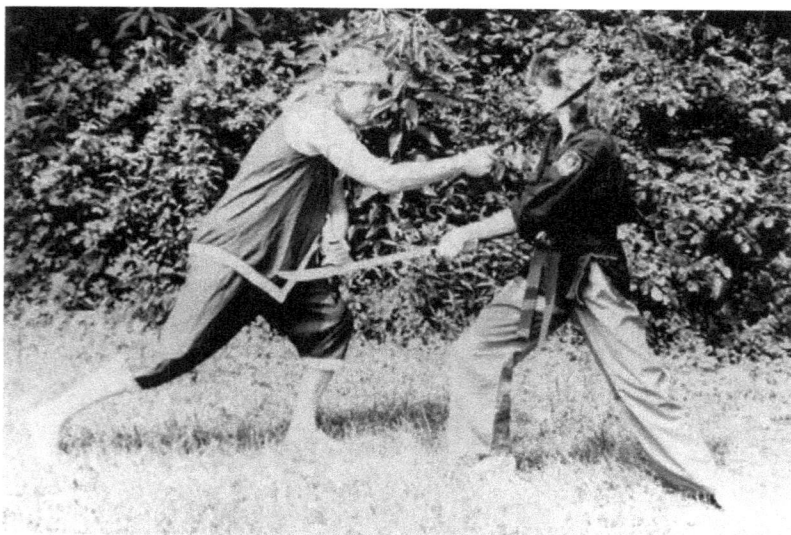

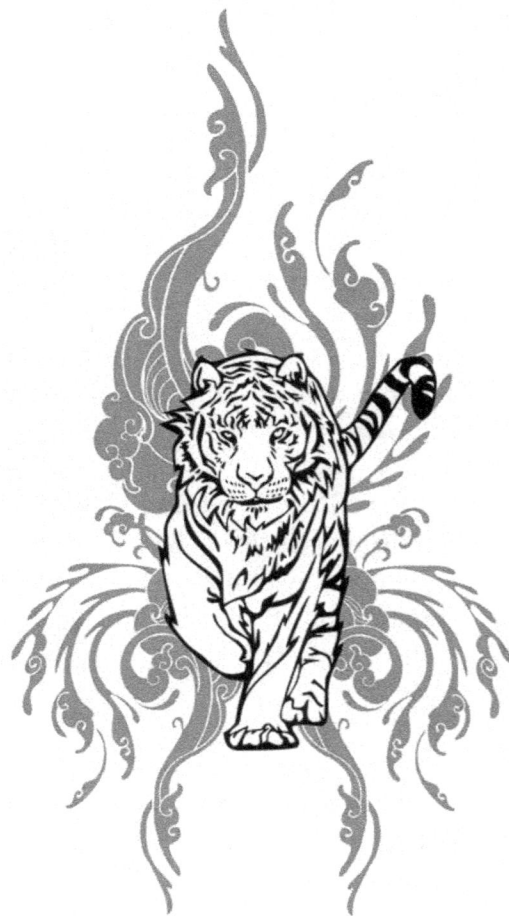

I find our way of crafting our Buddhai Sawan system cogent and in harmony with Sijo Bruce Lee of JKD fame's codification of the principles of mastery. These principles were first taught to me by GM Sijo Danny Inosanto when I trained with he and the other JKD Inosanto Kali Academy teachers Lary Hartsel, Alphonso Tamez etc.

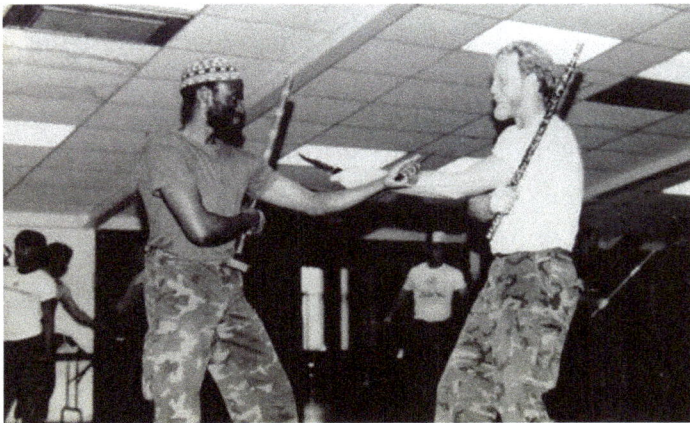

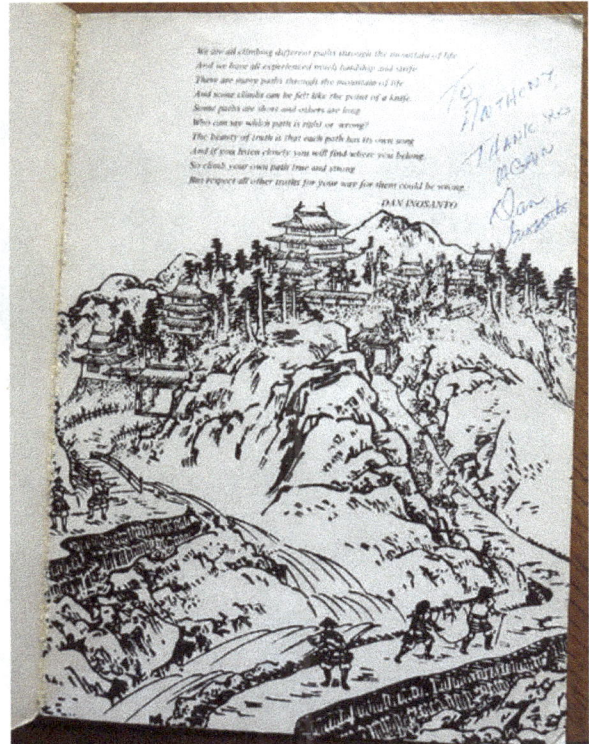

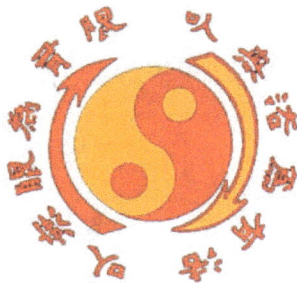

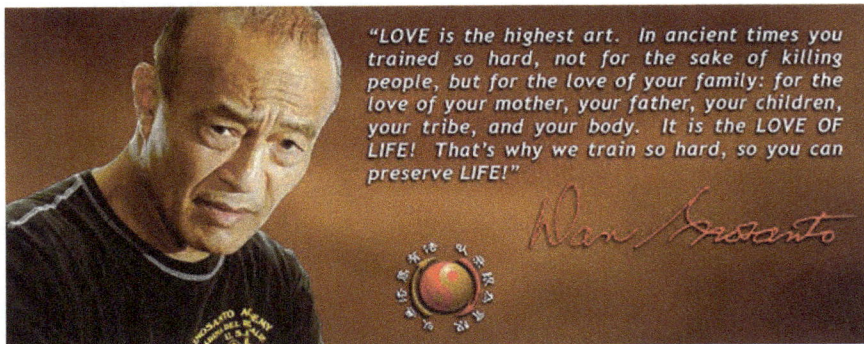

The principles of Mastery according to Sijo Bruce Lee

1) **Research Your Own Experience**
2) **Absorb What's Useful**
3) **Reject What's Useless**
4) **Add something specifically your own.**

In my opinion Sijo Bruse Lee himself would have appreciated Buddhai Sawan Krabi Krabong and incorporated it's methodologies into his JKD. Just as GM Sijo Danny Inosanto did after he joined Buddhai Sawan under GM Phaa Khruu Samaii in Nongkam.

Defensive Sword Fighting Techniques

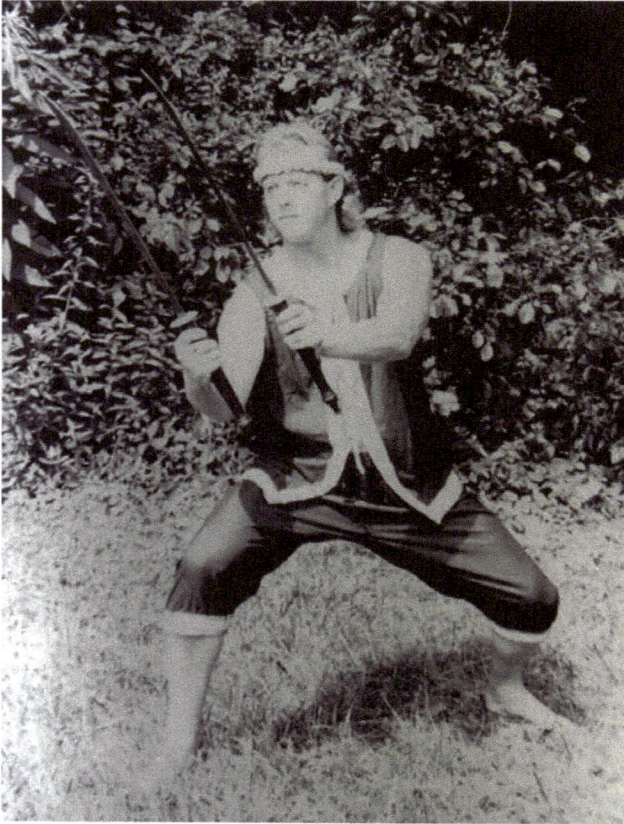

A. "*Rap*" (Double Wall Defense/ Double Sword Defense)

In defending against the Double Sword sweeping motion, you brace your elbows into the hips and hold both swords upright with a firm grip, and as you hit, back away rapidly in a circular fashion. There are major variations vertical, diagonal, horizontal, and downward.

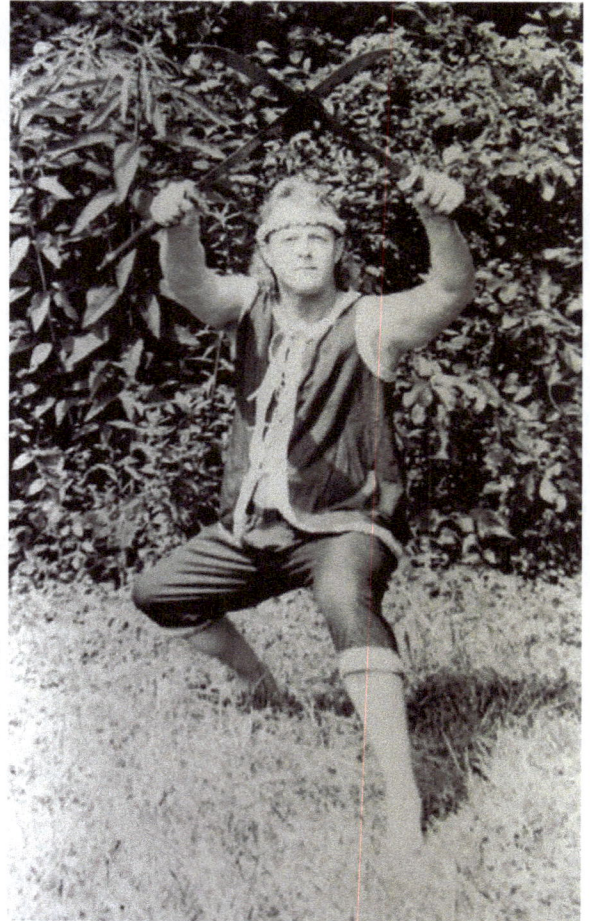

B. "Bata" (Cross Block)

In both the "*Bata*" and or "*Rap*", these elbows are locked.

It is better to be knocked down than to have your block collapse.

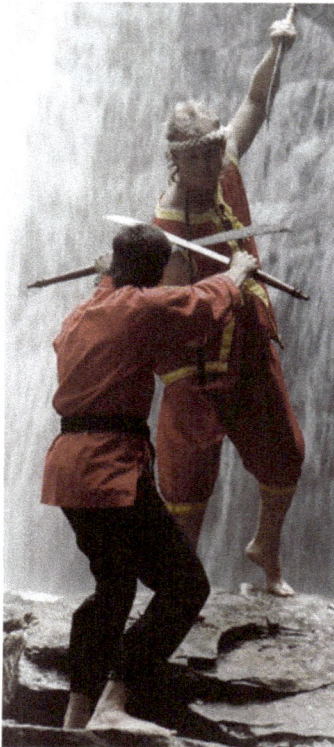

In Krabi Krabong, if your guard collapses usually that means that you have just been hit and or cut down.

Cross the swords, making an "X" and literally catch the blades. As you take the impact, thrust forward in a scissor-like fashion to hit what you are catching.

Muay Boran- Muay Chaiya Basic Training

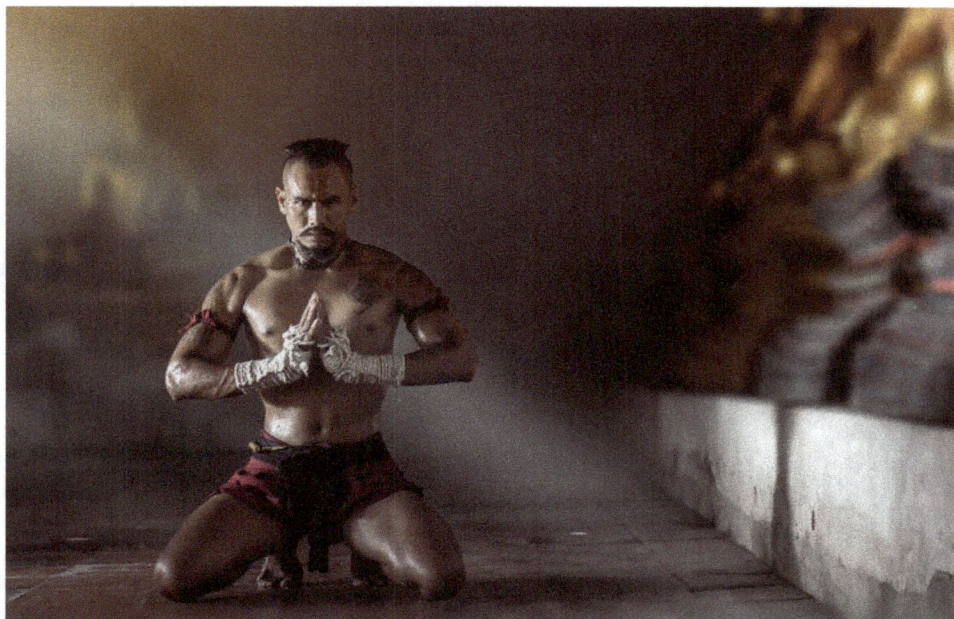

Every Krabi Krabong student learns the fundamentals of Muay Boran- Chaiya (*Buddhai Sawan Fan Daap*) fighting method. As GM Phaa Kruu once said, it is what you do if you either need a weapon or lose a weapon. It would not be your first choice in combat or self-defense as that would obviously require you to be armed. Every trained warrior will always prefer to have a weapon as the first line for attack or defense.

If you lose or drop your weapons in a real fight… that might be the end of you. It is vital to recover your weapons, your opponent's weapon immediately or survive long enough to get away. To get to a safe place for obvious reasons.

The difference between *Muay Boran* and *Muay Thai* or Thai boxing is that Muay Boran has been traditionally practiced as a combat martial art and incorporates breaking, strangling, finishing and or killing blows and techniques. Muay Thai is a sport "*safe for babies, women and children*" as Phaa Kruu used to say.

Many of the weapon-based techniques are patterned after the weapon/ sword fighting skills and drills… especially in such as foot work and general body positioning. One idea is that even in the art and science of the "empty hand", we are told to always assume that the opponent is armed or could be armed. Just because they do not have a weapon to start with, does not mean they will not acquire it along the way!

Muay Boran is not fighting. It is meant to be finished. Quick, decisive and "on to the next" type of way of combat is emphasized and drilled. In the past the types of warfare the warriors were in were what we should call "melee" or group battle types of situations. Visualize a thousand warriors in one place at one time, running at each other, with elephants and in later years horse cavalry. All of which are armored, armed and fighting to the death. There are scenes of these battles in many Thai temples painted as freezes on the walls. Many carvings in wood and reliefs in bronze etc. depicting these ferocious battles.

It was not unusual for Phaa Kruu in the mornings before the real practice and drilling in the courtyard to line us up and have us dash and run back and forth as fast as we could go! He stated this was the way. A warrior can dash! A warrior can run. There were famous historical battles where the Thai warriors both those of the organized army and the "free" militias, would have to run all day to get to the area of the fighting. Imagine running several miles on the way to then fight for your life. This idea brings a whole new dimension to the Krabi Krabong conditioning.

My Burmese Bando teachers including Bando Master's, Sensei's Erol Younger, Joe Manley and Lloyd Davis with their teacher GM Dr. U Maung Gyi, spoke to me about this from the Burmese perspective as the Traditional Bando and "Lethwei" training also included running and dashing with weapons in hand. By invitation of these Grand Masters of Burmese Bando, I presented the Buddhai Sawan Krabi Krabong Wai Kruu and Sword dance and weapon demonstration at the "Bando Nationals" in Prince of Prussia, Pennsylvania in 1986.

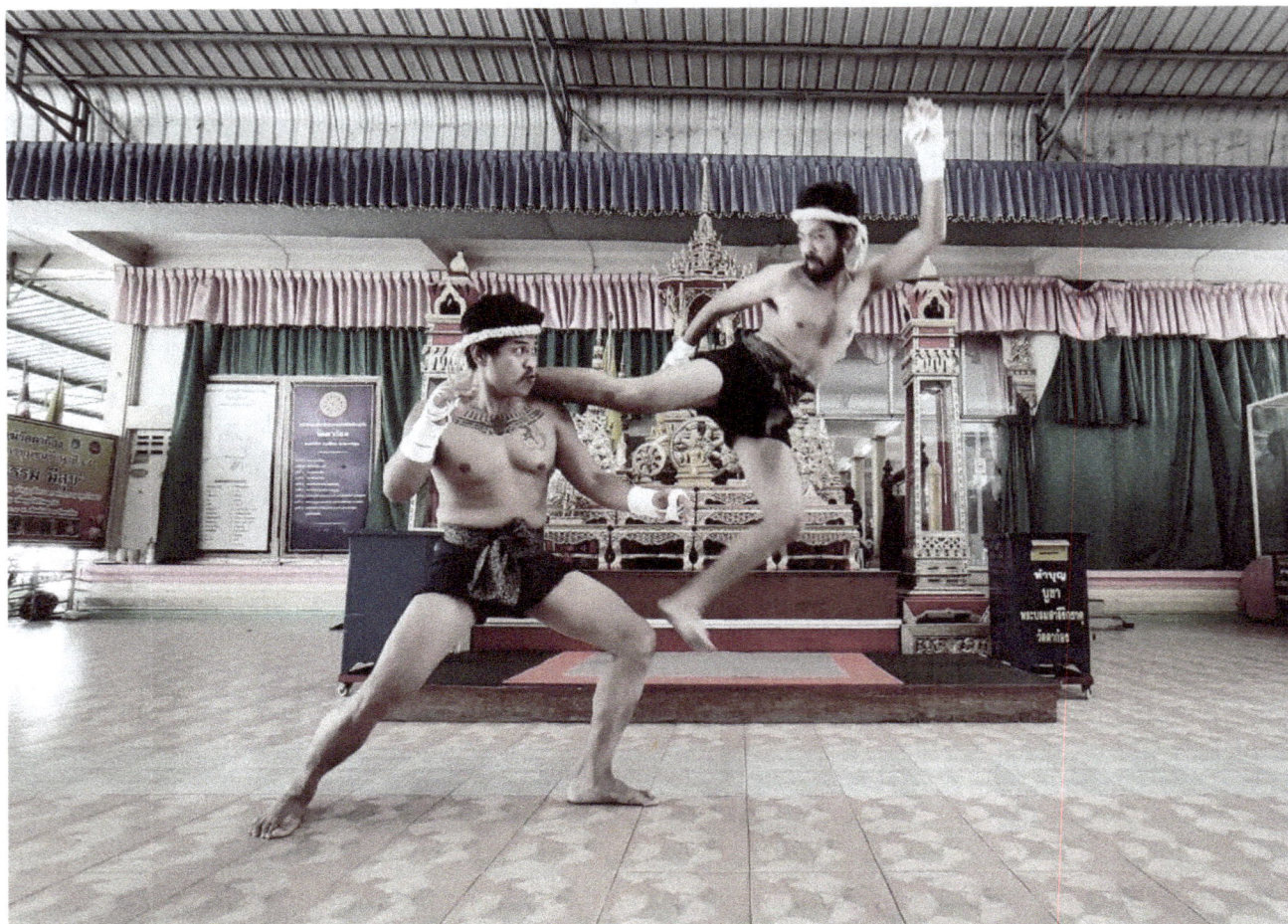

Muay Boran Wai Kruu (*Lu Rom Muay Thai* & Buddhai Sawan Krabi Krabong)

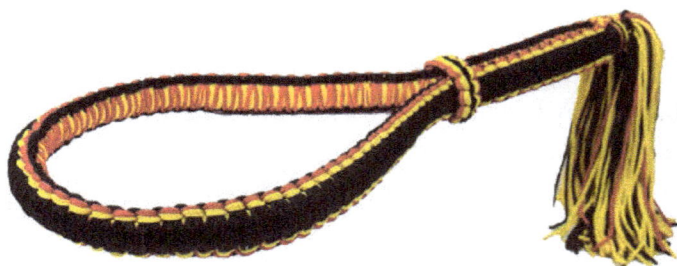

For Muay Thai or the sport of Ancient Thai Fighting "Muay Boran '' and Sport Thai Boxing "Muay Thai '', the "*Wai Kruu*" is not done just for meditation or for exercise. It becomes significant as a will or even a last testament.

Usually made of hemp, the *"Mongkhon"* or sacred head piece is elaborately decorated and extends over the head and down the back between the shoulder blades, ending in a tassel.

This, the most sacred of all Muay Thai ritual objects, is treated with great reverence and is never placed on the floor and always left hanging on the shrine when not in use. It will have been blessed by the monks and each camp has its own *"Mongkhon"*, often being passed down from teacher to teacher. The Thais believe that the older the *Mongkon*, the more powerful its influence over the boxer. We have in collection *"Mongkgon"* from *The Wat Buddhai Sawan Temple* that is over 200 years old!

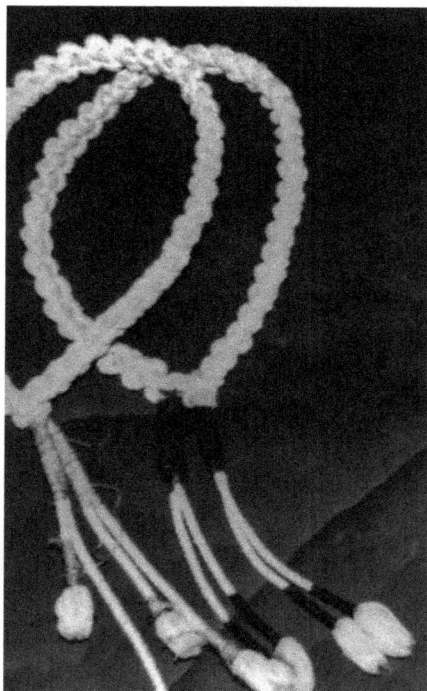

Photo Left: Two Mongkhon personally made by GM Phaa Kruu Samaii: 1984

Once placed on the head of the fighter, a short Pali mantra or prayer is chanted over the student. It said that this prayer or Pali Mantra is to serve as a reminder to the boxer that he is not only representing his teacher and camp but his family (both living and his ancestors) and Buddhist beliefs.

The fighter will now climb onto the apron of the ring and deliver three bows then climb over the top rope. When wearing the *"Mongkhon"* a fighter must go over the ropes and never under! It's considered very bad luck to go through the ropes wearing a *"Monkon"*. He now turns to face his own corner and gives three Wai's or bows while performing the *"Namaska Mudra"* (*Namaste Mudra* in Classical Indian Yoga tradition). In Thailand this signifies paying respect to *The Buddha, The Dhamma* (Teachings) and *The Sangha* (Community of Monks).

Once the Thai Boxer climbs into the rising and accepts the *"Monkon"* (blessed head band in the specific style of the school) from his teacher, he is literally ready, or becoming ready, to die at the hands and feet of his opponent. He makes an agreement or pact with his teacher, his god, his family, and lastly with his opponent that should he be crippled or die in the match all is forgiven. For the time being it is a similar concept of that of the Native American Warrior who cries out "Hoka Hey" i.e. "Today is a good day to die!". All in. Nothing was left not on the table.

It is not necessarily the intention of the Thai Boxer to kill his opponent, it is just that once in the ring and wearing the *"Monkon"* he is ready for war and death. Whatever the inducement was for originally getting into the ring is forgotten; he is not there for personality, ego, entertainment, favor, or money.

In addition to the wearing of the *"Mongkhon"* the wearing of a *"Kruang Ruang"* or *"Praciet"* on the upper arm. This is usually a blessed amulet or talisman blessed by a favored monk or teacher wrapped in a piece of fabric and tied to the upper arm. Both the *"Mongkhon"* and the *"Kruang Ruang"* are blessed and serve to give the boxer protection against his opponent. A fighter would never wear the *"Praciet"* for ordinary dress purposes as it is an object of spiritual importance and should be treated with great respect.

The whole world becomes condensed into 576 square feet of canvas. There is no "What do we do after the fight?" At the conclusion of the *"Rom Muay"* (*Wai Kruu*), the Thai Boxer has paid proper respect, he has made an offering to his god, and he is fully concentrated to the task at hand--to put his opponent down or, even better, to make him beg for mercy. The highest art in Muay Thai is to control your opponent through pain and cause him to voluntarily retire. If you simply knock him out, he doesn't know who won or why. But, if you cause your opponent to think that if he continues, he might not survive and make him quit, he will not want to fight you again.

Maybe never again.

The *Wai Kruu* of *Lu Rom Muay Thai* varies a little from that of the Krabi Krabong in that it is for the empty hand and there is not necessarily a reference to a weapon. There are, however, several recurrent themes commonly seen regardless of the style or school represented.

Most schools of Thai Sword and Thai Boxing have at least two different *Wai Kruu*. One is the formal school exercise and is quite lengthy, taking as long as ten or twenty minutes. The other is the ring or competition *Wai Kruu*. It is just as noble and serious; it is just not as long.

In the empty-hand form, the Boxer usually kneels and *"Wai's"* or bows to the ground to pay respect to the Buddha. Most of the time he does this three times, as three is considered a lucky number; a perfect number. He may then go through a ritualistic bathing routine where he (or she) appears to be washing his whole body. When finished, he throws the dirt behind him. He is then ready to face the spirits and his opponent.

The fighter may circle the ring, with one hand on the top rope (this is to seal the area of combat from evil spirits that might seek to harm him). It is bad enough that the opponent is going to try to harm him, no need to encourage the spirits associated with the opponent to climb in the ring as well! This very traditional spiritual concept also refers to the "ancestor Spirits' or deceased family members of the enemy!

He will roll his hands to show his opponent that he will hit him many times. He will lift his knee or kick out and or swing his elbow to show how he will destroy his opponent using these mighty weapons. He will stamp and or stomp the canvas three times with a fierce look or expression on his face to signify patting the dirt on the opponent's grave. He may initiate or simulate drawing an arrow on a Bow, drawing the Bow and then releasing the arrow to flay at his opponent's heart to weaken the enemies resolve.

Contained also in the *Wai Kruu* is a highly developed strategy for warfare with examples of both attack and defense. The sophisticated technical means of weapon handling and use are also found.

The Krabi Krabong *Wai Kruu* is a form or method of meditation and GM Phaa Kruu Samaii would say "one can be closer to the self, the Buddha, and the God by practicing with the right spirit". At some point it is no longer practiced but becomes an expression of the spirit within. This may be especially true when practiced with the formal breathing cadences and rhythms (Indian Sanskrit lang. *PranaYama*).

The Buddhai Sawan Sword Dance *"Wai Kruu"* is quite long, having over one hundred moves and is good all-around exercise.

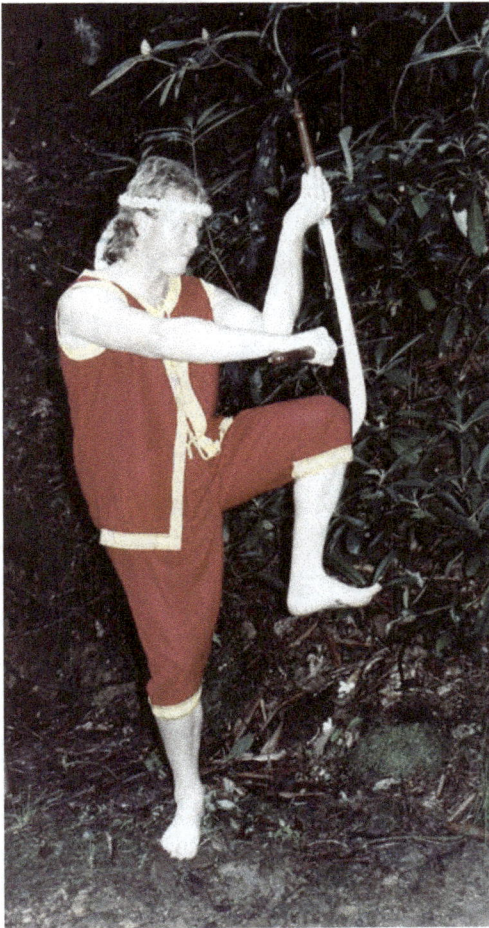

Historically, it was used by the Thais to develop stamina and power for battle. When done slowly, it belongs to the same category of exercise as Chinese Tai-Chi. Once this ablution- ritual is finished, the swords are taken firmly in hand and guided through the Four Directions. A salute is made to each major compass heading.

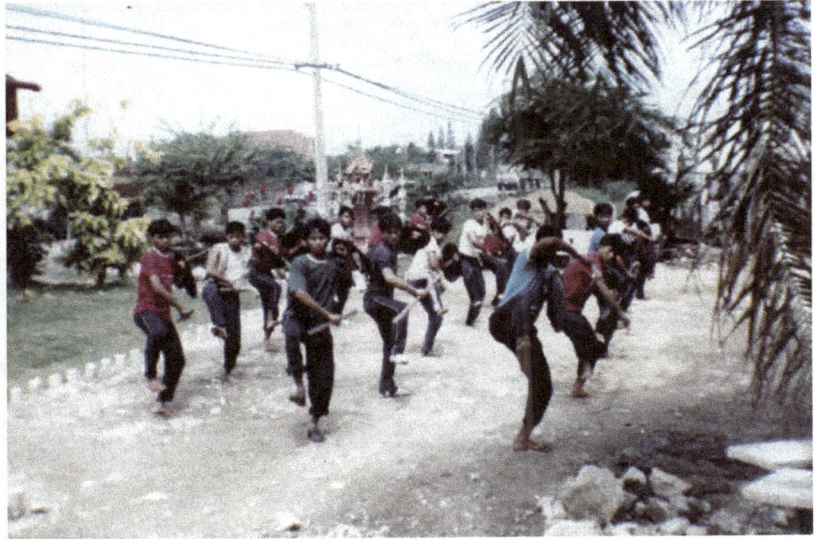

Wai Kruu is not restricted to swords or empty hand. It may be performed with any weapon!

It is also quite common to practice the BS Krabi Krabong Wai Khruu/ Sword Dance to music! Phaa Kruu Samaii taught that practicing to music was a traditional way to practice and would have students take turns learning the cadence and playing the drums.

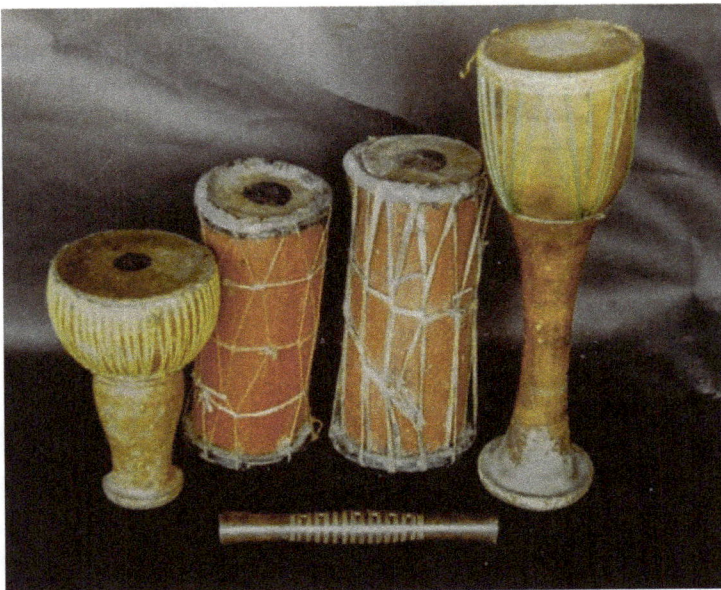

Especially he preferred the "Chinese" war style drum. This type of drum historically would have been carried into battle and used to coordinate the movement of Thai Armies.

Drums and instruments commonly used during training practice at Buddhai Sawan, Nogkam in the 80's.

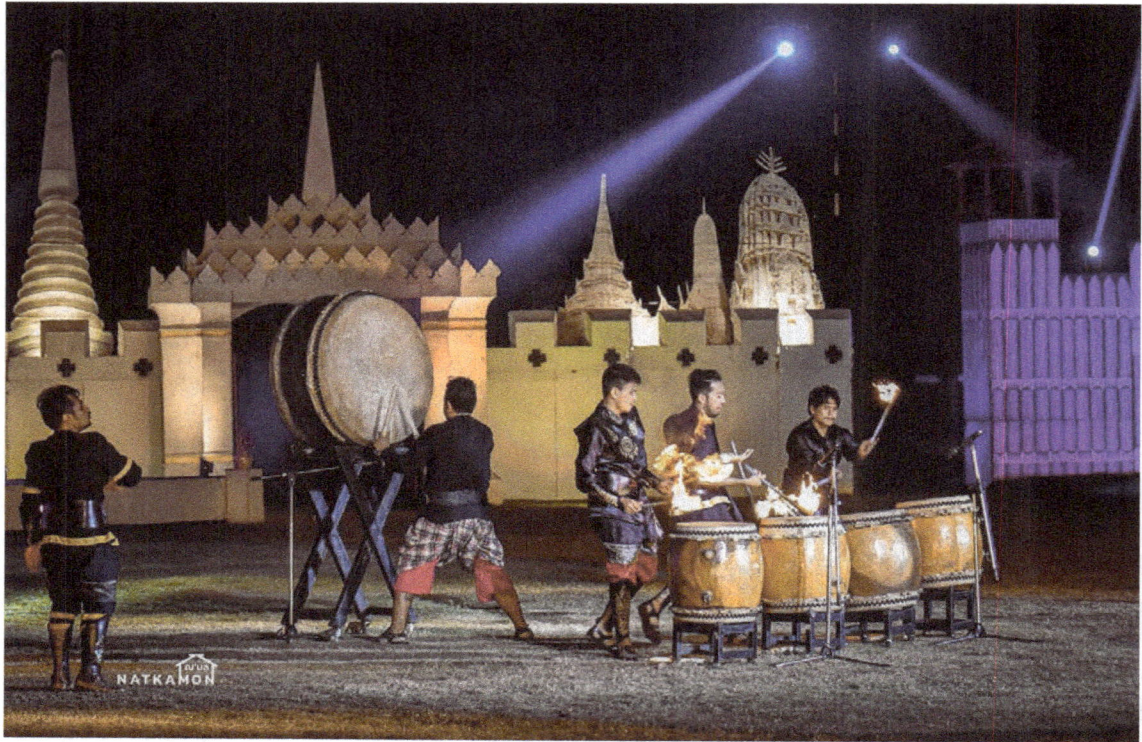

Example of "Chinese" style Elephant Battle or War drums used during Buddhai Sawa Krabi Krabong demonstrations in Thailand. Photo courtesy of Kruu Jira Mesamarn.

After the Four Directions are completed, the Dancer moves through performing the additional sections such as the "*Erawan*" or "Elephant" and "Bird's Wing", the walking and the spring back, The "Tiger" etc. finishing with the dramatic fighting sequence putting the dance like walking postures into motion with a partner or two!.

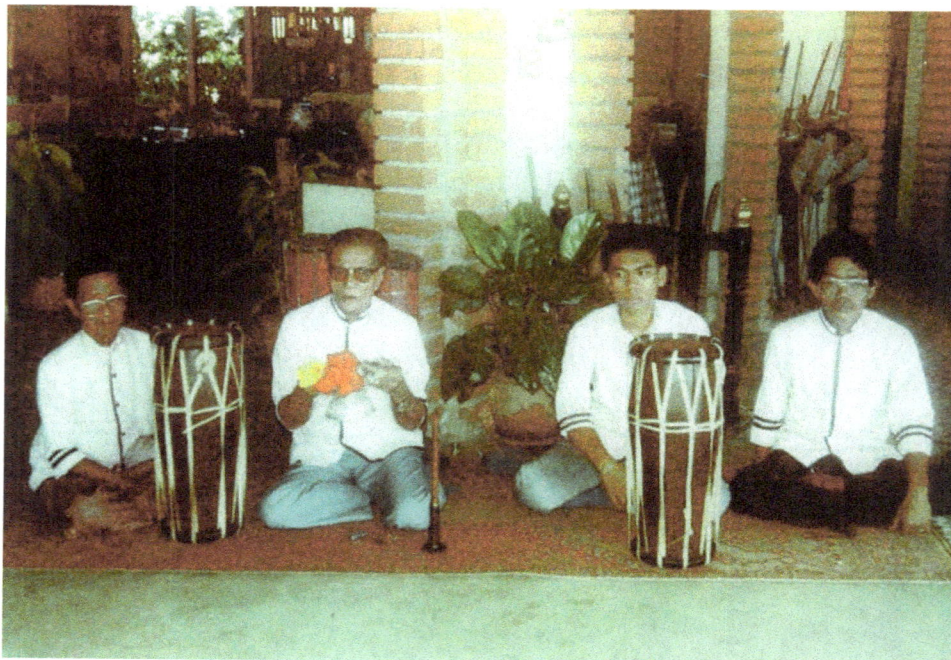

Special occaision! Buddhai Sawan Nongkam Band! This is very traditional sounding traditional Thai Music with Javanese flute and Tabla style drums,

In the fighting sequence, various striking and defensive postures useful in actual combat are demonstrated. If the pace was previously slow and methodical, it now becomes fast; furious. The fighting may or may not finish with empty-hand technique.

The Basic Muay Stance "Lu Rom Muay"

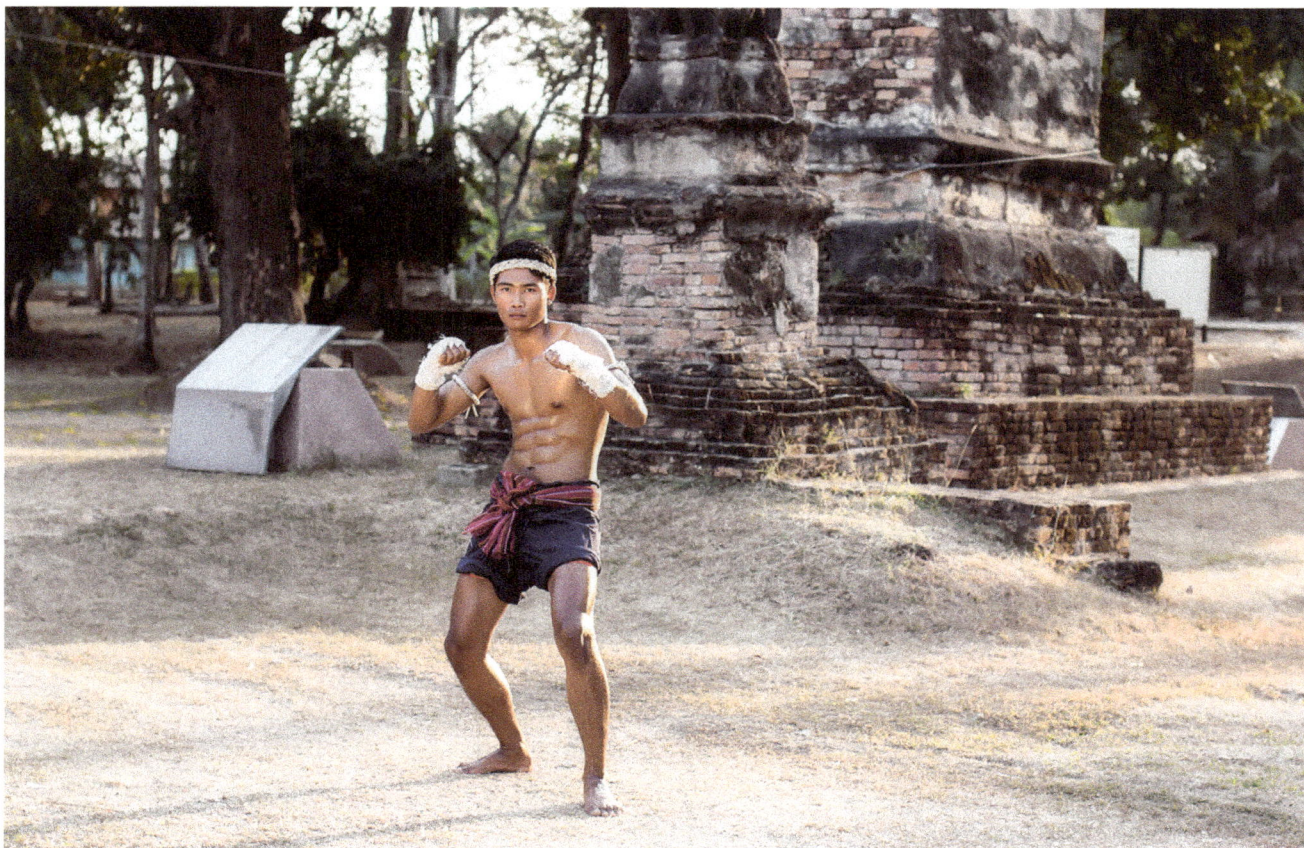

This stance is also referred to as the forward fighting stance. The basic fighting stance is the most s uitable all-purpose stance. It is balanced with great possibility for offensive as well as defensive capability and maneuvering. The left or right shoulder is forward with the hips following at approximately the same angle. The legs are placed about 1 shoulder width apart, comfortably spaced, and slightly bent or relaxed. The forward or leading foot is angled toward the opponent as is the back foot. The heel of the back foot is slightly raised.

This position is not held rigidly by any means. The shoulders are relaxed, and the body is ready to move in any direction.

The hands are held at the height of the shoulders, in front of the face, between you and your opponent. The forward shoulder determines the lead hand. The arms are comfortable and relaxed. The elbows are kept down and close to the side of the body. The rear hand or guard is held 1% or 2 hand widths from the face. The lead hand may be found that much further additionally. The weight of the body is evenly distributed onto both legs. This makes fast weight shifting and spinning possible. Both hands are kept constantly in motion, though not enough to open or to allow a possible attack.

The head is kept close in with the chin down. The chin is guarded by, but not pinned to, the lead shoulder. The overall posture is upright and erect. Most height change is accomplished by bending the knees. The rear foot is not directly behind the lead, on the same line, as in a side fighting stance. It should be placed on a tangent of about one foot's width.

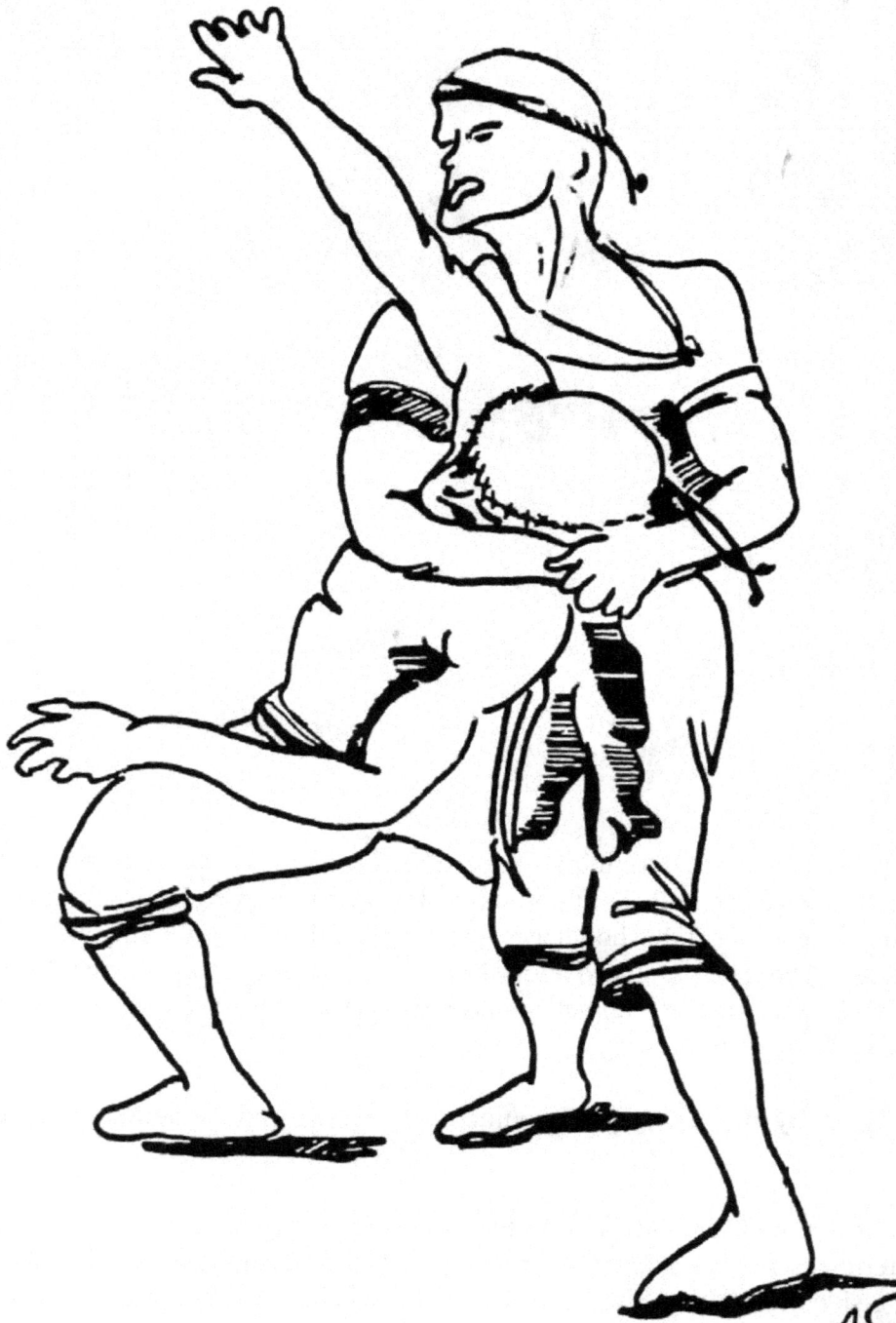

How To Toughen The Shins

The Shins when conditioned and used for attack or defense are devastating. Adding a program of periodic shin toughening may well prove to be one of your most valuable conditioning aids. It has been documented and utilized extensively in such fighting arts as Muay Thai (Thai Boxing), Bando (Burmese Boxing), Arnis de Mano (Filipino Stick Fighting), and others. In most of these systems, when the application of a shin kick or blocking method is utilized or demonstrated, they are referred to as brutal. Why is this? Why is the picture of being hit with a developed shin so devastating?

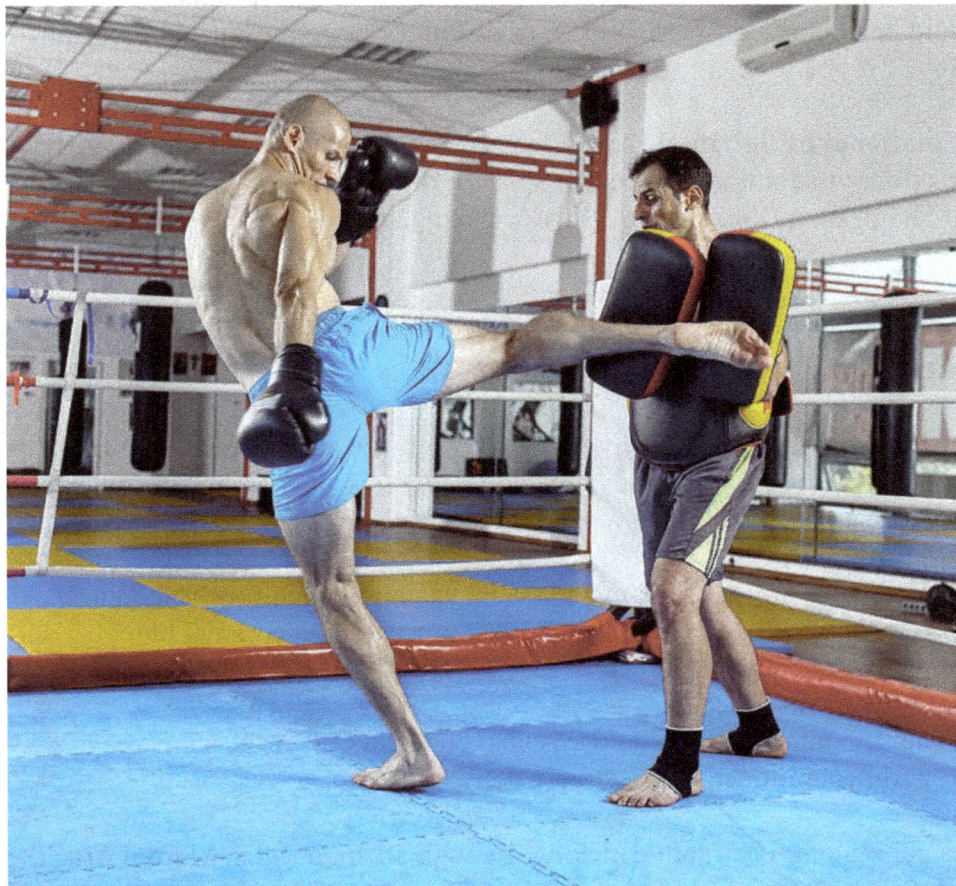

The "Tup" or Shin is a most powerful weapon and the strongest "shield" when conditioned and used properly.

We sometimes use Elephant or Buffalo Hide rectangular shield, which are quite hard or tough, for practive and conditioning. Warm up to their use gradually, over time to avoid undo bruising. But once your used to the contact... Bang away!

We don't see people cringing when they see someone punched in the head; in fact, western boxers seem to beat each other back and forth on the cranium for hours. But see someone who receives a shin to the head, and they don't bounce back.

The fighters of Thailand in their three major martial arts: *Muay Thai/ Muay Boran* and Krabi Krabong, have elevated the use of shin techniques and the conditioning of the shins themselves as a weapon to a high degree. This is one reason not many fighters have survived ring bouts with Thai style boxers on their feet.

The shin is the baseball bat of the body. When properly conditioned over a long period of time, it is capable of smashing 2x4's and/or a real baseball bat. This weapon is hard, has an edge, and is capable of large variations in height. The shin is as equally capable of destroying soft tissue or muscular areas of the body as it is of crushing bony areas, joints, or just about anything else which happens to get in the way.

The beautiful thing about incorporating the use of the shins in offensive, as well as defensive technique is the way it opens up possibilities.

For instance, in attacking, you may hit areas previously not considered vital areas and be able to disable. These areas could include the calf, thigh, hip, arm, shoulder, back, neck, and especially your attacker's own shins. This is especially great for those of us who either <u>don't like</u> to kick high or <u>can't</u> kick high.

Another aspect of this offensive invasion is the amount of damage and pain a shin attack is capable of producing. Usually, the pain is out of proportion to the actual damage, and the damage may be great! There are two ways to disable an opponent.

       1. Break Something Physical. Your opponent, due to a structural disability, is unable to continue. Examples of this would be unconsciousness, broken or dislodged bones or joints, or loss of blood.

       2. Break Something Emotional or Spiritual. This refers to the will that drives or motivates your opponent; your opponent's desire to continue. Once that spirit or desire is broken, or the opponent becomes afraid, he is disabled. Sharp, traumatic, and suddenly occurring, as well as long lasting, pain can do this.

Offensive Use Of The Shins

If you imagine the worst "Charlie horse" that you have ever had and you face an opponent who can create or duplicate that sensation at various points on the body, you begin to see what I mean. When kicked in the lower leg you may lose a portion or all of your ability to walk or run.

When hit in the thigh, front, back, or side, you may not even be able to stand, much less kick. When kicking to the body, a conditioned shin will simply cut through most types of conventional blocking and wreak havoc on whatever is hit, be it arm, hand, shoulder, or face.

Let me qualify this statement. The shin attack will only do this "havoc wreaking" if the shin area of the aggressor or martial artist is properly conditioned to effectively deliver that attack.

The use of shin kicking is not a panacea for destructive kicking. As with all concepts in Martial Arts, the concept is only as real as the person using it.

Defensive Use Of The Shins

Defensively, the shin's use is amazing. The shins become shields for and against all sorts of attacks with a very special benefit. This shield is not a passive deterrent.

It has a tendency, an inclination, to injure the weapon whether it be hand, leg, foot, etc. The developed shin is a true shield in that it is hard, long enough, and mobile enough to cover a wide area. The idea of a tool which protects the user and damages the offender or aggressor is a progressive concept.

It is progressive because by design it makes your defense more efficient. You accomplish two objectives simultaneously with the same motion! The Thai Boxer defends attacks from his lower leg to his head with his shins!

Examples of this two-fold benefit of the conditioned shin is in the defense against a traditional round kick or hook kick. Before the opponent's attack lands, the defender's shin is raised strategically in place. The kick lands against the defending shin instead of its intended target. Usually, this situation happens by accident with the result being the aggressor and the defender hopping about holding his foot or leg and howling about the pain. The tough guy will simply start limping. We would like to negate or avoid the accidental consequence of this type of encounter. We do this by blocking or shielding with a conditioned shin area. This leaves only the attacker limping, hopping, or howling.

With a little more contact it is not unusual for the attacker to end up with a severe bruise or contusion wherever the attack was made, or even fractured or broken bones.

Many Martial Artists kick with the foot, especially the top of the foot near the toes. In reality, this is a fragile area requiring very little in the way of pressure or contact to cause an injury.

When defending with the shin, the following three postures should be followed:
    1. Angle the shin so as to meet the opponent's aggressive extension head on with the leading edge of the shin. This sometimes means turning the shin slightly outward before impact.

    2. As you block with the knee, cock the leg inward tightly while flexing the foot. This does two things: a) it prepares the lower leg for contact, and b) it prevents a rising kick from extending into the groin area.

    3. Raise the knee high. It is possible to protect areas previously selectively guarded with the hands, like the ribs and the head.

Remember, you not only may cause an injury to the aggressive extension or weapon, but this in addition allows the hands to remain free to deliver counterattack or protect as necessary. This is an example of having one technique applied perform two objectives simultaneously.

Destroying The Enemies Foundation

The Thai Boxer feels that you begin to defeat an opponent by destroying the foundation of or for his attack (i.e., his ability or desire to move). One way this is accomplished is by directing the attention of the shin to the lower body, the thighs, and the calves of the opponent. The opponent progressively loses his mobility and footwork deteriorates as he is bruised. He becomes reticent or cautious with his attack as he hurts himself banging into the "steel posts" of his opponent.

Obviously, this constructive and destructive capability can run two ways. An objective in conditioning the shins is to protect against or prepare for an attack by someone who utilizes the shin in their arsenal also.

Offensive Benefits of The Shin

Offensively, the shin is a great weapon. Having a relatively narrow area of contact, about an inch, and a much larger mass than the hand or the foot, the shin already has more latent destructive potential. The average fighter who simply begins to incorporate the use of the shin into his arsenal will notice surprised expressions on his opponent's faces. It is the rigidity and extra mass or weight of the lower leg behind the shin which allows it to be so effective in attacking large body surfaces. These surfaces, like the thigh for instance, are not always considered targets.

Yet, a well-placed shin laid across the mid-thigh area can fracture the femur!

When attacking with the shin, care should be exercised in several areas. These areas include:

1. Make sure the hips rotate freely so as to allow the knee to align directly with the angle of attack of the shin. This does two things, it makes sure you hit with the hardest portion of the shin (i.e., the front as opposed to the side), and it prevents unnecessary lateral stress on the knee joint.

2. The ankle and foot of the leg with which the attack is made should be slightly tensed, as a relaxed or floppy foot can result in a whiplash-type injury to the ankle. Also, when kicking with the shins, the feet sometimes encounter elbows, belt buckles, and more.

3. Use more follow-through than would normally be expected. Lead with the hips and drive through your target. To use the analogy of the "baseball bat" again; to bunt every time at bat would be a waste of energy as the bat is capable of knocking out home runs. After you hit, experiment with not snapping out of your target but allowing the weight and impact of your leg to carry you through it.

Building Your Foundation

Conditioning: Traditionally, the Thais conditioned by kicking young banana trees and as their shins toughened went to more mature trees until they could kick a mature tree with full power!

The best bet in utilizing or properly defending against a shin-concept-based attack is in preconditioning. The following examples demonstrate a variety of practices and methods which are commonly used to develop the shin area of the lower leg for contact.

A. Rolling and/or Rubbing Method. Using a round object, a bar, a broom handle, a bundle of chopsticks, or similar objects, press lightly and roll upward and downward along the leading edge of the shin area. Press at different angles both center and off-center. A bunch of chopsticks bundled together with rubber bands makes an excellent device. The edges of the chopsticks dig in and create a conditioning effect as you move them back and forth. At first you will find this is uncomfortable, even painful, as this area is initially quite tender. The pain and discomfort will decrease in time as it does increase the amount of pressure and the speed of your movement.

Train with moderation. Although short-term goals are viable, it takes years of progressive conditioning and training to fully develop iron-hard shins.

Moderate, regular conditioning over a long period is preferred to hasty, irregular training. There should be a goal to involve yourself mentally and emotionally in this process. The small pain associated with training is analogous to the real potential for pain found in combat and in life. Do not so much try to forget these small pains as to welcome them as real friends; the kind of friends whose criticisms bring as much growth and inspiration as their admonishment and praise.

B) Tapping. (Iron Skin Technique) With the conditioning tool, stick, or whatever, make little tapping motions up and down the shin area, all the time varying the angle. Do not concentrate on one area too long as a large bruise may develop. Over time, progressively tap with more vigor. Once you are thoroughly tough, use a heavier or harder instrument. The tapping creates a similar effect as that of being kicked, an actual impact. This similarity creates specificity in your training. And as you control the tool used, there is complete safety.

In actually kicking against objects, there is an element of uncontrolled or improperly moderated impact. This chance could cause bruising or pain severe enough to halt training. This is undesirable as you wish for consistent and moderate training which is progressively more intense and difficult over time. Long-term training gives the body's mechanisms time to adapt to the stress of training.

There is some bruising associated with almost all forms of exercise or physical conditioning. This bruising is the result of small tears in the muscles, connective tissue, or vascular systems of the body, and in moderation assist in the developmental processes. The stress applied to these elements of the body increases circulation, thickens connective tissue, and stimulates thickening of bones, all favorable.

C) Heavy Bag or Shield. Begin with light kicking in the middle portion or softer area of the bag. Do not blast the bag as you wish to acclimate your legs to taking the shock in a new way. Especially considering the knees and ankles. Vary the area of impact so as to allow the widest portion of the shin area to land, from ankle to knee. Next, begin hitting lower on the bag, into the harder part of the bag but away from the edge. Over time, progressively hit harder. Lastly, swing the shins upward into the bottom edge of the bag in the same manner.

The results of training accrue during the inactive periods between workouts. Train hard and honestly when you train and then rest well when you rest. If a specific bruising or injury develops, take one or two days off to recuperate, keeping in mind that you begin to lose the benefit after three or four days. Initially, a good balance may be arrived at by training every other day or once every two days.

Use the R.I.C.E. method for treatment of any severe bruising or strains incurred while training. R.I.C.E. is an acronym for Rest, Ice, Compression, and Elevation of the injured area. Of course, competent medical advice is recommended in the event of any severe injury, though I recommend seeing one familiar with the injuries of athletes.

D) Toe Raises. To develop flexibility and build strength in the muscles in the area of the shins, primarily the Tibialis Anterior and the Extensor Hallicus and Digitorum Longus. These muscles primarily lift the toes and foot upward toward the knee. There are variations: 1) while wearing shoes, balance on your heels and flex your toes upward as hard as you can for ten seconds; 2) you can provide some additional resistance by hooking a bicycle inner tube under something and stretching it over the toes. Then, flex your toes against it; or 3) have a friend pull on your toes while you resist.

E) Overall, be sure to move through a full range of motion to maintain and enhance your flexibility. Work at your own pace. If you develop soreness, stop. If you are improving, continue. Do not compare your progress with other persons. Experiment to find what works best for you. The best teacher is in your own heart.

The "Shins"

THE SHINS

"TUP"

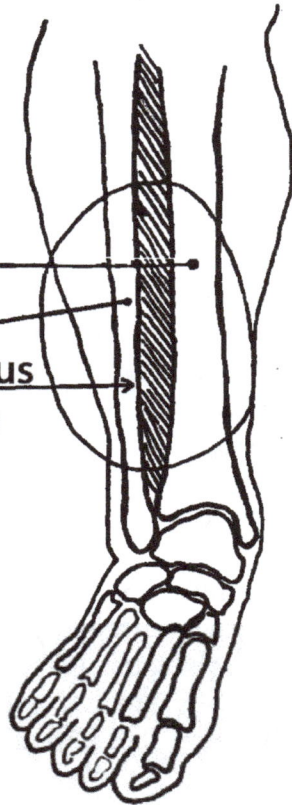

Tibia

Fibula

Interosseous
Membrane

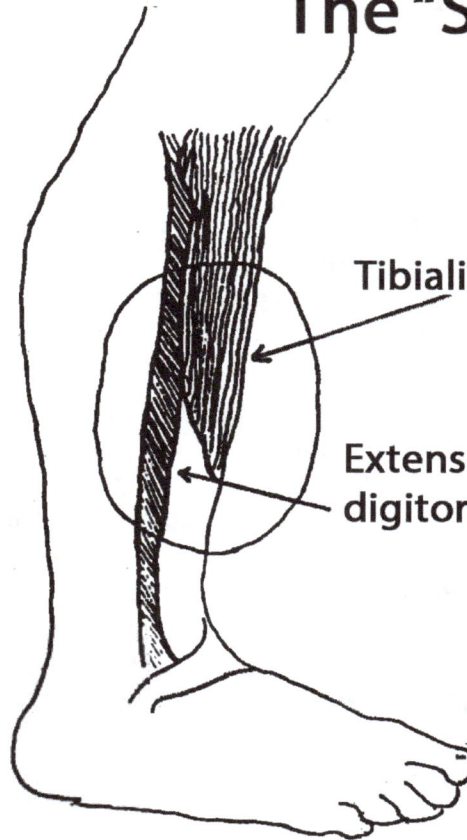

Tibialis Anterior

Extensor
digitorum longus

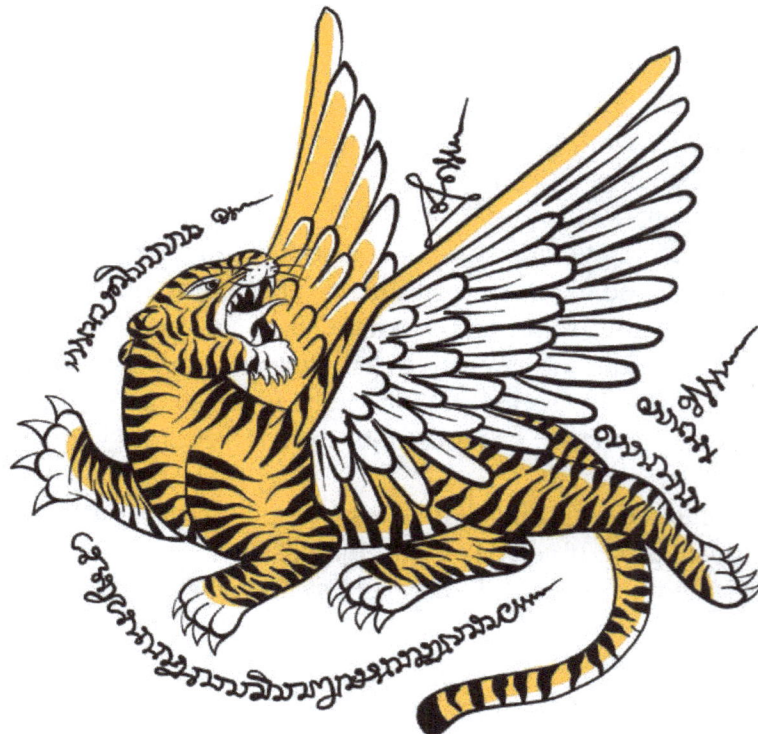

Center Line Theory and Application

If you draw a line down the center of the body, you will find most of the body's vital points residing along that line. In human anatomy terms this represents the Medial or Sagital Body Plane, one of the three primary planes of the body along with the Coronal- Frontal, Transverse- Dorsal. We imagine or visualize this Medial Plane or Center line extending from our center mass to the center mass of the attacker.

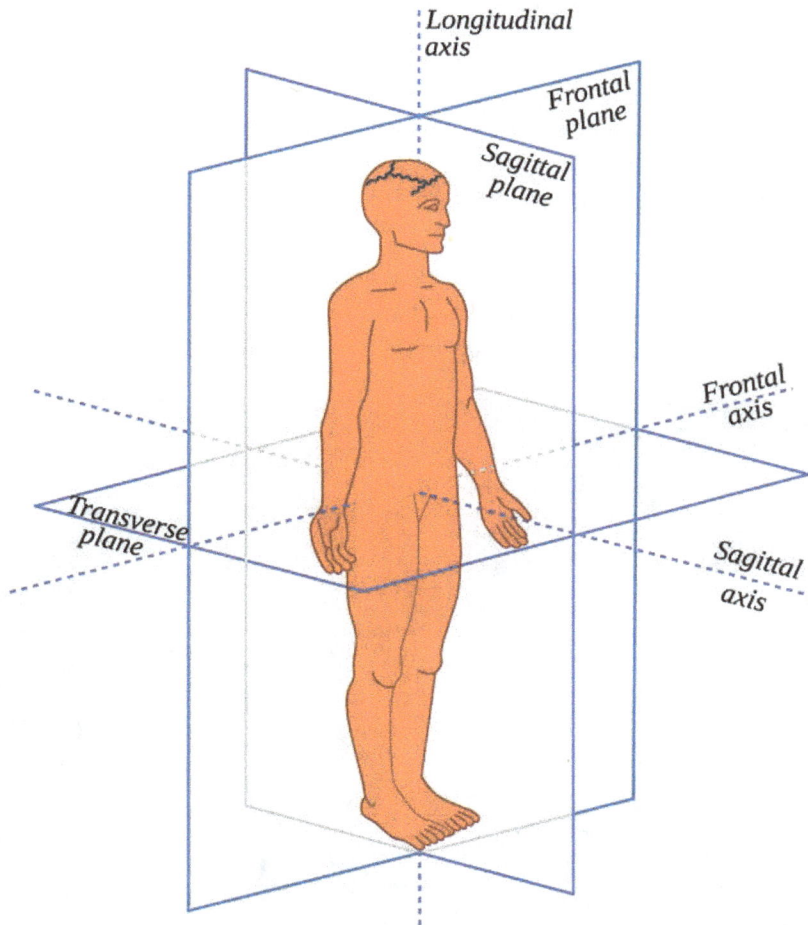

The eyes, nose, mouth, throat, solar plexus, and groin name are just a few. This line also marks the body's central axis, and as long as you keep this line as straight as possible, you will have the greatest possibility for strength, balance, and speed.

If the "Center Line" represents the greatest number of vital points on the opponants body, then it follows to reason that ones defensive maneuvering and attacking techniques and procedures should concentrate on this line.

In defense, you should guard this area at all times, being careful not to open a path or allow the opponent to gain access to the centerline. When one hand is extended the other is guarding. You need to keep the elbows in close (don't "wing" them up and out) avoiding a drawing back motion whenpunching. Recover from each technique as quickly as possible.

Recover meaning to return to guarding or moving from the center line. Always face the opponent more or less directly but do not stand completely square or sideways.

In offensive motion or in attacking, your purpose is to gain access to violate your opponent's centerline without exposing your own to attack. You do this either by moving faster initially and scoring first, or out-faking and hitting at will, beating down his guard and scoring as in a combination, or drawing him into a hyper-extension movement and scoring as the opening appears. The point is that whoever controls the centerline of his opponent is the stronger opponent strategically.

Seven Ways Of Moving Back

Defensive movement is the art and science of retreat while under pressure without sacrificing the integrity of your defense while maintaining opportunity for countering and decisively ending the fight at any time. A well executed backward or side step may set up a finishing strike in your favor. You can use the opponents attacking pressure to your advantage.

1.   Step back with your rear foot.
2.   Step back with rear foot then let front foot slide back to a fighting stance or further, but not as far back as the rear foot (see #3).
3.   Step back with rear foot then slide front foot back to rear foot.
4.   Slide front foot back to rear foot.
5.   Slide front foot back then step back with rear foot into a fighting stance.
6.   Step with the front foot directly through to the rear, actually changing sides.
7.   Spring back. Without stepping, jump up and straight backwards.

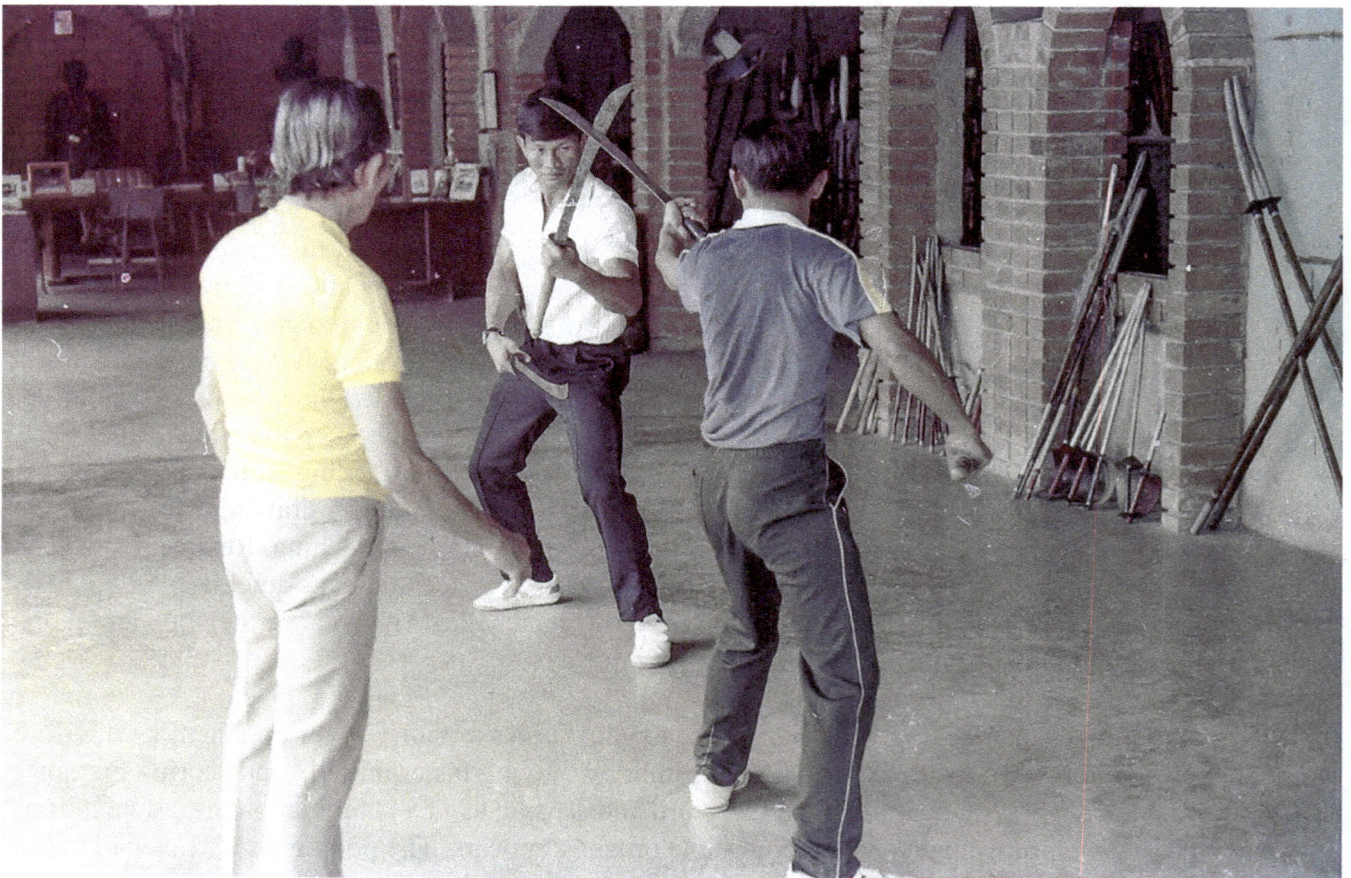

GM Khruu Samaii coaches proper defensive and counter offensive techniques

Striking Techniques: Hand

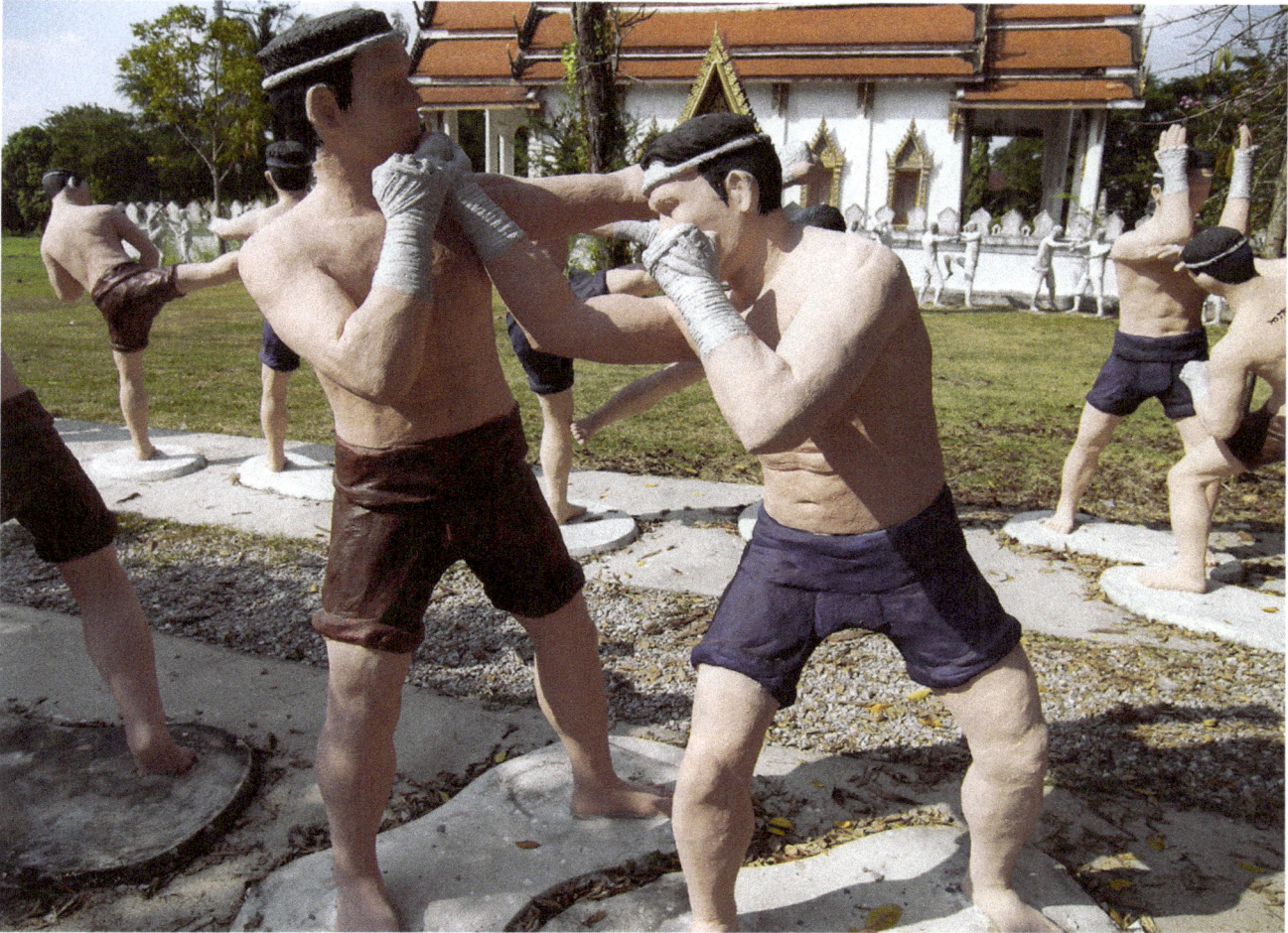

1. *"Mat Drong"* (Straight Punching- The Jab Punch)
2. *"Mat Drong"* (Cross or Reverse Punch)
3. *"Mat Aat"* (The Uppercut)
4. *"Mat Tong"* (The Hook)
5. The Lead Hook
6. General Block

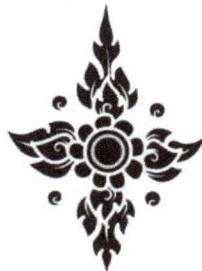

"Mat Drong" (Straight Punching)

1.   The Jab

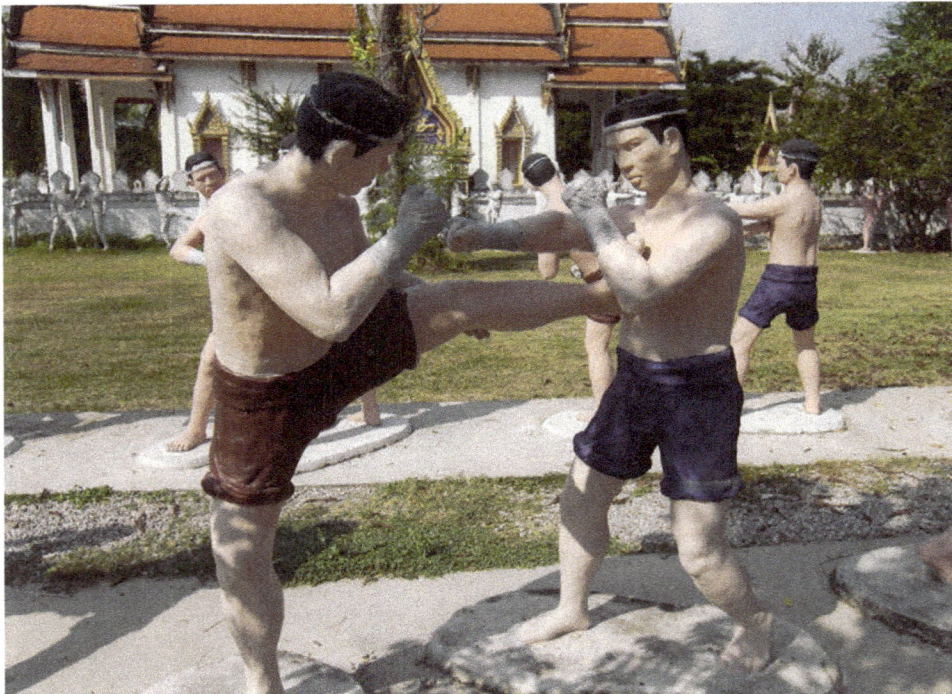

The jab is the quickest most direct offensive/defensive hand weapon. From the fighting stance, the leading hand (front) pushes straight into the target, the hand rotating palm down. Once the technique is thrown it is withdrawn sharply. The jab is light, quick, snapping in and back. It derives its power from its speed. The idea of using a sharp, fast punch is that it does not give the head of the opponent time to adjust, therefore causing concussion.

> **The targets for the jab are:**
> **a)**   Point of jaw.
> **b)**   Side of jaw.
> **c)**   Maxilla (below nose, above mouth).
> **d)**   Solar plexus.

The jab is a good offensive weapon. Use it to open opposite centerline combination opportunities or use it defensively to keep your opponent from scoring on retreat. The shoulders must be relaxed to throw properly. Do not lock out the elbow. On contact, the body weight should be going to the front foot.

On impact, the hand and arm are tensed. Variations: **a)** step out; **b)** slide up; **c)** step back; **d)** slide back (see Seven Ways of Moving Back).

2.   "Mat Drong" (Cross or Reverse Punch)

The Reverse Punch is so called because it is thrown with the reverse or back hand. Unlike the jab which develops most of its power impact from its speed, being a percussion punch, the Reverse Punch is dependent mostly on the twisting of the hips and body moving behind for power. It may be used high, middle, or low.

Generally speaking, the hand travels in a straight line to the target. If to the body, use a vertical fist; to the face, roll the hand palm down just before contact.

From a fighting stance with the left side forward, both hands held at shoulder height, drop the right (rear) knee while rolling the rear heel upward. This is simultaneous with the right hip swinging (pivoting) forward, squaring up or a little farther. The right shoulder follows, and the punch is thrown.

The hand travels straight into the target then comes straight back returning you to your original position. Execute the entire movement as one motion. Overreaching will cause a loss of stability.

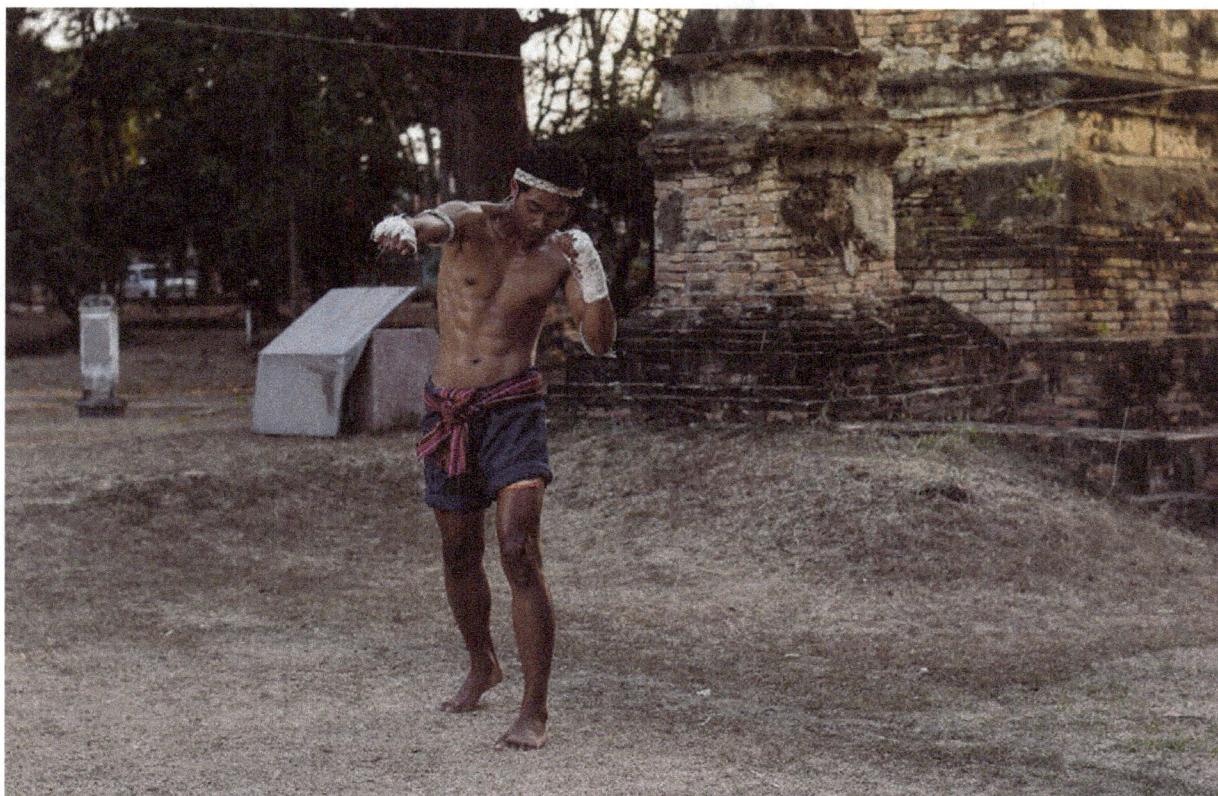

3.   "Mat Aat" (The Uppercut)

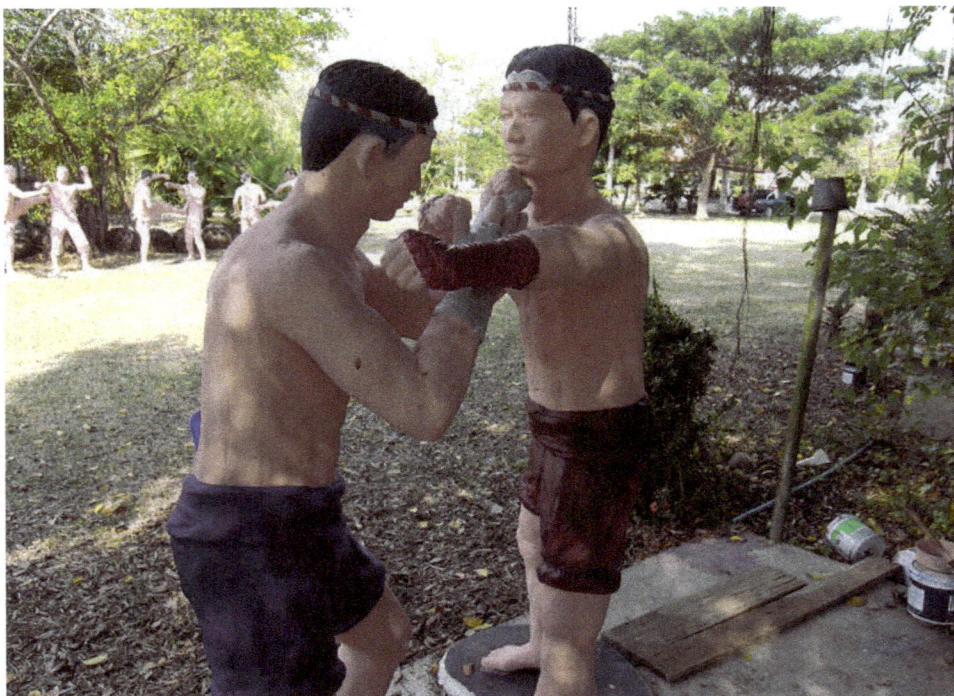

The Uppercut Punch is best suited for close quarter or in-fighting (Puno in Kali). At the outer limit use the elbow range as a gauge. At the inner, if you can get your arm between your body and that of your opponent, you can do it. This punch is well suited to an opponent who spends much of his time hooking or swinging his punches wildly from the side.

The trick to throwing a really powerful Uppercut punch, is to generate most of the hitting power from the knees. Keep the arm bent well and held close to the body before extending and then add a short snap to the punch at the last minute. Let's say you begin from a left side forward stance. That means you will have a right lead. To throw the Uppercut from the right hand, begin by dipping or bending at the knees. Then pivot inward, bringing the punching hand from a position just outside the centerline to one directly on the line. The palm should be facing you. Now spring upward driving with the knees trying to get onto your toes. Lean back slightly. Immediately, before contact is made with the target, snap the hand upward into the target. As you hit, continue to drive through with the knees as a follow up.

This punch may be thrown freely with either hand. The only difference between the lead and the rear hand being that a greater pivot is required of the rear hand.

4.   "Mat Trong" (The Hook)

The Hook is so called because the hand travels a pathway shaped like a hook into the target. Although the basis for scientific punching is the development of effective straight-line punching, there must be an ability to hit strongly from the side or the off angles. The Hook provides this counterpoint. Although it is simple to learn, it is difficult to master in that the punch, in a sense, mimics the natural swinging type of punch that all untrained fighters tend to throw. On closer inspection, however, we find that there are many differences.

Beginning from a basic "Lu Rom Muay" forward stance, you throw the "lead hook" to a high target by first raising the elbow to the same height as the target. The height of the hand may or may not change very much, depending on whether or not it was high or low to begin with. Once the hand and the elbow are in line with the target, pivot outward with the front heel. Allow the torso to turn as far as it can before bringing the hand into the target. This stretches the muscles and tissue of the chest and shoulder to their fullest just prior to actually throwing the punch. Keeping the thumb up and the arm flexed at about 90 degrees, snap the first into the target with a loose, easy snapping motion. The punch begins from the floor and proceeds to the knees and hips, then to the shoulders before the hand even moves.

The hand snaps inward as it comes into play. The idea is to tighten into the puch just before contact and add that concentric torq . The Hook can be done with ease and snap or it can be the hay maker taking the opponant out. Most commonly used in combonation with Jap, Cross, Hook tuype of combo just as in western boxing. However, one big difference with Buddhai Sawan Muay Boran/ Muay Chaiya, "Fan Daap" application and use is that it is like all the other "punches" ... It is meant to be delivered Bare Knuckle and or with some kind of weapon held in the hand! When throwing punches bare knuckle or no gloves or wraps, you have to be especially careful and or precise in delivery so as to avoid breaking your fingers, especially the 5th metacarpal (finger bone of the little finger). When using with a sword in hand it can be especially devastating as you can make use of the handle to make the fist harder and then continue the hook contact into a follow through cut!

The "*Mat Tong*" Hook punch although more often thrown from the lead or front hand is also thrown from the rear or cross hand. When thrown from the rear or back hand it is a "knock out" punch if it connects and the whole body pivots and drives it home.

5.   THE LEAD HOOK

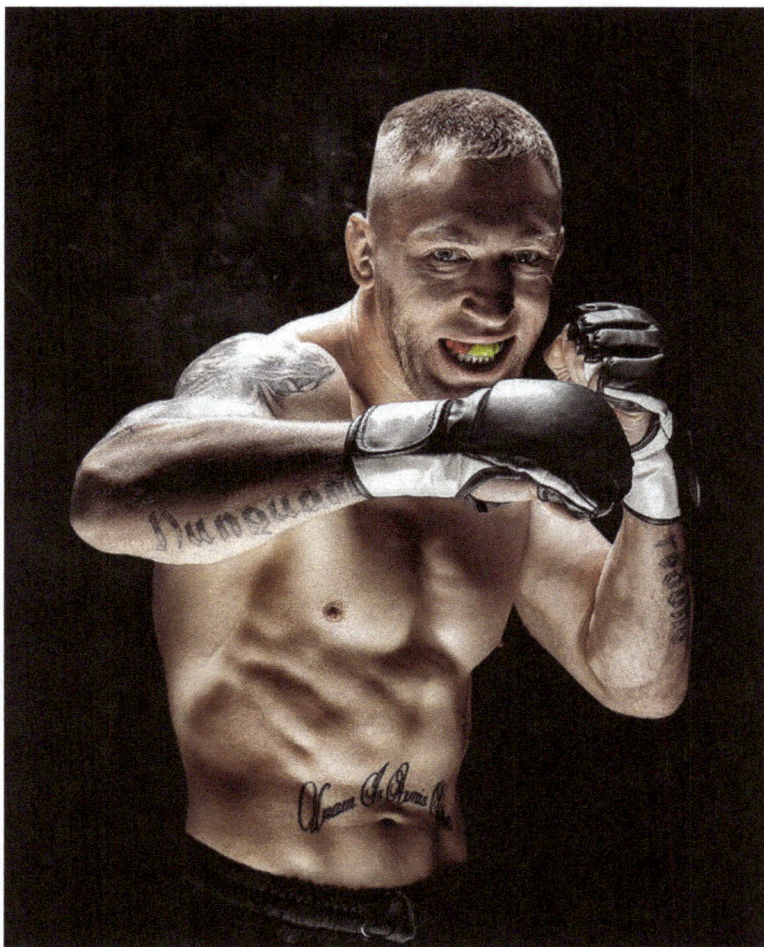

The Lead Hook is mostly suited for close range or infighting. When properly thrown, the punch is hard to see and correspondingly hard to follow. It should basically be used with caution, primarily when going in or moving out. It is absolutely essential to keep the rear guard up when executing this punch as the counter is a hook.

#6: General Block: Hands & Arms

This is the active form of the *"Lu Rom Muay"* or Basic fighting stance. Active because the idea is to raise the forward knee on the side being threatened or attack to make contact or near contact with the bent arm and elbow on the same side. This creates a "Shield" top to bottom: Fist (with weapon in hand?), forearm, elbow, front knee, shin, ankle foot. You present this right into the opponents attack. The opponant bangs into to this shield and may sustain a disabling injury as a result. So, although it appears defensive it is an attack! An attack to wear down or detroy the opponants weapons of punching and or trying to kick you. They might as well be trying to puch or kick a tree.

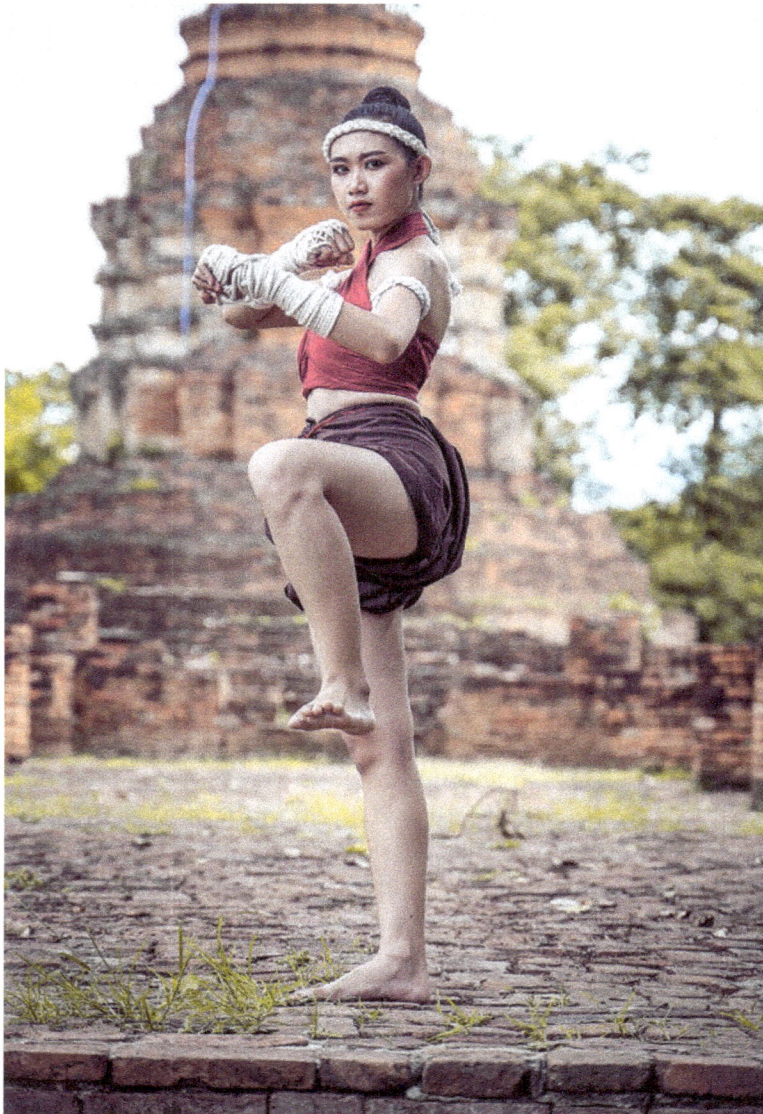

In today's world as in the past, women warriors are a vital and important part of our "fighting arts" community. On many levels our schools can not function without them! We welcome them and their amazing fierce spirit and creativity as they work with us to be our partners in passing on traditions to new generations. All hands on deck!

From a fighting stance, say left side forward, both hands being held approximately shoulder height, drop the lead hand down until it is approximately five or six inches above the lead knee (left; both hands in relaxed semi-cup form, the right palm facing inward, the left palm staying generally in front of the face, facing the same direction. The elbows of both arms are tight, close to each other in front of the centerline.

The function of this particular block is to guard the high gate and the low gate (face and groin) simultaneously.

When using this block and changing from one stance to another, it is very important that at no time do you open your centerline to attack.

This is accomplished by:

a)   Rolling the leading hand inward and upward to a middle or high position forearm block.

b)   Dropping the upper rear hand inward and upward to a low position block, palm facing outward.

(The intermediate position, while changing from one side to the other, keeps the elbows in and close, the centerline completely protected).

Striking Techniques: Kicks *("Chung Tao Tiip")*

1.   ***Back Leg Front Kick***
2.   ***The Arc Kick (Thai Style Round Kick)***
3.   ***The Cut Kick***
4.   ***"Tiip" (The Straight Kick)***
5.   ***Drop Spinning Sweep***
6.   ***Sliding Kick***
7.   ***Defensive Kicks***

#1: *Back Leg Front Kick ("Tiip")*

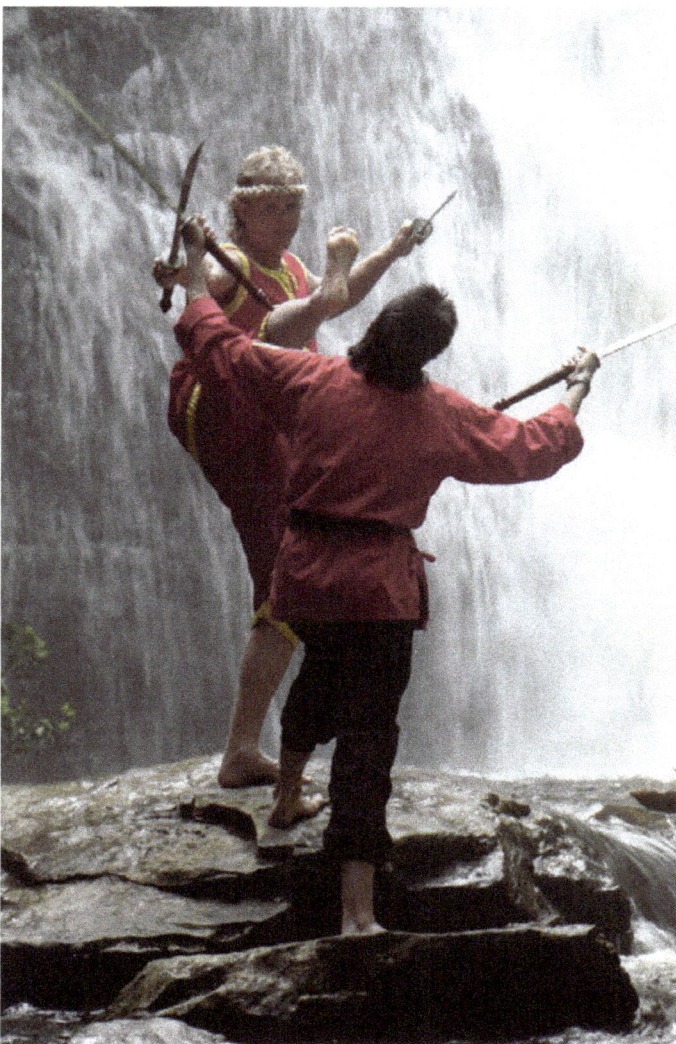

The Back Leg Front Kick develops its great power from a combination of accelerating levers, the hip and the knee, as well as the mass of the body moving behind the kick. The movement is a linear one directed toward the target.

From a fighting stance, left side forward, pivot on the ball of the left foot turning the heel of the foot inward. Bring the hips square as you draw the right leg directly up by the left to a forward position. As the right leg moves forward it almost brushes the supporting leg. With the leg cocked, continue to raise the knee high, even if the kick is to be a low one.

Push the heel or bottom of the foot straight into the target. Just before contact is made and continuing through the contact, thrust the hips forward strongly. Bring the leg back by pulling the hips rearward and drawing the knee back toward the chest. From this position an additional kick could be executed, if necessary.

As the kick develops, the right or rear shoulder comes to a forward position. At the time of contact, that hand becomes the leading or alive hand. On recovery, the hands also return to their original positions.

As time goes by and familiarity increases, you will be able to put more and more weight into the kick. By involving the whole body's mass, you generate more power.

#2: The Arc Kick ("*Manop Len Ka*", Thai Style Round Kick)

The basic foundation of Krabi Krabong and Muay Thai kicking (Thai Kickboxing) is the Arc Kick. The Arc Kick is a Round Kick type of motion. Most styles of Martial Arts have some variation or type of a Round Kick; however, none appear to have mastered this particular kick as well, or to have developed it to such a height of destructive capability. In fact, the Arc Kick appears to have become the trademark of the Thai Martial Arts. It is their single most readily recognized technique. This kick is quite capable of breaking bones or tearing and spraining muscles and ligaments when

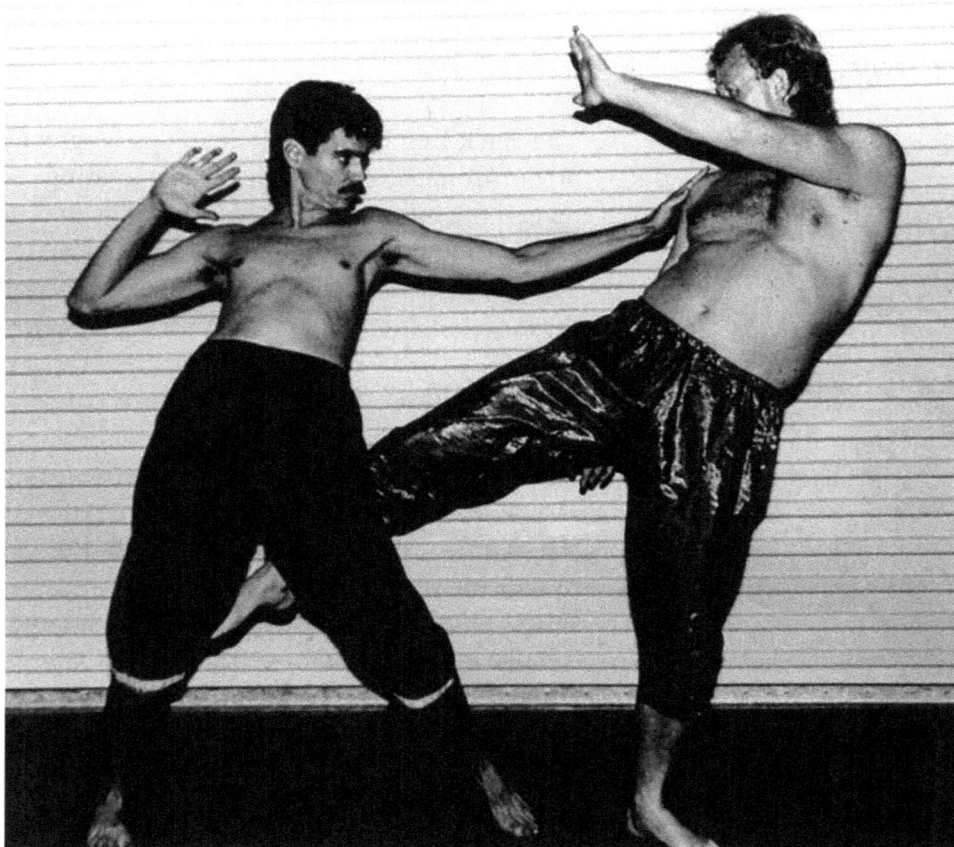

The difficult part is to kick every time as if it is the last kick you will ever throw! Even if you throw hundreds.

When properly executed, one of the most salient features of this particular kicking motion is its adaptability to changing ranges. It remains effective and dynamic from very close range to extreme long range.

If your opponent begins to back away from you as you kick, you can literally open up and chase him, stretching into the kick, still hitting with great power. If he closes in, you may hit with the middle and upper shin by keeping the knee well bent.

The Arc Kick is one of the most powerful kicking motions. Anyone who has had the fortune or maybe misfortune to hold a shield for a Thai Boxer can attest to this. The impact is incredible. Rather than knock you or push you away, there is just a tremendous teeth-rattling shock which appears to go right through you. In actual contest or combat applications, this kick is rarely intentionally blocked by the defender as often severe sprains or broken bones result.

The idea is to hit through the target area with the whole man behind it. The kick is executed from either leg, back or lead. The upper torso leads or initiates the movement followed by the forward or the inward motion of the hip and then the leg literally swings into the target.

There is no pivot, per se, but the supporting foot is allowed to drift or to turn with the kick, giving the necessary freedom of movement. Generally, the kick proceeds directly into the target. The weapon varies from a conditioned instep to the toughened shin.

As the foot leaves the ground, the knee is cocked slightly. Do not kick with the knee stiff or locked out. Just before impact there is or may be a snap added from the knee; however, it is not essential to a hard-hitting kick. Upon making contact, you sink into the target and let the leg drop to the ground in a controlled fashion. Some Round Kicking methods emphasize snapping the foot out after making contact; however, the Thais feel that this would take something out of the kick.

It is possible to throw many of these kicks in quick succession, four, five, or even more. The following kick is thrown from where the foot lands with no further preparation. To help visualize the type of impact involved here, think about a sock filled with sand and swung into the target. There is a definite sense of sinking into the target. As the kick comes into contact with the target, the foot is flexed at the ankle with the toes pointed. If the foot is not flexed, there is a possibility of injury. The foot may twist or snap at the ankle causing a sprain. Also, as this kick is often targeted into the mid-section, you might encounter a shin or an elbow.

Initially, train by executing light and easy air kicks, not hitting too hard. Work on simply swinging the leg forward. Avoid any intentional pivoting of or on the front foot. Shift the body weight and swing. Go well- past the point where you would normally contact the target. Practice hitting through the target. Relax! Keep the elbows down and the hands high, especially the opposite hand from the kicking leg. For example: if you kick with the right leg, hold the left hand high to protect the face.

Have a sense of keeping on the balls of the feet. Before initiation there should be a certain springiness in the stance. Many Muay Thai/ Muay Boran instructors, such as GM Phaa Kruu Samaii Mesamarn, stress the importance of being lively in your attitude, light on your toes, not flat-footed and sedentary.

Do not lean when kicking even if the target is very high. Leaning is a way of cheating on your natural range of motion. It also slows down the introduction of the hands and recovery in general. In many cases, an elbow technique follows the Arc Kick; it becomes more apparent why the torso should be more upright.

This uprightness provides a centralized base from which to work from whether the intention is to throw or to deliver several Arc Kicks in quick succession or some type of combination attack using the hands and the feet.

Thai fighters stretch regularly to improve and to augment natural flexibility. Another way they develop the effective targeting range of this kick is to drill and practice it with an almost maniacal persistence. It is very common for a Muay Thai practitioner to drill on the Arc Kick alone for several hours a day, five or six days a week. Aside from just having a technical competency, this type of drilling leads to a familiarity and expertise seldom experienced.

The philosophy of Muay Thai is not so much to develop a variety of different techniques as it is to take one or two practical and sound ones and bring their execution to the highest possible state.

Once you have developed a fluid delivery in Arc kicking, practice on shields, or air bags, or whatever light hand-held pads that may be available. Keep your kicks initially in the low (thigh) to mid-range. This type of practice is good because it allows you to develop a sense of range and timing while developing the technique.

Also, it is perfectly important to condition the body, especially the legs, knees, shins, and the ankles progressively to the impact. It is no good to be able to do the kick essentially correctly, but to in the process sprain the ankle or damage your knee when you hit. It takes time for muscles, ligaments, and tendons to condition and to become durable enough to withstand sustained hitting with this kind of kick. This is not even in the same world with what it takes on the receiving end!

Next, proceed to the heavy bag. Again, it is important to remember to go light and easy. Keep the hands high and stay light on the toes. Do not blast the bag. If you work up to it gradually, you will eventually be able.to throw a kick which will fold a one-hundred-pound bag in half! Work on developing a good rhythm on the bag, hitting it on the return swing. Be sure to always work both sides of the body equally. Try not to go too fast as speed will come as your familiarity increases.

There are basically four angles in Krabi Krabong in the delivery of the Arc Kick:

> **1)** Low Rising
> **2)** Straight or mid-level
> **3)** High Falling
> **4)** Low level

In example 1), the foot or shin's trajectory is directed to a medium height or higher angle on a rising diagonal line into the target. This allows the kick to get under the defending elbow position to land effectively. We are keen to avoid the point of the defensive elbow as if improperly impacted it can break bones.

In example 2), the weapon (foot or shin) is laying into the target area on a perfectly even or level plane. This is the workhorse of Thai kicking, generally thrown to the head.

In example 3) is used with a chopping motion. The high falling kick begins by going to a high position and then dropping downward into the target area. Many times, this kick is aimed at the opponent's supporting leg in order to knock it out from under him. When used in this fashion, it is called a "cut kick."

The final variation, example 4), is a straight kick starting low and ending low.

This kick is usually aimed at the calf region or to the ankle of the opponent. It may sweep or simply create a "Charlie Horse"- type severe and debilitating cramp in the leg making it difficult for the opponent to maneuver effectively.

#3: The Art Of The Cut Kick

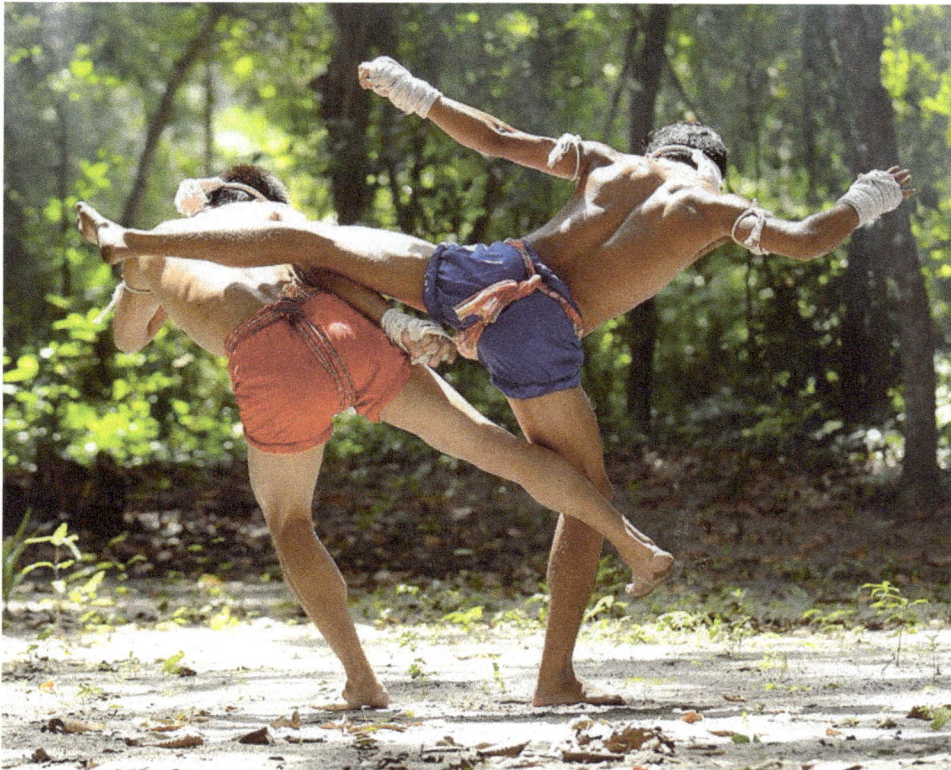

Essentially, the Cut Kick is an Arc Kick or knee attack; however, it is used in a very specific fashion. It is in line with the Krabi Krabong/ Muay Boran philosophy to "destroy the foundation," which in this case refers to the supporting leg. Many times, instead of blocking or checking an attack, the defender simply goes right in and cuts his opponent down with a Cut Kick.

Technically, the kick is very simple. As the opponent begins his attack and has one foot off the ground, bang the supporting leg with an Arc Kick or knee attack. The attack, or counter if you will, may be anywhere on the supporting leg as long as it is thrown wholeheartedly. The counter is thrown under the attacking kick or in front of it. It may go to the inside of the defender's leg or to the outside. This is a devastating counter — it removes the stable base the opponent is using to launch his attack from and is a uniquely Thai concept. This works well with the sword as it leaves the hands free.

There are several variations and uses of the "Cut Kick".

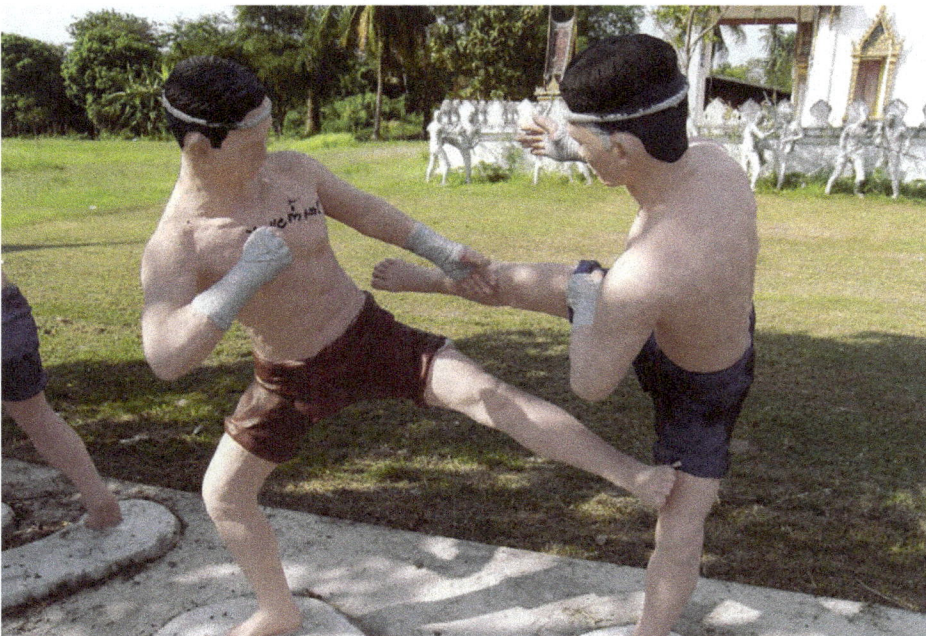

A variation is based more on timing. The opponent attacks with a Forward or Knee with a step in, backleg or slide up motion. You block, check or destroy the Knee Attack with your front Elbow… As the opponent places the attacking leg down on the ground, you pivot sharply into them hitting the not quite settled landing leg with a hard Inside Cut Kick to the medial lower leg (inside Shin)… this knocks that leg out and or causes the opponent to stagger, creating an opening to exploit.

#4: "Tiip" (The Straight or Front Leg Push Kick)

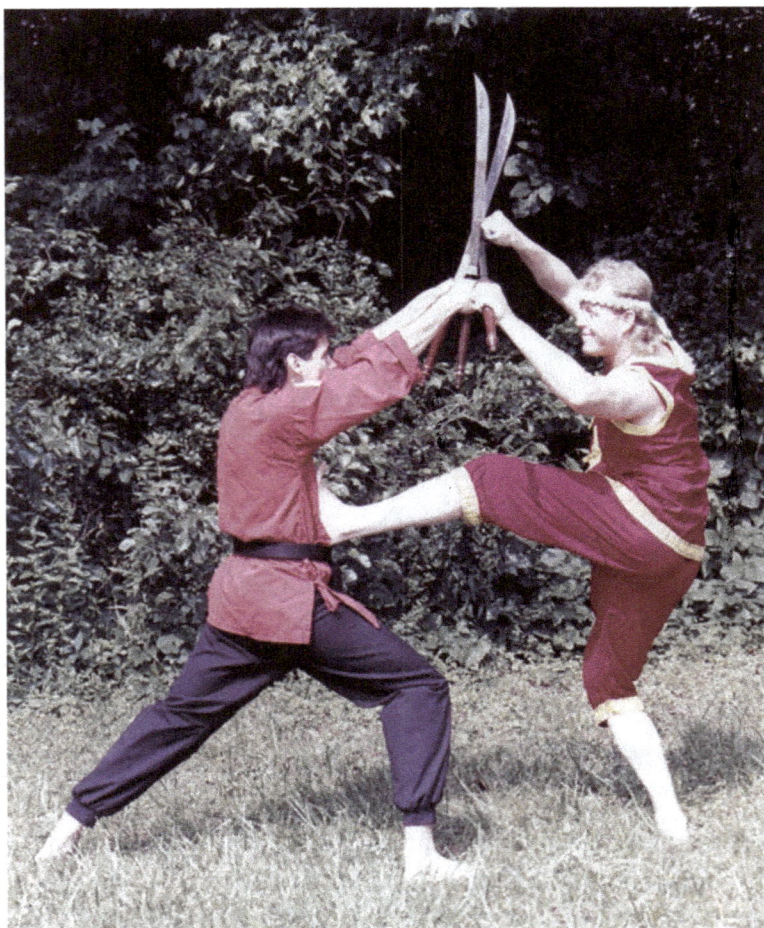

This technique can be used with bare hands and or with virtually any weapon, swords, staff, spear, knife etc. Used to stop or create space. Perfect for decisively interferring with the opponants charge or aggressive forward movement.

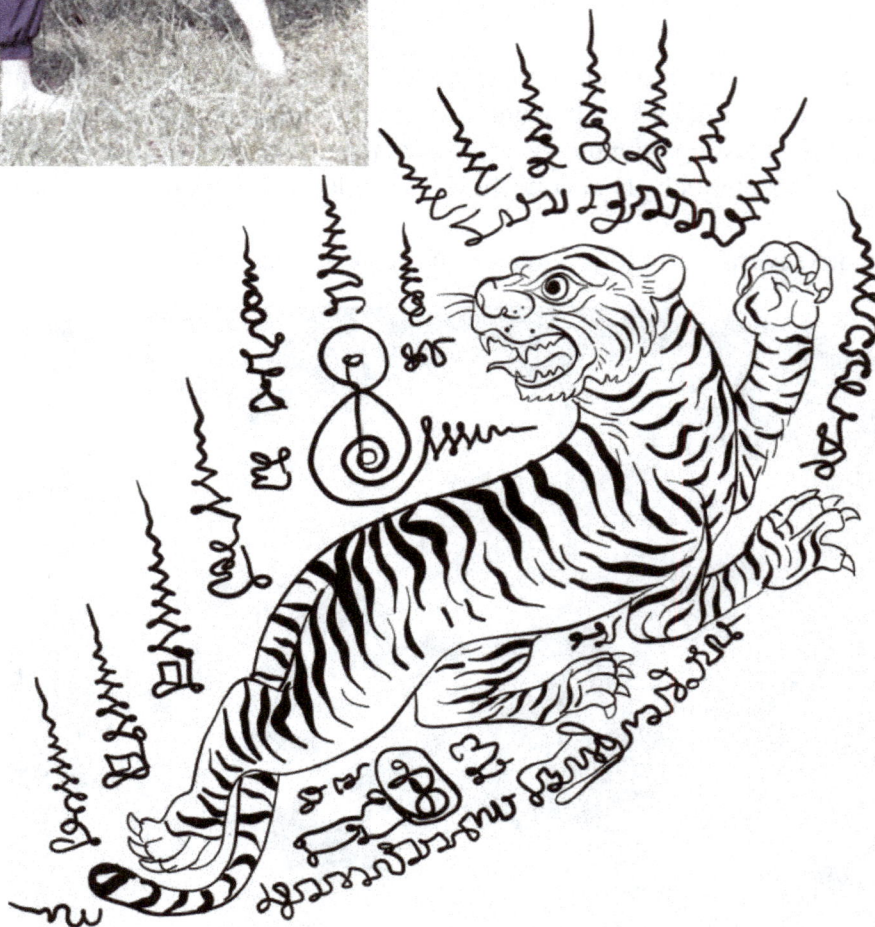

#5: Drop Spinning Sweep

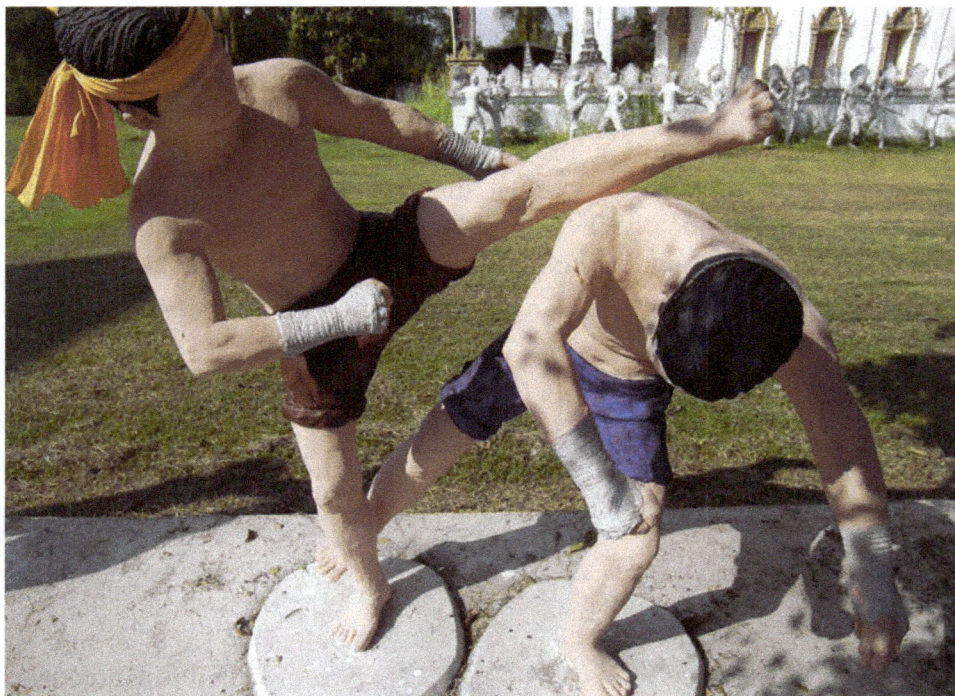

PLEASE NOTE: Risky! Timing is everything! This technique may be used against kicks which are waist high or above.

Kicks which are overly committed or those which are unintentionally slow in developing.

The Drop Spinning Sweep may also be used against various long- hand techniques. It is important to keep the guard up in front of the face as you drop and turn as your face is waist level or lower and especially vulnerable. This sweep is generally executed against the back side of the opponent's leg," however, with good placement and timing it may be successful to the front as well.

Break Down: First, on count one, pivot the lead heel as far forward as you can and kneel, turning the back toward the opponent. Second, turn around and face the opponent. Third, whip the rear leg around in the sweep while resting on the bent knee. Use a swing kick type of motion to kick through the opponent's position. The sweeping leg should just graze the ground.

The Drop Spinning Sweep may also be used more offensively by hitting the back of the opponent's ankle or calf. Done properly you will knock that leg out and up. I've seen fighters turn the opponant upside down by hitting with this tricky kick. It is always about timing and opportunity and it is a big gamble.

As the opponent falls, follow through with the sweep and either rise to the feet and counter or counter on the ground.

The foot is bladed in the side/swing-kick type of weapon. Depending on the range, you may strike with the whole leg from the heel to the hip area.

When practicing, drop and execute a 360-degree spin and recover smartly to your feet in a fighting stance. Drill or practice "squat rotations" backwards and forwards as a great way to condition for Spinning Sweeps.

#6: Sliding Kicks

Sliding kicks represent more advanced kicking techniques than slide-up kicking methods for the following reasons. One entire step in the kicking process is eliminated. An example would be in a slide-up motion, the rear foot is brought up to the front, the front foot is raised to ready position, and then the kick is executed. In a sliding-type kicking motion, the kick is executed while the rear or supporting leg is brought up. Because of this combined movement, the kick takes less time to perform, and there is less tendency to telegraph the move. Ideally, the kick should land as the supporting leg finds its balance point. Possible variations are numerous and include Sliding Side, Sliding Front, and Sliding Round kicks.

#7: DEFENSIVE KICKS (*"Bud Tawan"*)

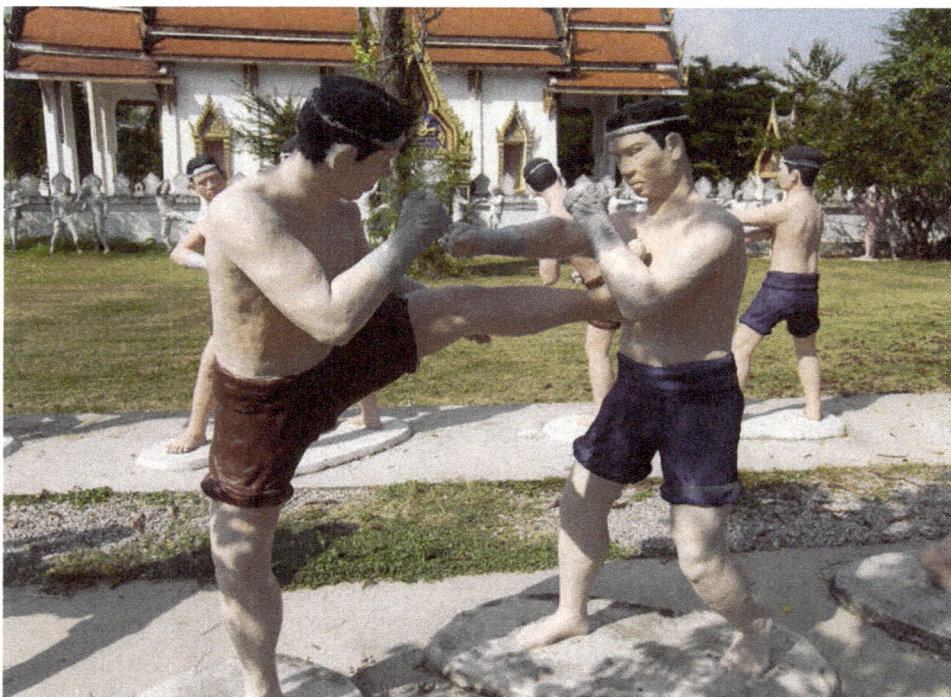

"Bud Tawan" or Open The Door! By definition, a "Defensive Kick" is any type of kick thrown or executed with the leading or front leg (without a step). The main advantage in using a Defensive or Front Leg Kick as opposed to any other type of kick is that a kick thrown with the front leg takes less time to perform. The reason for this is obvious. The technique will reach the target faster because it requires little preparation, and the front foot is closer initially to the target.

The kick itself presents a huge and formidable barrier when properly used. It is off putting and hard to get around when used skillfully.

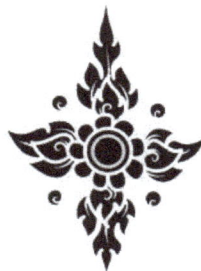

Defensive kicking technique is characterized by the following traits:

1.   The kick is executed with a minimum of preparation.
2.   Balance remains essentially neutral throughout the execution. It is not necessary to lean either to the front or the back to perform the kick.
3.   Defensive kicks are "fast" kicks because they are done without committing the body.
4.   They generally travel directly to the target with a minimum of unnecessary travel.
5.   Executed with a "snap", simplest and most direct delivery possible.

As far as actually doing a defensive kick is concerned, you should keep the aforementioned four points in mind and also these:

1. **Know the kick**. (You must practice the individual technique until it is natural).

2. **Relax for Speed**. (Universal rule: the more you relax, the faster you move, the faster you move, the harder you hit).

3. **Simply throw the technique**. (Do not be overly concerned with the stance, etc.).

4. Be prepared for the opening that a well-timed (see times to attack) Defensive Kick will create.

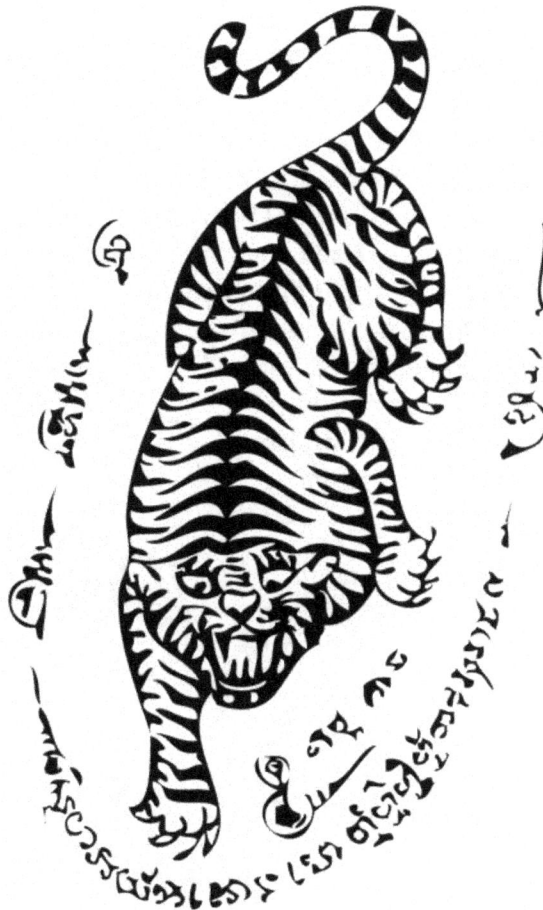

Thai Knee Attacks

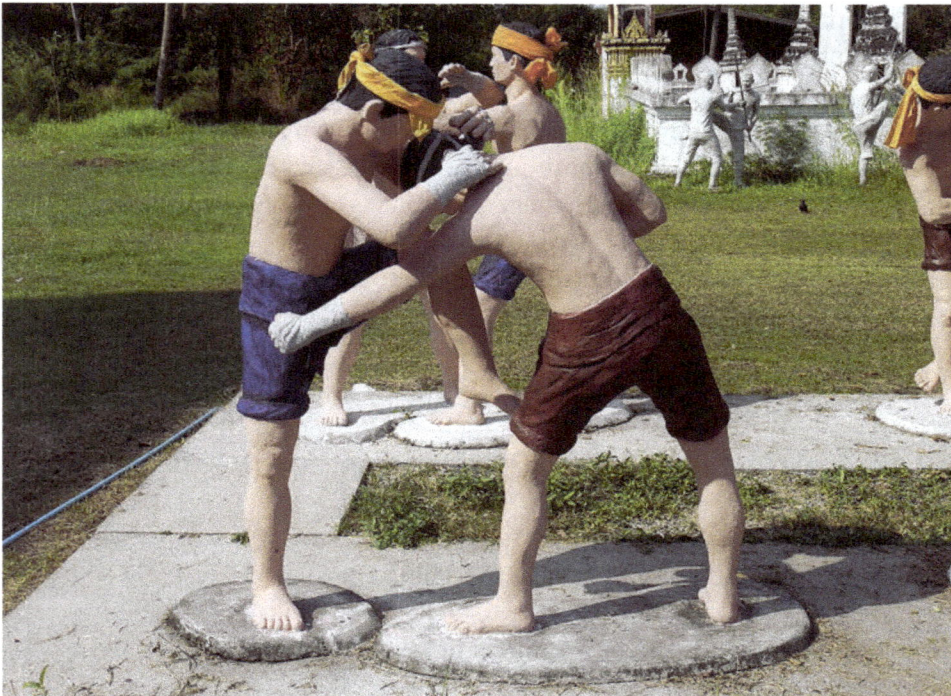

Wat Bang Kung Muay Boran-Muay Chaiya ststues illustrate in lifesize details. Photo's from Wat Bang Kung temple, Amperwa District are from the authors personal photo collections.

There are no less than nine major variations of knee attacks:

1) *"Kheun Kao"*/ Defensive Knee (Rising Front Knee).
2) *"Kheun Kao"*/ Full Rising Knee (Back Leg Rising).
3) *"Kao Drong"*/ Defensive Forward Knee (Forward Thrusting Knee) .
4) *"Kao Drong"*/ Full Direct Knee (Back Leg Thrusting).
5) *"Sawing Kao"*/ Swing Knee (Upward and Outward).
6) *"Wang Kao"*/ Arcing Knee (Upward and Inward).
7) *"Dtai Kao"*/ Angle Knee (From the Side).
8) *"Kradot Kao"*/ The King's Knee (Flying).
9) *"Narasuan Kao"*/ Monkey Knee (Climbing)
10) Side Shin Defense (Outside Shin Block)
11) *"Book"*/ Inward Shin Block

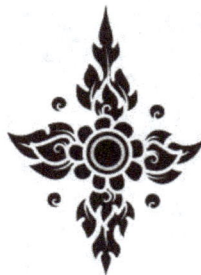

1) *"Kheun Kao"* (The Full Rising Knee) **The Defensive Knee**

Consider this technique from both the perspectives of as an empty hand technique and as appropriate while holding one or two swords or other weapons such as the *"MaeSowk"*.

The Front Leg, Defensive Knee, or the Rising Knee, is ideally suited as a tool to use in "close-in" fighting. At the grappling range, it is devastating. This knee technique or concept is the natural complement of most elbow actions. Requiring little in the way of preparation, it may be thrown at the last minute and can be quite hard to follow. The damage incurred from a well-placed knee is all out of proportion to the real effort and time it takes to do one. At the grappling range, it may be thrown repeatedly with little or no visible loss of power. When we say, "destroy the base," this is the kind of concept envisioned. Not only is the Defensive Knee a weapon of attack; it is also a great and versatile defensive tool.

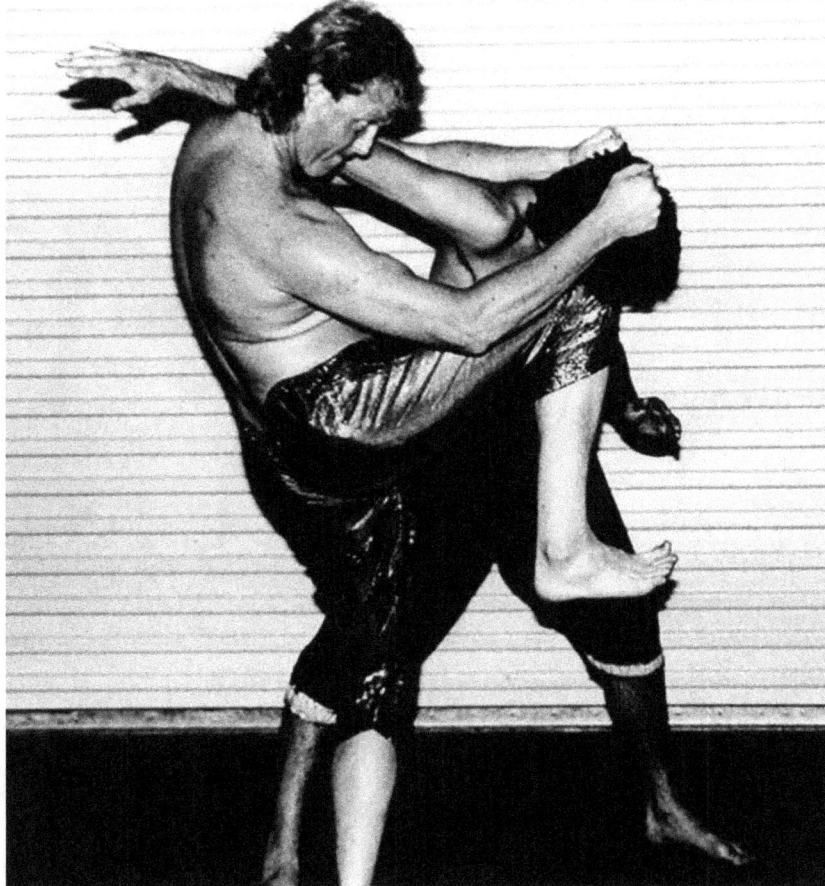

When used in a blocking or checking fashion, it allows you to intercept the opponent's attack while maintaining your own position. Certainly, one of the most powerful applications and used as a quick finishing technique.

Whether receiving a kick or a hand attack, you can leave both hands free and unencumbered. Used in this fashion, the knee takes on the characteristics of a shield.

With the guard extended and the elbows close in, snap the front knee upward as high as you can.

Remember that "front" means "between." Make sure the legs are well bent and the weight is on the balls of the feet before you go.' As the knee approaches chest height, spring upward with the supporting leg giving additional momentum and drive to the kick. Allow yourself to come all the way up onto your toes.

As the kick reaches its highest point, bring the elbows downward and inward. With the hands held high it should be easy to touch the top of the knee with the rear hand. In drilling, simulate hooking the hands behind the opponent's neck and jerking his head inward and downward, smashing the head right onto the rising top of the knee. This practice actually compounds the impact of the knee as it crashes into its target area, whether the target is the head, torso, or whatever.

Drop the knee and land lightly on the balls of the feet while re-extending your guard. As the lead foot touches the ground, be ready to immediately return with another one. To return, pull and spring into the next knee strike. It is incredible the amount of damage this can do. It is related to the shortened lever and the heavy, concentrated massof the upper leg when the knee is well bent. Drive upward through the opponant. Aim for the sky!

Please note: The Full Rising Knee Attack can be used with almost any weapon. For example instead of using the hands to pull the opponant into the knee? Use the handles of the Deo- Sword/ swords, Mai Sok, Stick, knife or pole arm to hook and control the opponant. This will be true of all hand and or foot techniques.

2) *"Kheun Kao"* (Back Leg Full Rising Knee)

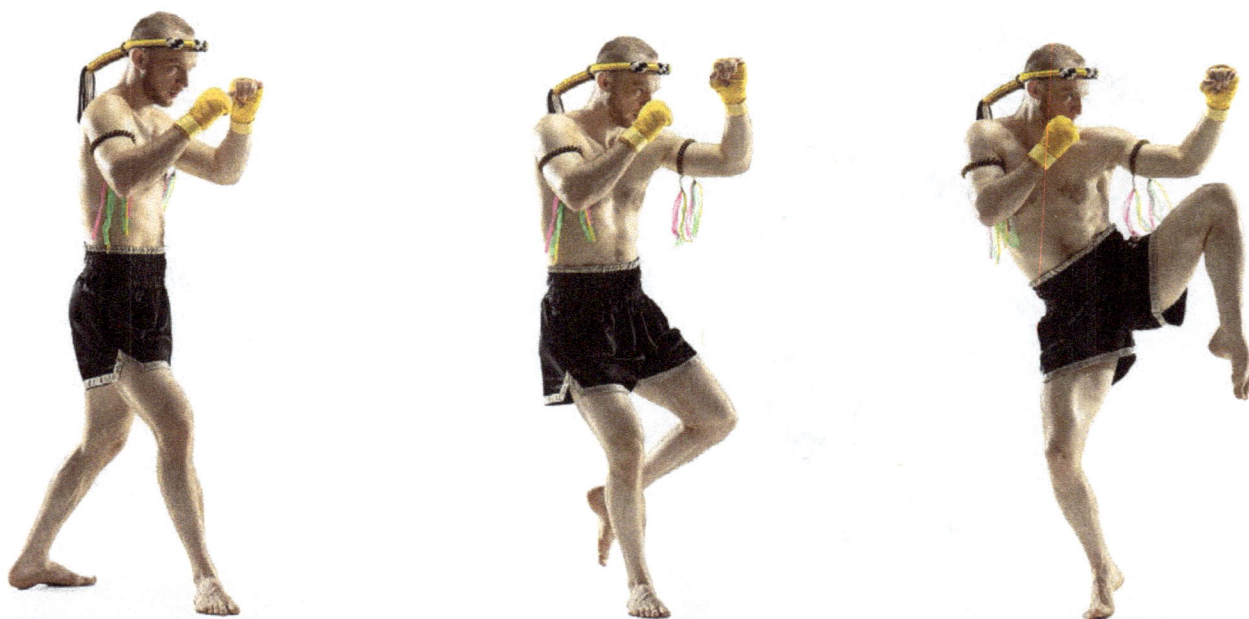

A small step is made forward with the front foot. After this step, the rear or back leg is brought forward and upward. The leg is cocked tightly to reinforce the knee joint and to protect the groin. As the first step is made, the hands are stretched toward the opponent, grasping him tightly. The opponent is jerked roughly into his face, chest, or ribs. Usually once the Full Rising Knee lands, a series of Defensive Knees or Forward Knees are thrown to continue the attack. Remember to spring from the toes at the moment before impact.

3) "*Kao Drong*" (Defensive Forward Thrusting Knee)

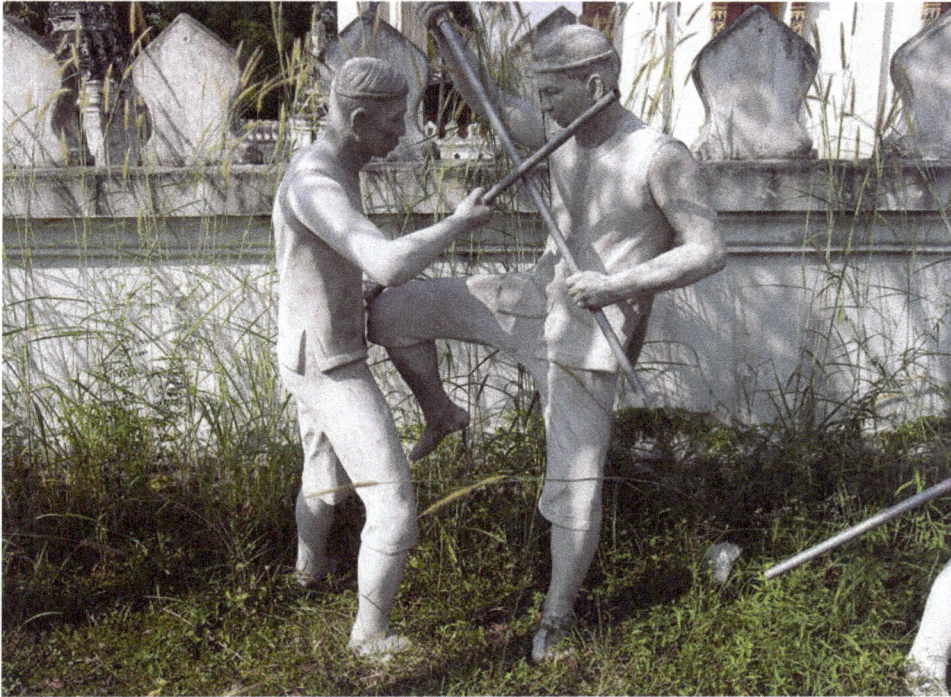

"Kao Drong", Defensive Forward Thrusting Knee with Plong vs. Plong

The "*Kao Drong*" Defensive Forward Thrusting Knee is a close-range fighting technique and is based on the basic Defensive Knee. Just as its name implies, it is thrown with a forward thrusting movement. This is to allow a greater forward or horizontal penetration. It may also allow for the rearward movement from the waist or hips of an opponent who is trying to get away.

With the guard extended, and the elbows close in, snap the front knee up and forward as you push off the rear leg and thrust forward from the hips as far as you can go. The knee rises up to about waist height as it moves forward.

When drilling, simulate grabbing and pulling or holding the opponent as close to you as you can. Use the "*Jut Sao*" or jerking type of movement.

Drop the knee and land lightly forward. Either slide the rear foot up or step back to recover.

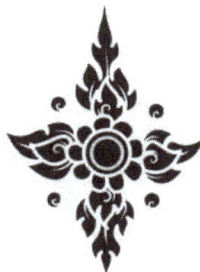

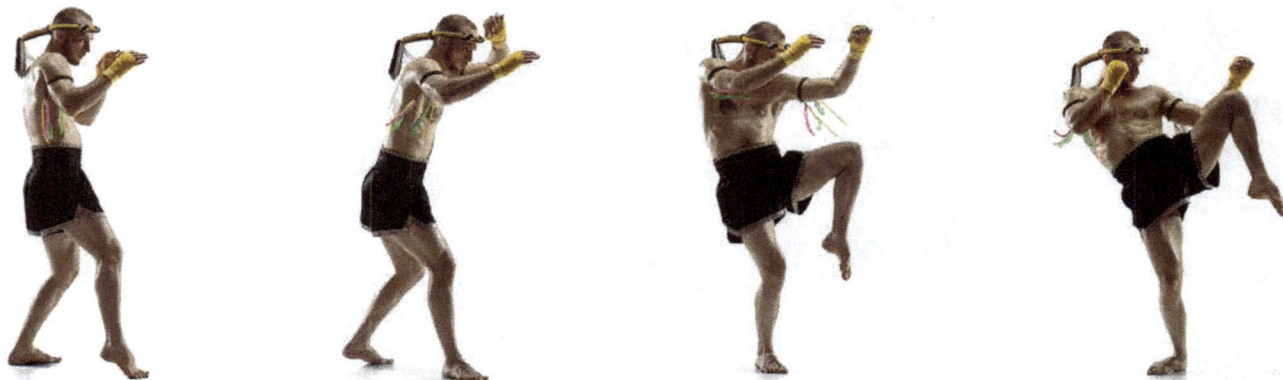

4) "*Kao Drong*" (Variation: The Full Direct Knee)

This knee begins in a similar fashion to the Full Rising Knee; that is, with a small step forward and the back leg moving through to the front. However, now instead of striking upward, the knee is thrust forward from the hips and pushed directly into the opponent as far as possible. The upper body leans back slightly to avoid the elbow counter, and the hands are stretched out forward ready to grab or punch. Think "stabbing" or driving through the target as opposed to "lifting" into the target. This is a big attack.

5) "*Sawing Kao*" (The Swing Knee)(Upward and Outward)

Very useful for when the opponant is situated more to your side or beside you and close. The Swing Knee moves in an upward and outward arc away from the body. This knee attack or technique may be performed with either the front or the rear leg. This knee technique is often desirable when the opponent is off centered or to the side of your body position. Begin by grappling the opponent's upper arm or shoulder, and then snap the knee up, outward and into the opponent's body or head, while at the same time pulling him forward into the knee. Arch the back as you pull and really stretch.

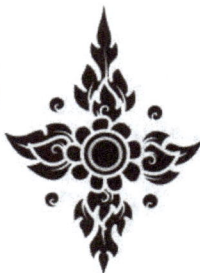

6) *"Wang Kao"* (The Arcing Knee) (Upward and Inward)

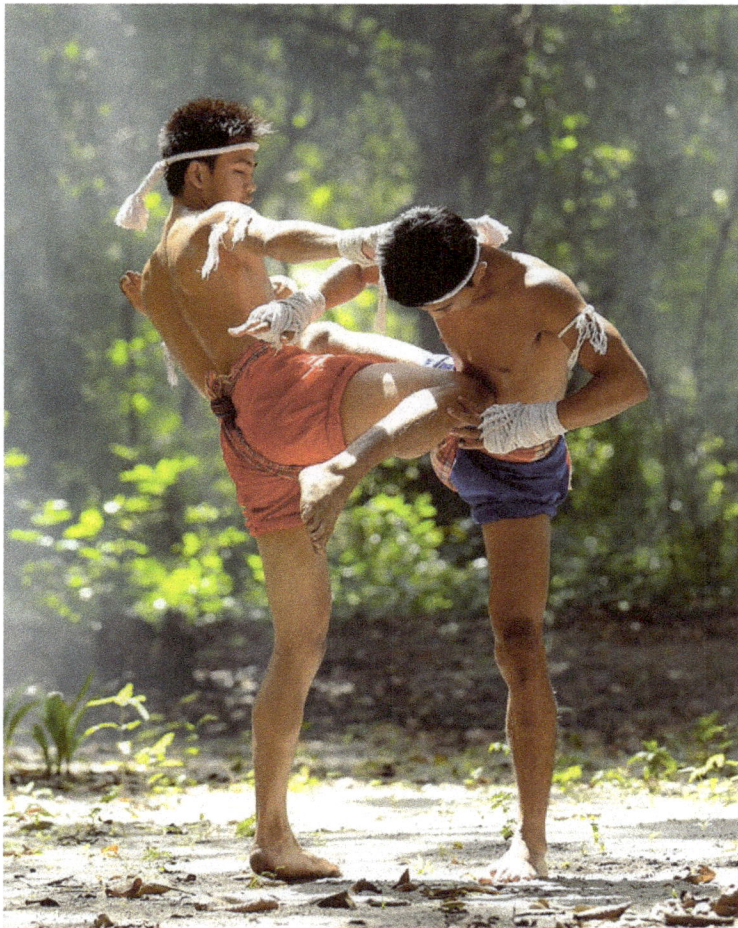

The Arcing Knee drives directly on a rising diagonal angle into the ribs or lower body, hips, or thighs of the opponent. It rises upward at about a 45-degree angle off either the front or back leg.

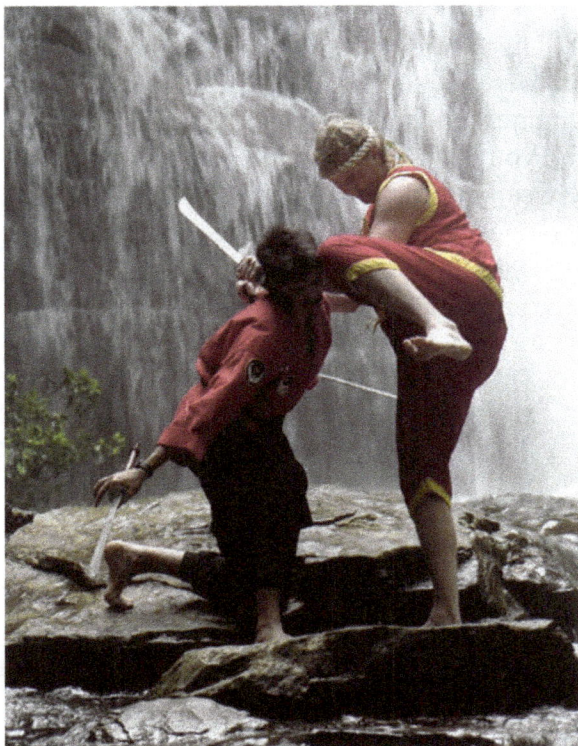

This knee is also used against the arms and head if they are brought low enough. For example when you hook the back of the opponents neck with your swords handles to jerk the head downward into the Arcing Knee.

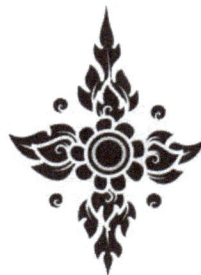

7) "Dtoi Kao", *"Takang Kao Yok Nang"*
(The Angle Or Side Knee- From the Side)

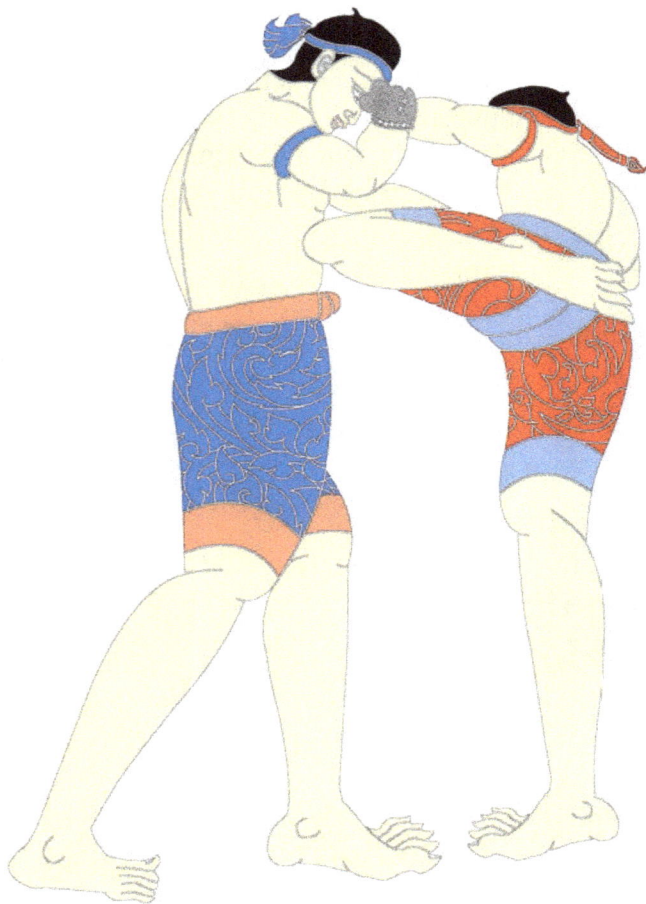

The Angle Knee is different from most of the other knee techniques in that you do not necessarily hit at the peak of height nor use the top or front of the knee. Rather, you get the knee to the height at which you wish to use it and slam it sideways into your target. The weapon is the inside (medial) of the knee joint. This knee is well suited to close quarter and grappling range, even when you're so close you hug your opponent. Simply snap up either knee to the outside and whip it inward. This knee is even done over the shoulder and into the head.

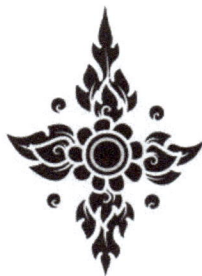

8) "Kradot Ka" ("The King's Ka" - Flying Knee)

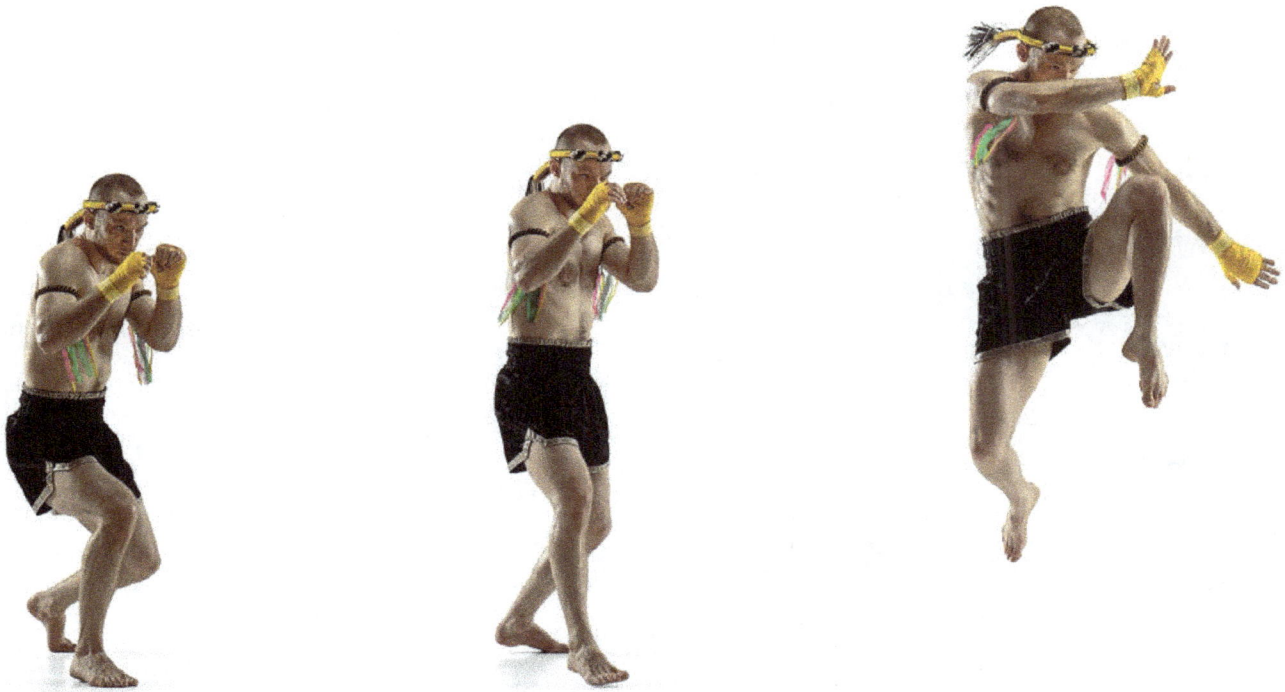

This knee was named after King Narasuan. Before becoming King, Narasuan was known as the Black Prince. He was famous as a boxer who had traveled widely and one of his most well- known techniques was the "Flying Knee". This technique is very aggressive and must be well timed to be effective.

Begin with a small step of the front foot and take off leaping with the rear knee at the opponent. The hips are pushed forward to get the maximum extension and thrusting power. The target is the chest or head of the opponent.

In Thai period docu-drama type movies such as in the "*Ong Bak*" trilogy starring actor Tony Jai, he is often depicted performing these types of the more spectacular "flying" and or "climbing" Muay Boran techniques. For kicks and giggles and some fair representation of both traditional Krabi Krabong, Wai Khru and Muay Boran, I recommend these movies.

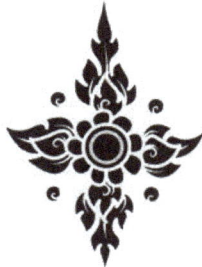

9) "*Narasuan Ka*" (The Black Prince Monkey Knee- Monkey Climbing Knee)

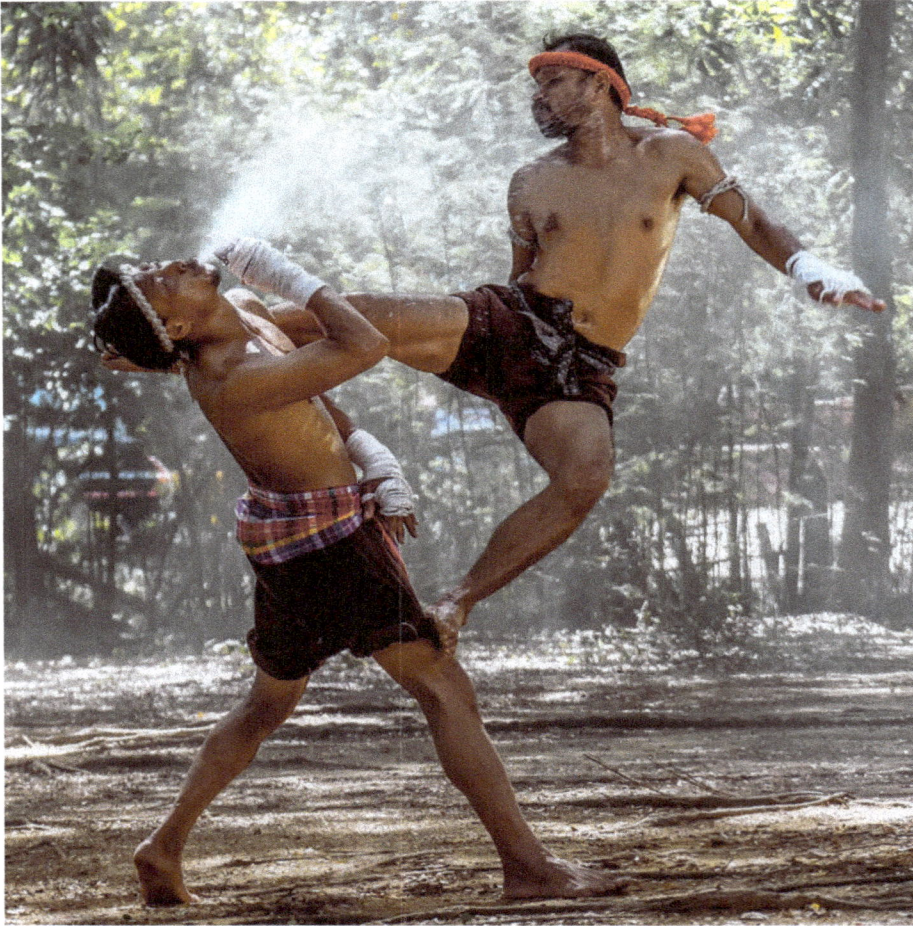

This knee is another famous technique of King Narasuan. In the Monkey Climbing Knee you climb your unwary opponent like a monkey climbs a fruit tree.

The Monkey Climbing Knee was used in open warfare when the attacker had to not only defeat his opponent but needed to continue forward rapidly. He literally climbed up and over his opponent.

Begin as always from the basic position and take a small step forward with the front foot. With a running type of motion, leap at your opponent placing your rear foot firmly on top of his front thigh. Get as close to the hip as possible. Make sure the foot being placed is turned with the toes pointed outward.

Without losing momentum, climb up the opponent's leg while hooking your swords or hands behind his neck. Just as if you were going to climb another step, bring the back knee crashing into the opponent's head. He will likely collapse totally while you land on your feet and continue forward. The hands may or may not be holding various weapons. If all you do is pile drive the opponent backwards to the ground as you crash climb him? Then follow to ground and finnish or keep going on to the next fighter... up to you.

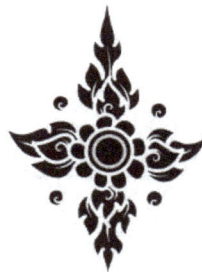

10) Side Shin Defense (Outside Shin Block)

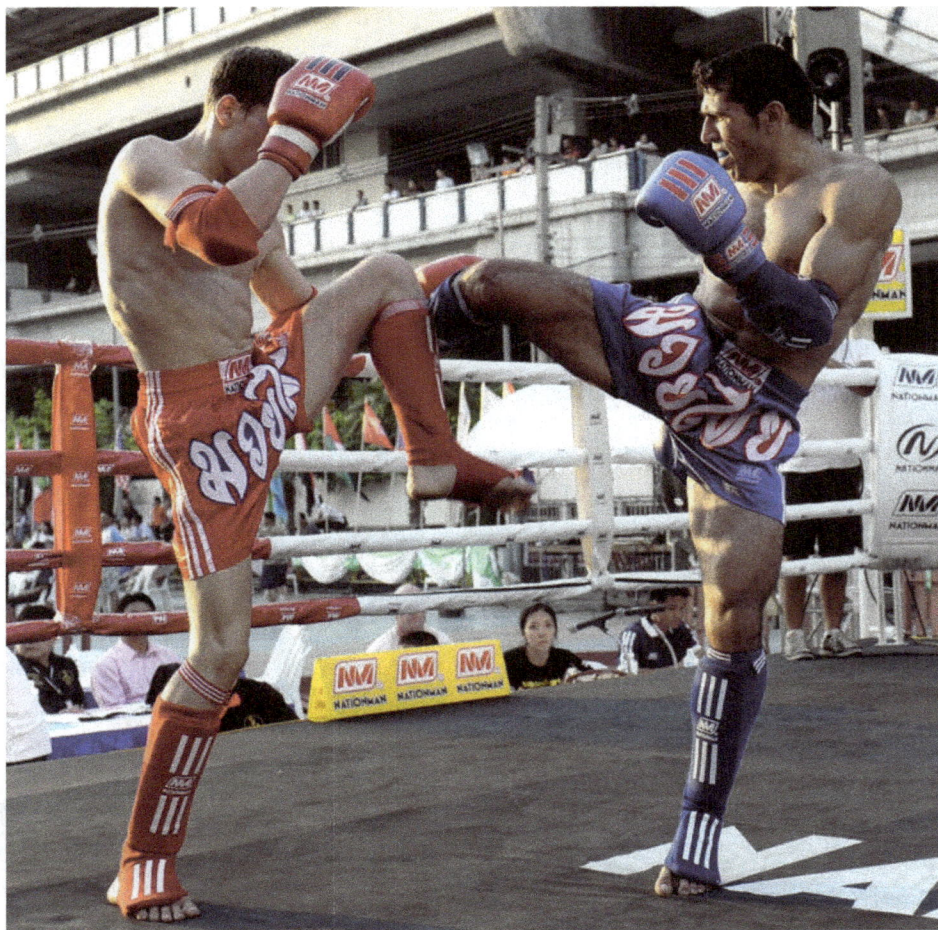

As the opponent attacks with an Arc Kick or knee attack, pick the knee up and catch the kick along the outside of the shin. Cock the lower leg inward tightly to flex the calf and support the shin. Try to disperse the impact of the kick along the upper thigh even to the buttocks.

This block is used for attacks from thigh to shoulder height. It is preferred to blocking with the hands, which are fragile.

Begin with a small step of the front foot and take off leaping with the rear knee at the opponent. The hips are pushed forward to get the maximum extension and thrusting power. The target is the chest or head of the opponent.

Eleven) "*BOOK*" (Inward Shin Block)

This block is only available to Krabi Krabong or Muay Thai people who condition their shins as you cut into the attacking leg or shin head-on with your front shin.

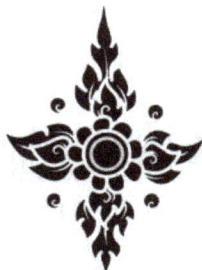

"*Ao Sok*" (Elbow Technique)

1. "*Sok Trong*" - Horizontal Elbow
2. "*Sok Kun*" - Rising Elbow
3. "*Sok Lon*" - Descending Elbow
4. "*Sok Won*" - Spinning Elbow
5. "*Sok Bin*" - Flying Elbow
6. "*Hong Peek Hak*" Broken Birds WIng

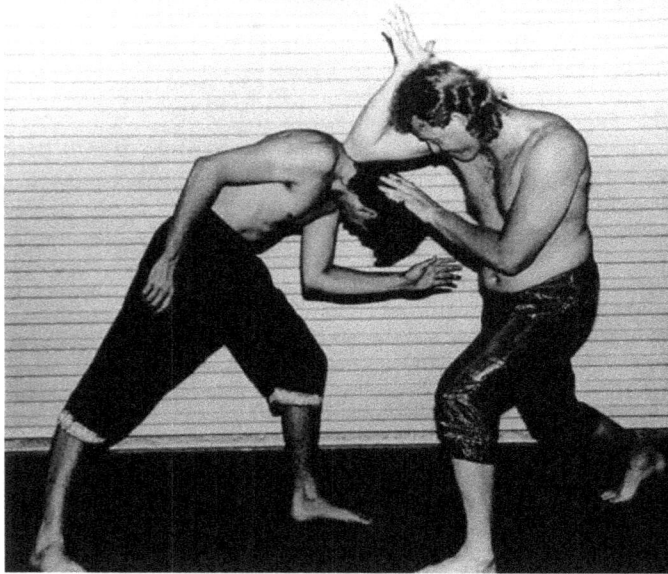

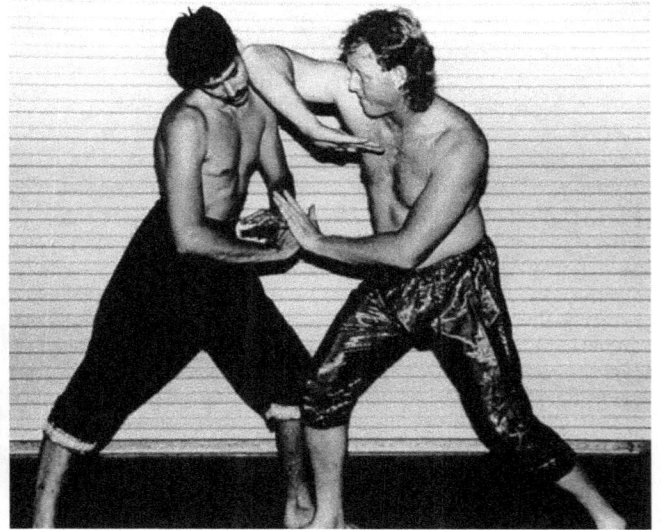

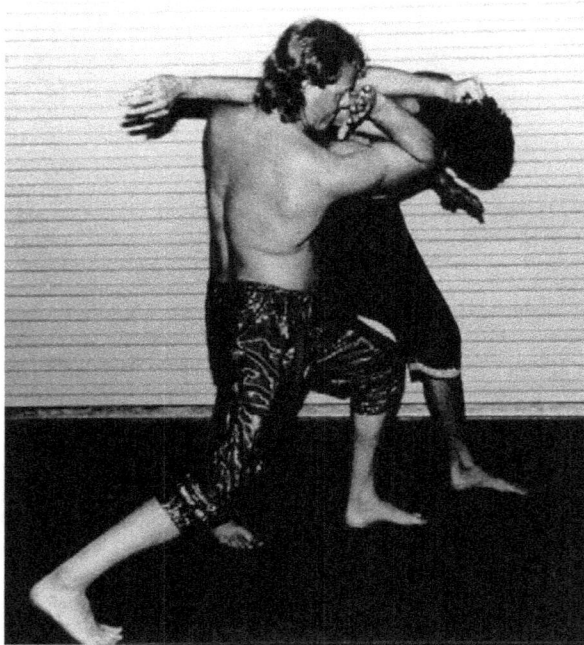

The elbow is as versatile and devastating a weapon as the hands and feet. It is used in a variety of ways and at varying ranges.

The elbow is well suited to the total commitment philosophy of Krabi Krabong. There are at least eight major types of Thai elbow strikes.

What is unfamiliar to many people is that the origin of the style of elbow techniques may be derived from a weapon.

That weapon is the "*My Sok*", which literally means first and elbow shield. The "*My Sok*", is a strong, fairly light shield running from just in front of the hand- fist to just in back of the elbow. The hand holds a forward grip, and the elbow end is secured by thong or rope. The "*My Sok*", were used singly and in pairs. When used in an individual fashion they were in conjunction with lance or sword. When used in pairs they were used in a sort of boxing attitude.

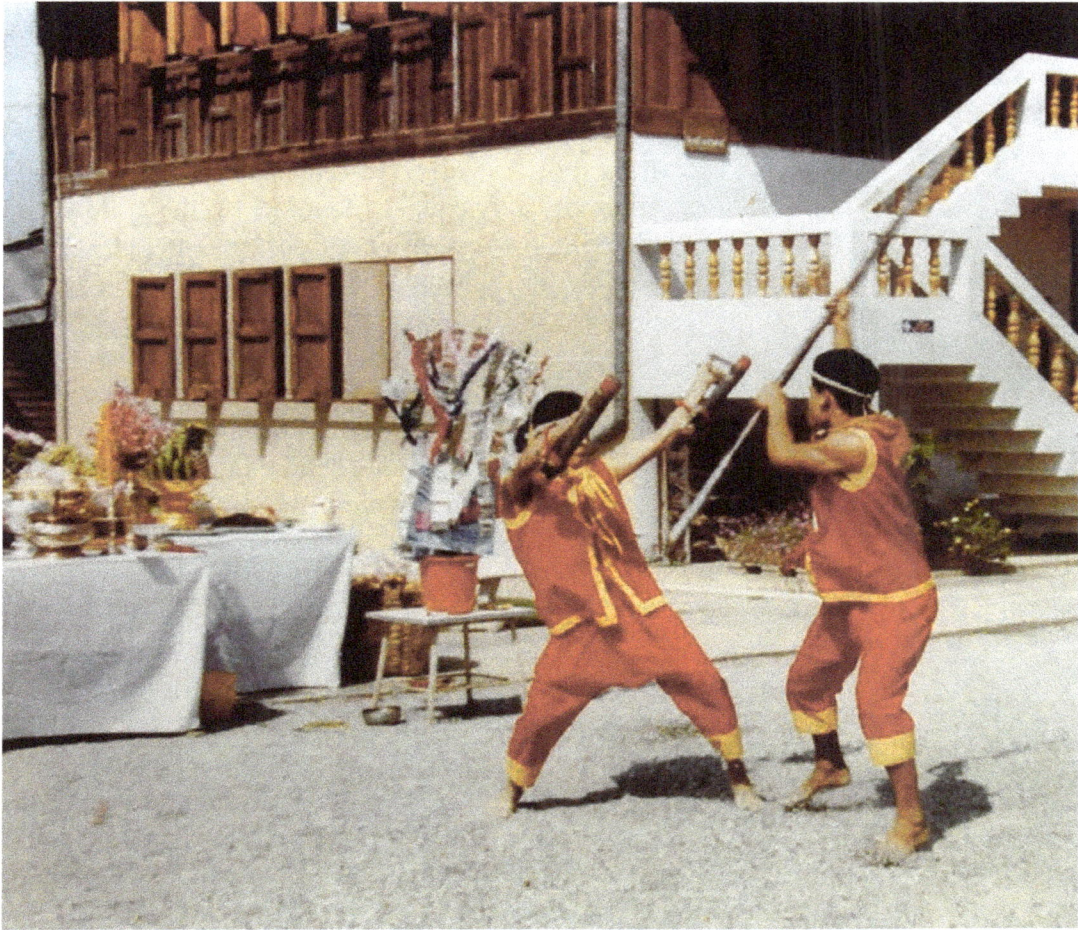

Mae Sawk vs. Plong

This boxing attitude is likely the forerunner of modern empty-hand Thai Boxing.

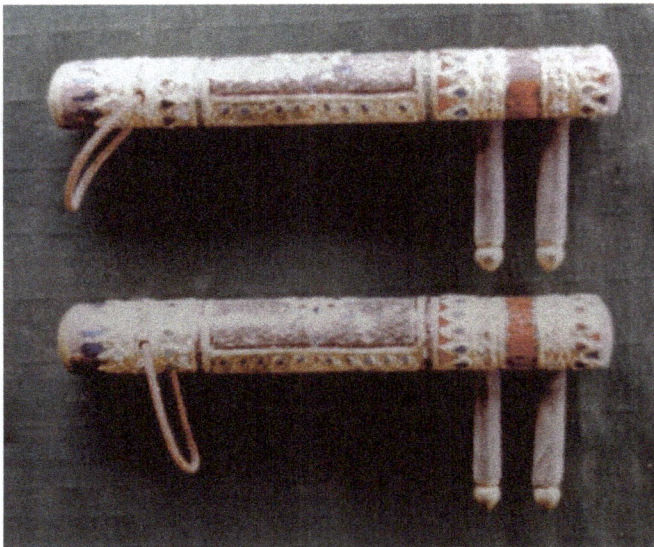

Old ornate "*Mae Sowk*" from Phaa Khruu's Buddhai Sawan collection.

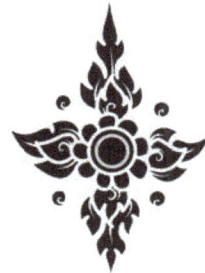

1) "Sok Trong" (Horizontal Elbow)

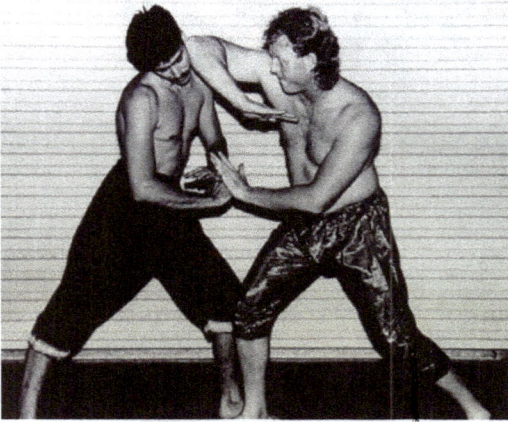

A)   Inward. Lead with a small step forward from the front foot. As you do this, raise the rear elbow to a height approximately equal to shoulder or higher. Make a clearing or blocking motion with the front hand and push the rear elbow straight through and hook across at the last moment. Pivot on the balls of the feet as you spring forward. Allow the rear foot to move forward to balance at the end of the strike. To strike with the lead or front elbow. Keep the hand centered while sharply raising the front elbow out to the side at 90 degrees, pointing the palm of the hand on the same arm towards the opponent, and then whip it sharply inward to strike.

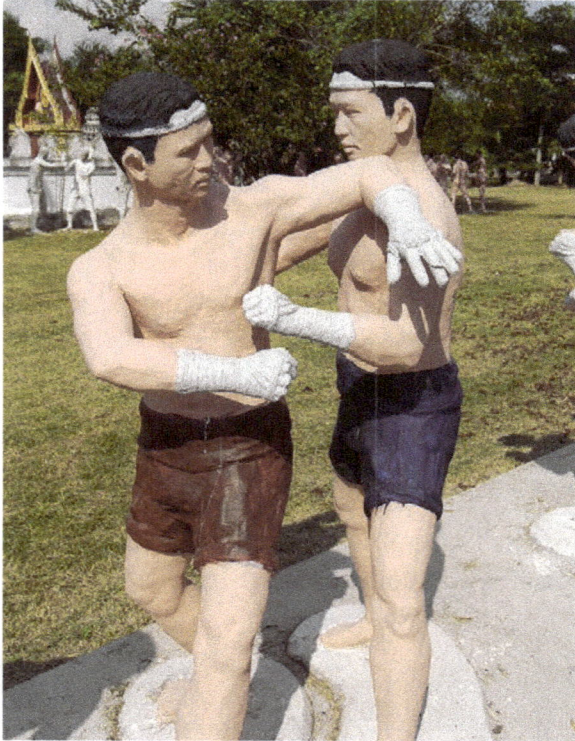

B)   Back-turning. (Reverse Elbow or Back SPinning Elbow)

There are two significant versions of the Back-turning Elbow. One is to defend against an opponent who is directly behind. This is done by reaching forward with the lead hand as if to grasp a hand full of air, then looking over the lead shoulder to the rear, driving the lead elbow straight backward. Spring off the feet turning into the direction that the elbow is moving in. Step through to the rear as you complete the turn. May be done with either arm.

The second variation of the Back-turning Elbow is for an opponent who is in front of or slightly to the side. Pivot the front heel forward and snap the head around so as to keep the eyes on the opponent. As the head is turning, load up the elbow by lifting the arm and again reaching for air. Spin to the rear and drive the elbow straight ahead. Allow the rear foot to follow through to keep from falling

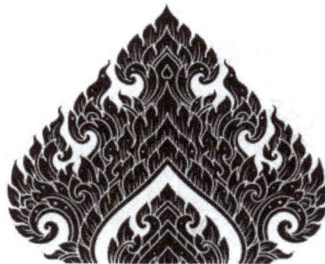

2) "Sok Kun" (Rising Elbow)

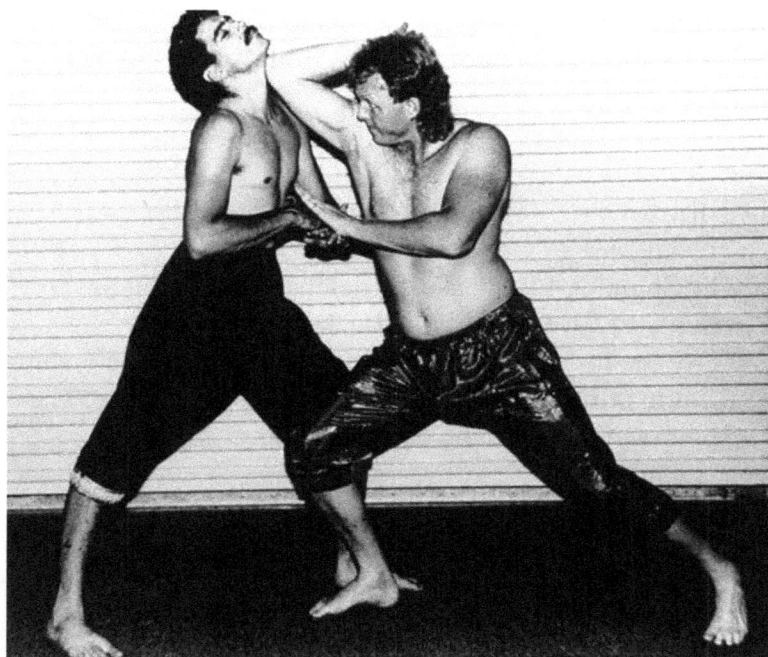

There are two major variations of "*Sok Kun*". The vertical rising and the diagonal rising.

A)   Vertical Rising. (*"Fhan Look Buab"*) From the basic stance, move the rear hand forward and upward. Make a motion as if to brush the hair on the side of the head. Continue this all the way to the back of the head. Of course, the elbow follows the hand upward and finishes pointed directly upward. As you do the hand motion, step into your opponent. Just before making contact, spring upward from the toes. It is never just an arm motion. Always hit with the whole body. Vertical Elbow can be done with either elbow.

B)   Diagonal Rising. Begin as if you are going to throw the straight punch from the rear hand (Cross). Bring the back of the punching hand to the opposite side of the face and circle around toward the back of the head. As you do this, pivot and twist the body in the direction of the turn pushing hard with the legs. Rising Elbow can be done with either elbow.

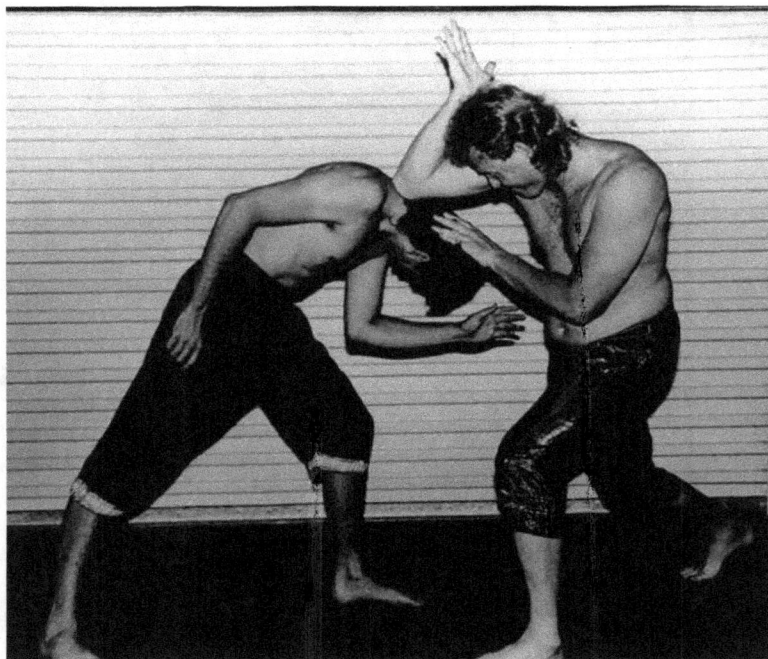

3) "Sok Lon" (Downward Elbow- Sinking Elbow)

There are two major variations of "*Sok Lon*", descending with the bottom of the elbow and descending with the front of the elbow.

A)   Bottom Elbow. Draw the rear hand back as if to throw something (palm out). Step forward rapidly and as you do this, rotate the hand back and the elbow inward and bring the elbow directly over the head and down in front. Time it so the body weight settles as the bottom of the elbow makes contact. Essentially the arm makes a complete circle with the highest point directly over the head.

B) **Front Elbow.** The front elbow is made with a cutting motion. Lead in with the forward foot. Raise the rear elbow while turning the palm of the hand outward. Swing the elbow up, over, and downward as you step through with the rear leg. Keep the hand tucked inward and downward, the opposite of the Bottom Elbow. Strike with the flat area just in front of the point of the elbow. As you make contact, allow the body weight to sink with it.

4) **"Sok Won"** (The Spinning Elbow)

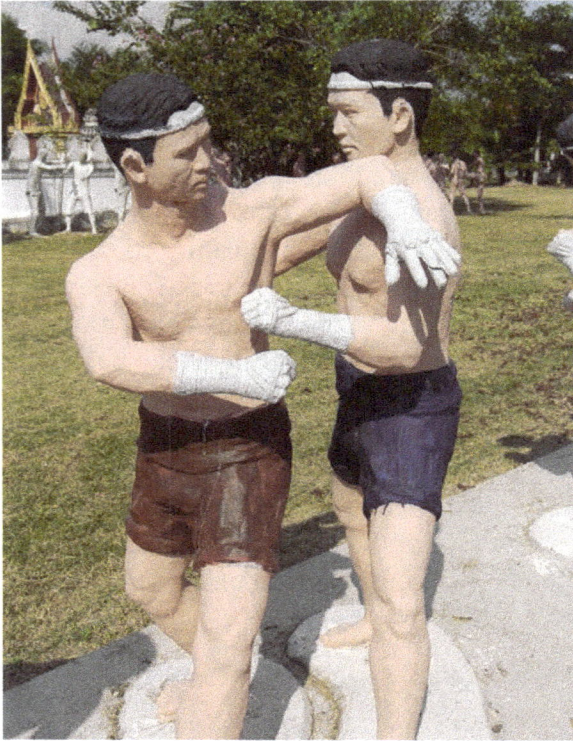

Hak Kor Chang Erawan (Flying Elephant)
using both elbows!

The Spinning Elbow is used defensively as well as offensively. Begin with the Back-turning Elbow; however, instead of driving directly into the target, whip the arm around and across with a snapping motion. The Spinning Elbow can be done with either elbow.

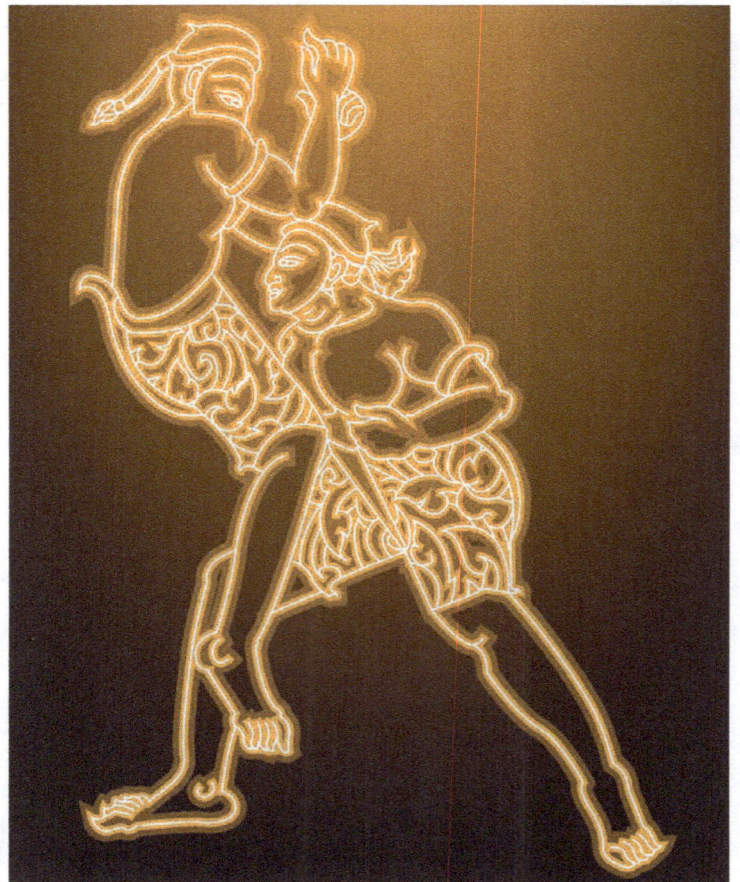

5)   "Sok Bin" (Flying Elbow)

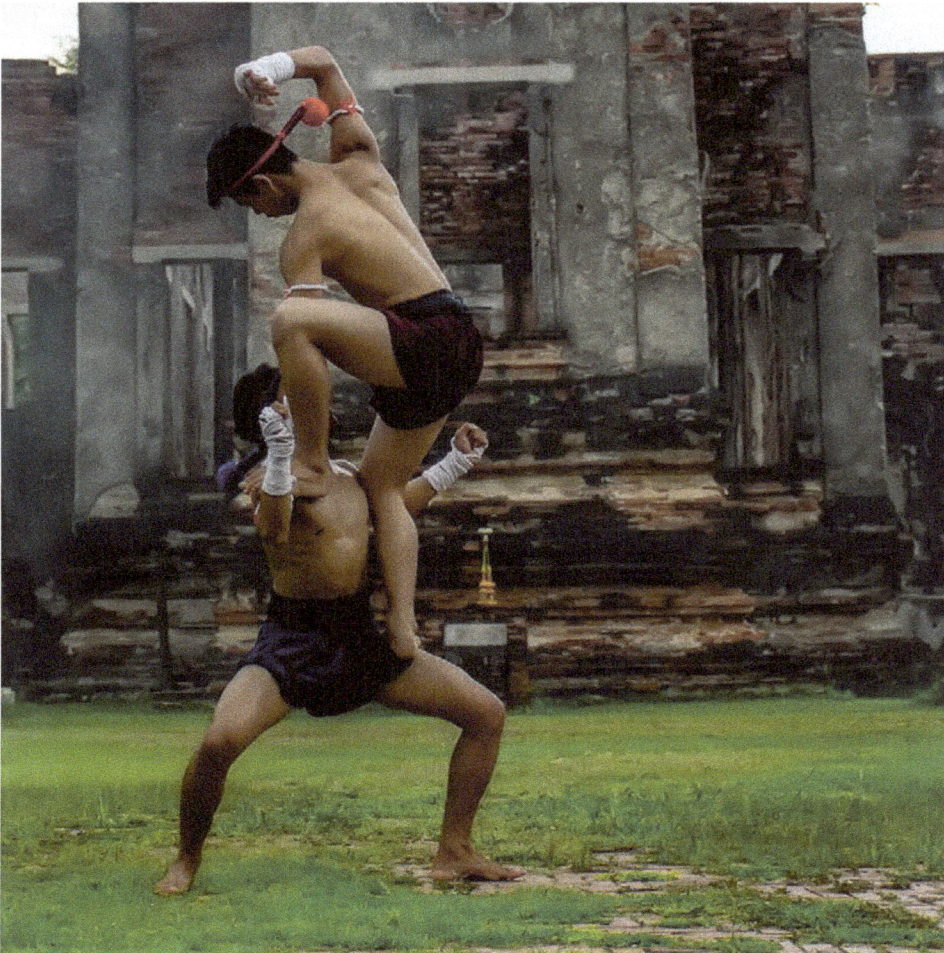

The "*Sok Bin*" is the most dramatic elbow technique. Virtually any of the basic elbows may be used as a flying technique. The most common, though, is probably the "*Sok Trong*" or "*Sok Lon*" as these lend themselves well to leaping or flying techniques. Simply add the elbow to the end of a running leap at your opponent to cut him down.

6) Hong Peak Hak (Broken Birds WIng)

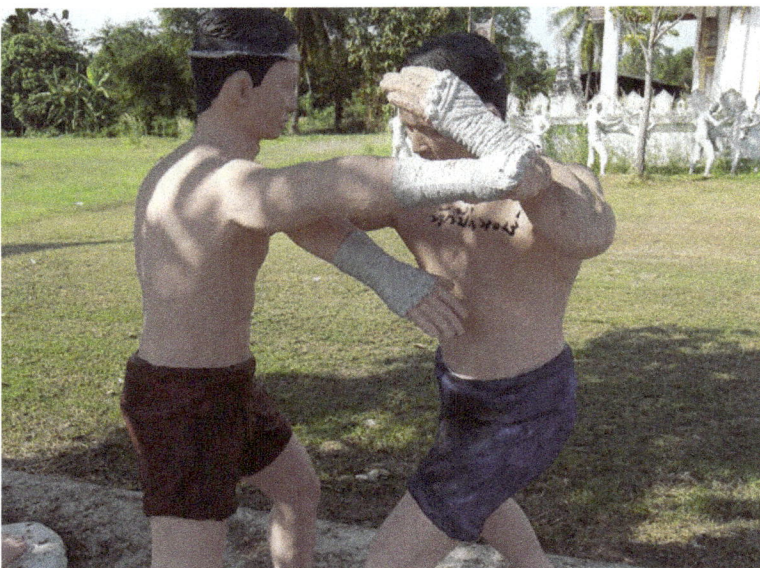

In general, the "*My Sok*" or "*Ao Sok*" techniques may be applied to any part of the opponent's body, including upper and lower leg, hip area, ribs, arms and shoulders, middle and upper back, neck, head, and groin, provided you are using a properly conditioned weapon. The procedure to condition the elbows is very similar to that of the shin.

The Basic *Muay Boran- Muay Chaya/ Fan Daap* Drill/ Flow Set

Part of the daily training routine at Buddhai Sawan- Nongkam, was drilling in Muay Boran and empty hand fighting. Once the students understood the basic techniques and footwork it was time to put them together and repeat until assimilated in muscle memory. Of course, there was also contact practice on leather shields and "banana bags" i.e., Heavy boxing bags.

The Basic Drill Sets or "Flows" are breakouts, many of which are derived from the Lu Ram Muay and or Buddhai Sawan Wai Kruu. By "breakout" I mean short sequences of techniques which are performed in a set or pre-arranged manner… Think, Short Kata! However, these short drills sequences (Yogic Vinyasa) are functional and practical as tools for attacking and or defending in real fights, in real life scenarios.   *No "Full Contact" in daily or Open practice!*

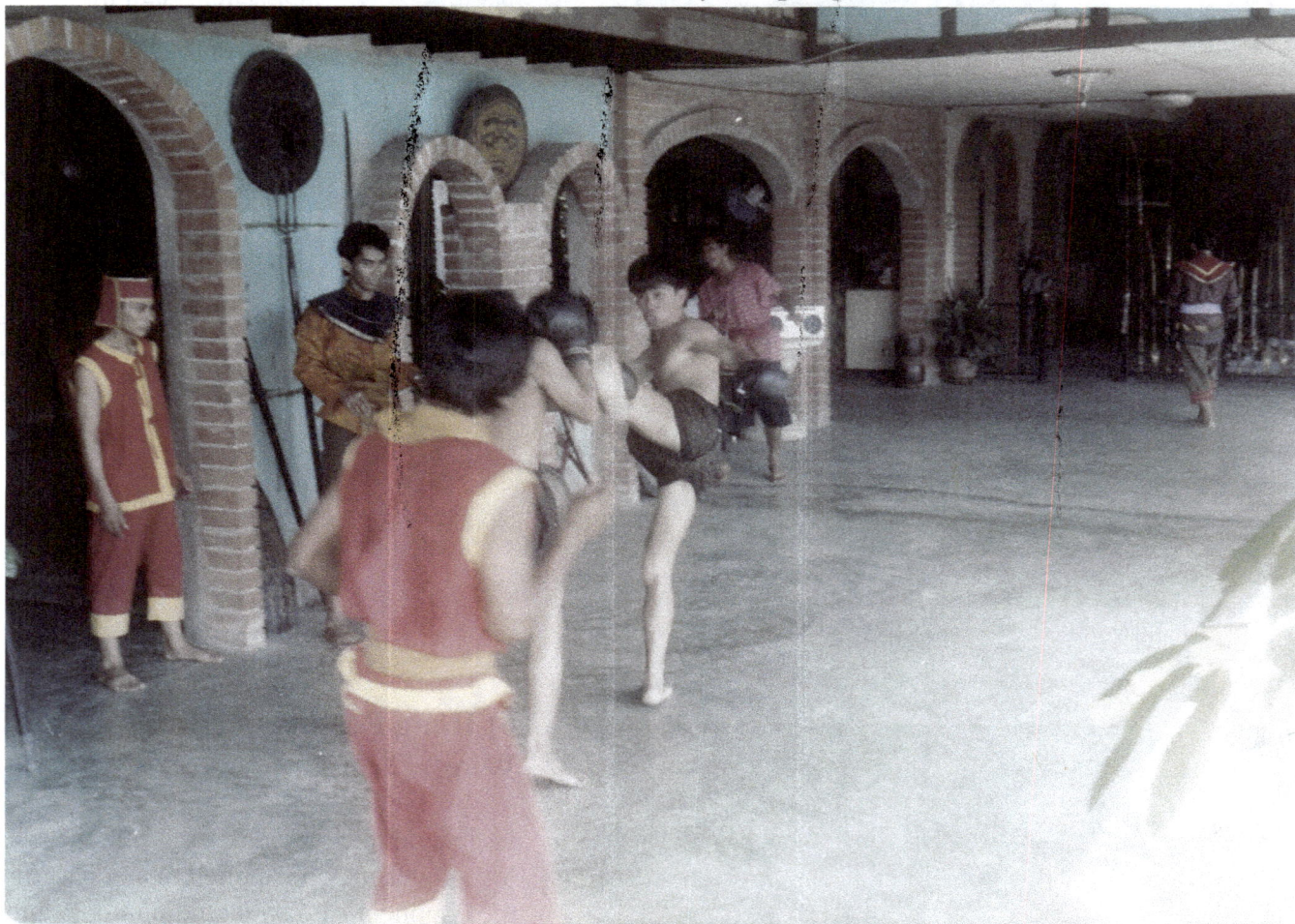

In daily practice we were instructed to not hit each other too hard. Why? Because it is hard to train hard every day when you are injured! Drills are usually set up on the weak side forward. Since most students are left-handed, this favors the weak side. Eventually the idea is to cultivate a NOT weak side. You want to develop a strong and a stronger side. I think of the term "ambidextrous"… able to freely switch and or use either side leading at will. After you step through and complete one drill, you turn and repeat the drill back to your starting point… ready to advance again or repeat however many times you need to!

We wear "Saftey Gear"! When practicing "Full Contact". We do recommend "Full Contact" for Advanced Students.

1. Jab, Cross, Back rising elbow, Hook, back thrusting elbow

2. Step Out Jab, Cross, Uppercut, Hook, back thrusting elbow, & step back

3. Step in upper cut/ forward rising elbow (lead arm), back rising elbow, horizontal inward elbow (lead arm), back cross elbow (rear arm), descending or downward elbow (lead arm), step in and descending elbow (rear arm), jump into vertical downward or dropping elbow (lead arm), jump into downward elbow off rear hand & step back

4. Step into "pull the head down" and upward thrusting knee, repeat opposite side with exchange step, repeat again with angle knee, repeat opposite side, step pull down into rising knee, step pull down into rising knee & step back

5. Back step with reverse elbow, back step with reverse elbow, back step with reverse horizontal elbow, back step with reverse horizontal elbow, back step with reverse high descending angle elbow, back step with reverse high descending angle elbow

6. Kicks:
    a. "Tiip": Middle target: Both sides stepping forward
    b. "Tiip": Low target: Both sides stepping forward
    c. "Tiip": Middle target: Both sides stepping forward
    d. "Tiip": High target, to spinning heel kick, Both sides stepping forward

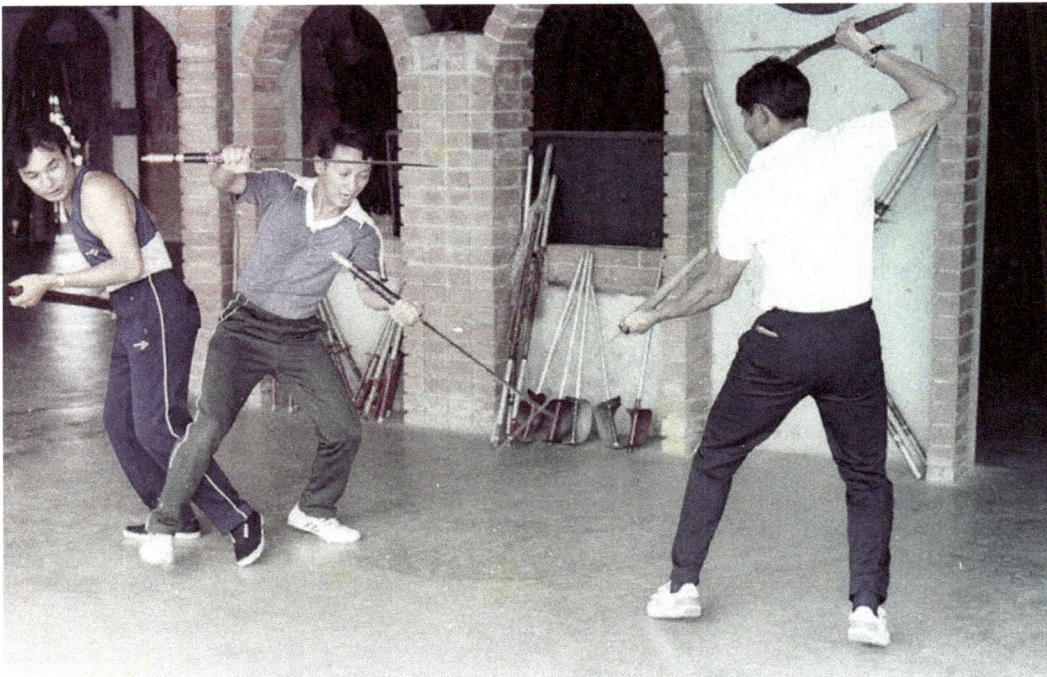

BS KK Drils were often with two or more attackers at a time with multiple and different weapons such as here in this photo... Two on One vs. Daap Song Myrr Deo (Double swords) and Plong- Heavy Staff. ANy combination of different weapons could be practiced or drilled.

15 TIMES TO ATTACK

1. When the opponent is changing sides

2. As the opponent initiates an attack. While it is developing (stop hit)

3. When you have actually landed an attack on the opponent (hit again to finish)

4. When the opponent falters in stride, either because of a miscalculation, confusion, stumble, or slip

5. When the opponent has completed an attack

6. When your opponent's resolve waivers

7. When the opponent is distracted due to outside interference

8. When your opponent makes a mistake

9. When the opponent cannot see or is falling

10. As the opponent lands or hits the ground from a fall

11. When the opponent is in the middle of taking a breath, especially if it is a big breath--say when he is tired

12. When the opponent is obviously tired and slow

13. When the opponent drops his guard

14. When your opponent turns his back on you

15. Anytime you can make a clean hit

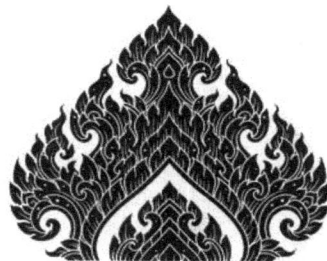

Footwork (Dancing)

Basic Dancing Steps:

1. Loke/Advancinq
2. Look Tronq Pai/Advancing with Thrusts
3. Toi/Retreating
4. Toi Tronq Pai/Retreating with Thrusts
5. Lokewan/Spinning
6. Walking Step- Basic Shuffle
7. Dancing Step to Kneeling Position

1) "Loke" (Advancing)

A) Slide Up and Step Out: The rear foot initiates by sliding either forward a half or whole step. The lead foot then steps forward. The advantagen of this movemnet is that the initial forward motion is not so obvious, as it is partially obscured by the lead foot. Both this movement and the step and slide may be taken in very small, quick motions also covering longer distances.

From the fighting stance slide the rear foot forward about half a step. As this is done, shift the weight of the body forward being careful not to rise up. Step forward with the rear foot all the way through into another stance. The end of the first step is the beginning of the next. This method of stepping is the most common and often used.

B) Step and Slide: The rear foot initiates forward or a lateral motion by taking a step. The rear foot follows by sliding an equal distance forward. This movement is beneficial in that it leaves one foot in contact with the ground at all times. While being one of the fastest and sureest stepping methods, it is still a conservative one. It allows you to react fast in either attack or defense as you are never far from firm footing.

C) Step Through: (Quick Advance) Just like it sounds. Step completely forward and through with the rear foot moving forward. This is the same motion used in "Dashing" and or "leaping" forward techniques.

2) "Look Tronq Pai" Advancing with Thrusts: Start from the "Ksum", basic fighting stance with the swords in the traditional ready position for fighting. Push off the front heel and land heel first rolling to the toe. As the toe settles, slide the back foot forward to its original relative position. The upper body is held erect and does not lean as you advance.

The swords are making a rotating type of movement while the feet are advancing. The hands rotate overhand or clockwise while the points are making straight thrusting attacks. The thrusts are timed so that the front hand leads with the front foot stepping out and the backhand thrusts as the rear foot slides forward.

3) "Toi" (Retreating): The body weight is shifted to the rear leg and the front foot slides back about 8 inches. Then, the rear footsteps directly back to the rear into another stance. The finish is at the beginning of another step— with the sliding back of the front foot. This little slide- up or preparation is characteristic of Thai footwork and is called chambering.

4) "Toi Trong Pai '' (Retreating with Thrusts): Similar to *"Look Trong"*- Advancing with Thrusts: Start from the "Ksum" stance with the swords in the traditional ready position for fighting. Step directly to the rear with the back foot. As you place that foot on the ground, slide the front, foot the same distance. The center of gravity should remain essentially the same throughout with the upper body upright and relaxed.

5) "Loke Wan" (Spinning): Advance a short step with the foot closest to the direction you wish to go. Drop low and sweep the rear foot around in an arc. This is done fast, usually as a counter-offensive step or even as a leg sweep to the rear, causing an unwary opponent to fall.

6) Walking Step- The Basic Shuufle Step: To simply take a step forward in a normal relaxed walking mode. The Basic Shuffle is similar to the common type of footwork in western boxing. The rear foot moves directly forward at the same time, the lead foot slides to the rear. The feet remain in contact with the ground at all times. The body's weight is just shifted enough to allow the balls of the feet to simultaneously slide.. Hense the "Shuffle". This is the fastest way to change sides or bring forward the rear foot. You can step, walk or shuffle so easy and quick that the opponent might not even notice that you have changed sides!

7) Dancing Step to Kneeling Position: Advancing. From the fighting stance slide the rear foot forward about half a step. As this is done, shift the weight of the body forward. Step forward with the rear foot all the way through into the beginning of another stance. At the last moment, drop the rear knee all the way to the ground. This gives a sudden change in height to accompany an attack or an evasive movement. **As Sijo Bruce Lee said "The essence of fighting is the art of moving".**

13 Ways To Bridge The Gap
(Advancing Footwork)

   1. Step in
   2. Step in, step out (Exchange step)
   3. Step and slide (Bring the rear foot forward)
   4. Step and slide, step again (Front foot leads)
   5. Slide up (Rear foot)
   6. Slide up and step out
   7. Basic shuffle
   8. Exchange step and advance
   9. Step through (quick advance)
   10. Spinning step through (to rear with rear foot)
   11. Lunge (Long Step, spring forward, push off rear foot)
   12. All of the above on any angle (ranging i.e., longer, or shorter step).
   13. Any of the above in combination. For example, #2 followed immediately with a #8…

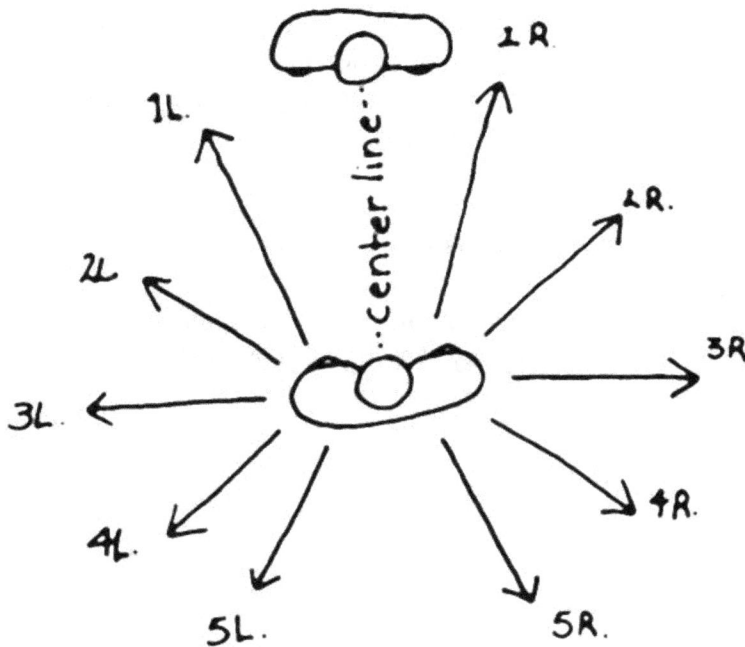

Ranging in Footwork

Ranging is a method or strategy to avoid the opponent's weapon and at the same time stay close enough to instantly counter attack. The step forward to off center is actually a li=unge. The rear leg remains where it is and as the front knee bends, the body inclines along the same angle as the initial step. You may return along the same line or continue with another step in any direction. We have a saying "Get off The Line!". This also means to control who dominates the center line.

Footwork #1 Illustration

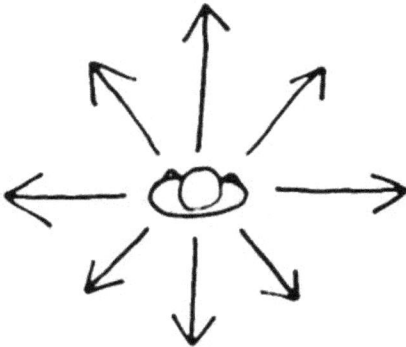

The advancing footwork patterns must not only move forward, but instead may move in any direction.

Footwork #2 Illustration

By alternating and combining steps, you have the ability to create a base from which to throw any form of offensive or defensive motion. This also gives you indirect attacking angles.

In defense, sometimes all that is necessary is to step out of the way.

"Mo": Indirect Step

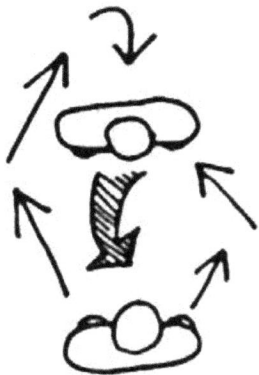

Step out in any direction.

Footwork #3 Illustration

A) Step out "off the line" (center line), then immediately step back in towards the line.

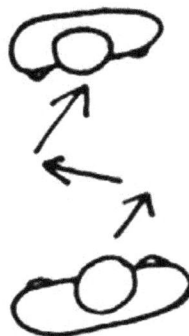

B) Front foot steps around, back foot slides and or shuffles and follows.

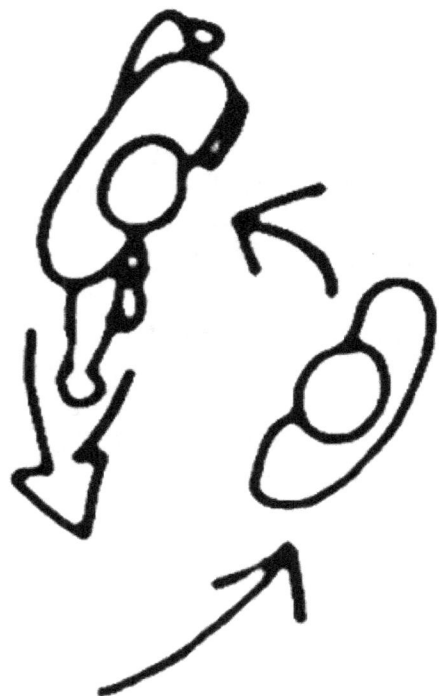

By alternating and combining steps, you have the ability to create a base from which to throw any form of offensive or defensive motions. This also gives you indirect attacking angles and in the moment adaptability.

Footwork #4 Illustration

In defense sometimes all that is necessary is to step out of the way! No big whoop! Just get off the line!

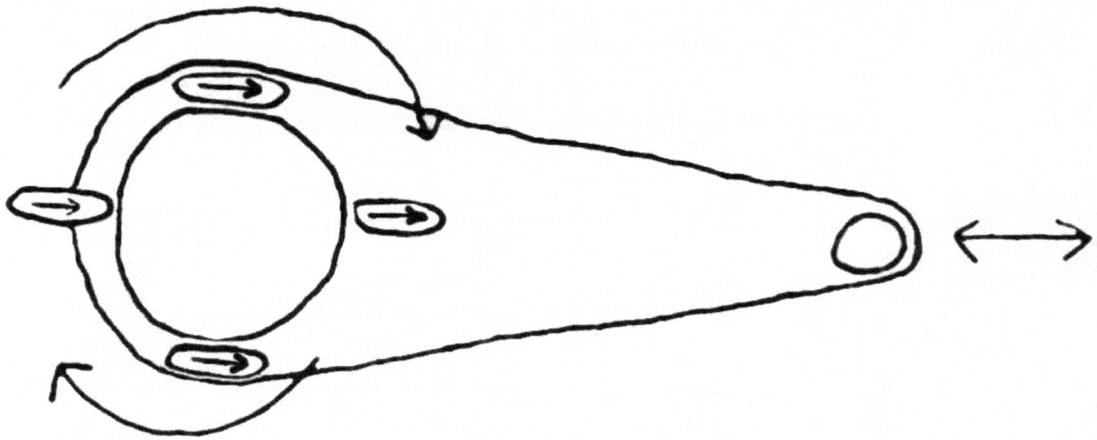

Footwork #5 Illustration : Hand motion while advancing with weapons.

So Many Weapons, So Little Time!

My Sok vs Plong

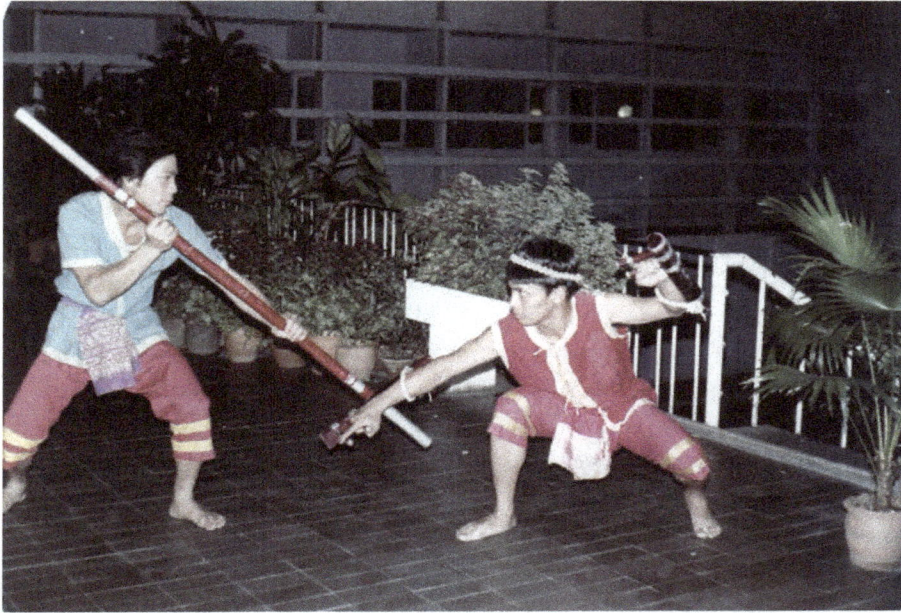

Proper Stance for *Plong Wai Kruu*

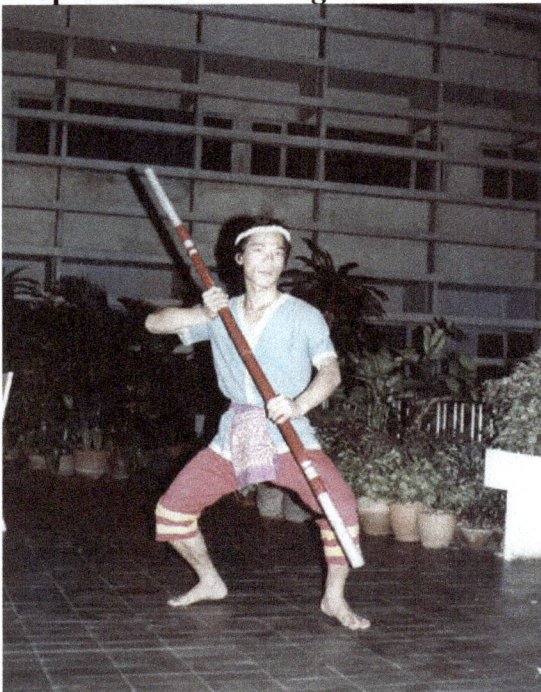

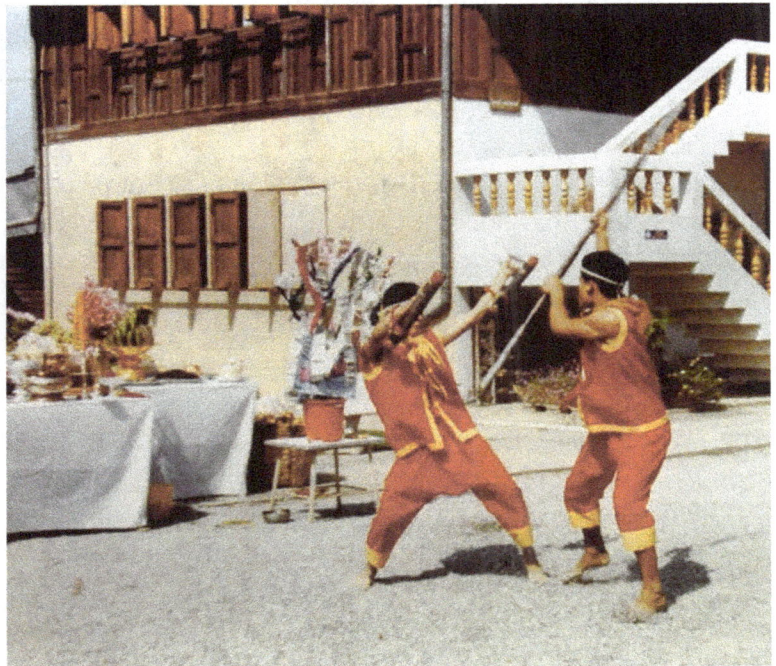

The Nine Weapon Systems

The Nine Weapons Systems are divided up into four main categories:

A)   **Offensive or Attack Weapons:** Swords (many kinds, types, lengths and weight, single and or double edged, including special swords that had a knife built into the handle!), Saber, Cutlass, Foil, Epee, Short and Long Lance, Rope Tied Lances, Spears, Halberds, Clubs, Hammers/ Mace, Sticks (Ratan and Hardwood) and Quarter Staves (Long heavy Staffs and Poles i.e. "Plong"), Long and short handled Axes and all Farming tools such as Rice Sickles and threshing tools common to farmers.

B)   **Defensive or Protective Weapons:** Leather, Wood, Rattan and Metal Shields of varying sizes and shapes as well as :"Mai Sok" or small hand shields. (please note: Mae Sowk can also be used offensively!), Flexible staff and Spears, including Naginatas (Japanese Style) and Chakri Spear (Three Bladed), Kris and Kalis (Indonesian Style), Bamboo Hidden Bladed swords and knives.

C)   **Projectile or Long-Distance Weapons:** Bow and Arrow including crossbow & bolt, Throwing spear or lance, Whips, Throwing knives, Throwing Axes, and Spikes, Rocks, and projectile weapons: Guns, Rifles, Pistols and Canon. Firearms and cannon in use go back to their invention!

D)   **Armored War Elephants and Horse Calvary:** The weapons and tactics appropriate for them, (Mostly reserved for elite, noble and or royal persons and their retinue/ bodyguards etc.)

All of these weapon classes represent an individually unique system as the specific weapon calls for its unique and peculiar nature in its respective use and handling characteristics. All of these may, depending on circumstance, be combined creatively. For example, the round shield and rope tied lance used together, or a combination of a long and a shorter weapon. The possibilities are only limited by the skill and creativity, availability of the warrior.

Additionally, to the above list… which is not complete by any means, we will also have to add ANY Indian, Burmese, Lao, Mon, Khymer, Cambodia, Javanese, Malaysia, Indonesian and or Japanese, Chinese versions of the above! All of these countries were in active warfare with the Thai for 1000 years, give or take. Their weapons and tactics would have been seen and experienced on the battlefields over the years. For example, let's not forget the Thai Kings adopting Japanese Samurai and their weapons from the Ayudthaya and later period! That means some Krabi Krabong warriors would have been seen sporting *Katana, Wakizashi* and *Tanto! There was a two-way influence between Japan and Thailand… There is speculation by me and others, that the Samurai Miyamoto Musashi's famous' "Nai Itto Ryu" or "Two Heavens", double sword fighting style may have originated in the Japanese Samurai who fought in Thailand being exposed to Krabi Krabong on the battlefield.*

We would also have to add the fighting styles and influence of the French, Portuguese, Dutch and other "want to be" colonial powers wrestling with the Thai over centuries as well. We see the style adaptation of the European Saber and "Espada y Daga" of the Portuguese into Thai Krabi Krabong.

Today it is easy to locate old weapons of these different cultures in many of the regional and or national museums of Thailand. Two that especially come to mind are the Royal Pavilion Armory attached to the Grand Palace in Bangkok and the Sukhothai National Museum in Old Sukhothai, Thailand.

Krabi Krabong Is More than about fighting with weapons!

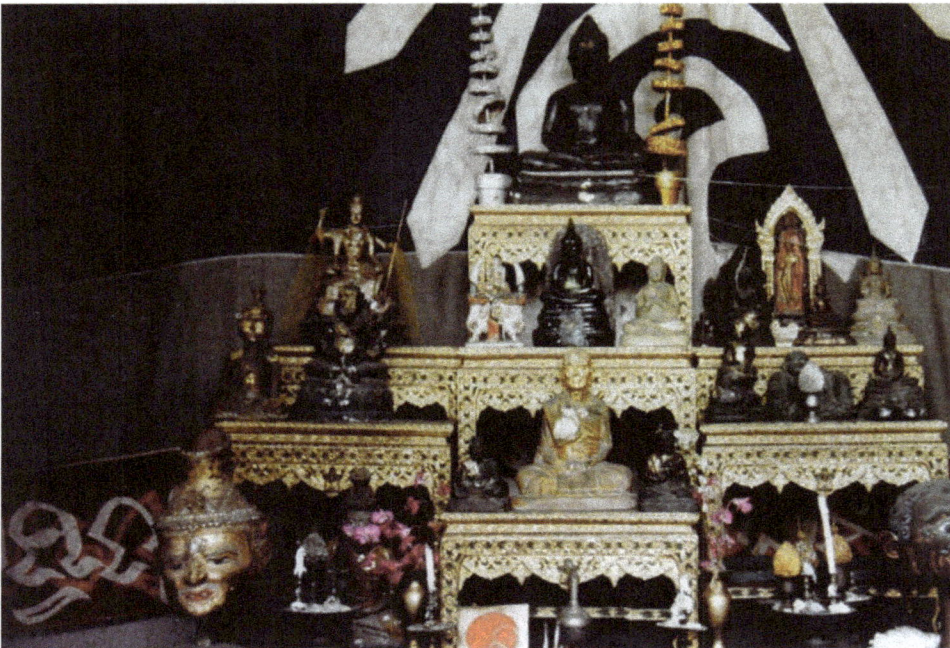

Krabi Krabong is clearly not just about the sword (*Deo*) or the two swords' techniques (*Dap Song Myr Deo*). Buddhai Sawan style traditional Krabi Krabong is a comprehensive sophisticated system and discipline.

It incorporates training which can enrich every area of life based on teachings and practices emphasizing development of spirit, mind, and body.

The "Up Stairs" Alter at Buddhai Sawan Institute, Nongkam, Thailand, 1983

It incorporates protection and defensive strategies for dealing with both internal and external pernicious influences.

It incorporates fighting strategies and techniques for open warfare and combat to more up close and personal self-defense using bare hands or knives. It teaches us to face our enemies with integrity.

It incorporates meditations and sacred dances to Thai Traditional Medicine, "*Reussi Dottan*" Thai Reishi Yoga to "*Ryksaa Thang Nuad Phaen Boran Thai*", sacred tattoos (Yak Sen) to magic amulets and head dress (*mongkon/ mongkol*).

It incorporates ritual blessings, chants, mantra and prayers with a moral code and principles to guide one to cultivate and experience a good life and reduce harmful karma or energetic blockages which interfere with the ability to be a good person and have ethical, moral way of being with integrity.

It incorporates music, community and family. It is not just a "Martial Arts" it represents a community of purpose and consciousness, preserving an ancient legacy and heritage emphasizing independence, freedom, spiritual expression, art, culture and spiritual understanding.

I personally feel that this is a deep well and I am constantly learning, seeing, and experiencing new energy from the well. This is especially true as I strive to integrate the Buddhai Sawan Krabi Krabong principles into my daily life and work. Too much for one book, I invite other knowledgeable persons in our BSKK community to contribute more documentation, books, videos from any and all of the traditional based schools.

Combat Systems of Krabi Krabong

Every weapon individually represents a system and peculiar approach all unto it's self. Individual weapons are to be mastered individually if possible before combining or using in tandem with other weapons and systems. The Espada y Dagga fighting systems of Spain and Philippines offer a comparative. However, now use or blend in conjunction all possible combinations. Ancient Thai Warriors would commonly carry a brace of different weapons including fire arms when available so as to be able to choose the appropriate weapon system according to circumstances in the field.

Bai Oi - Long, straight double-bladed Thai spear

Bai Pai - Small broad-bladed spear

Dha - Thai Long Handled Wide Bladed sword. Meant to be used with two hands.

Dhap Song Myrr Deo (Daab Hua Bua) – Matched Double Thai Sword (Slung and worn across the back crossed like an X)

Dhap Deo - Single Thai Sword

Dhap & Scabbard – (The scabbard is also used as a shield or club)

Dhap Naa Look Ka – Long handled, long blade, leaf shaped, semi-rounded in scabbard) Popular with Royalty. Blade sometime forged with appearence of a flame or flames. May also be known as "Dhap Sri Gun Chai Dha"

Dang Deo - Narrow rectangular hand shield and Thai Sword

Eee knep – 11+ inch blade, Jungle knife/ Thai Farmers Long knife or machete.(Various sizes, shapes and weights. Also used for cutting- trimming Bamboo)

Haw Phoo - Long lance for horseback

Hok Bai Pai - Large broad-bladed spear (Elephant)

Got Tuan - Short lance for horseback

Kalis - Southern Thai style mixed wavy- and straight edged knife

Kaw Spa Chang - Elephant mace (Used against armor)

Ken - Rectangular shield

Kheīyw - sickle, scythe, hook farming tool with a semicircular blade, used for cutting grain, lopping, or trimming.

Kong Ao - Elephant spike (Used against armor)

Krabi - Long Thai Saber (European Style)

Krabong – Long bladed weapons included both original "Thai" and other types such as Japanese Katana, both single wielded and two handed "great" swords.

Kris – Southern Thai style wavy-edged knife. Blade shape found throughout SE ASIA from Thailand, Malaysia, Indonesia to Philippines

Kwan - Long-handled Axe

Lo Deo - Round shield and Thai Sword (Deo)

Lo Deo Gottuan - Round shield and short lance

Mae Sowk - Hand and forearm shield with arm loop

Nao Ciin (Ngao) - Chinese-style broad spear for Elephant or Horse

Nao Kabrong - Thai spear, Special and rare Knife, and sword combo

Plong - Heavy staff, Possibly with iron ends.

Thai Cooking Knives and Square tipped or pointed Choppers!

Thai *"Laap"* - "Jungle" Knife (Machete with wide V shape and square end… Quite heavy and some times called a "Bamboo" knife used for building and construction.

Meet Ting- Double Throwing Knife

PLEASE NOTE: The above list is NOT complete or all inclusive!
There could be hundreds or thousands of variations of many types of weapons used over the centuries.

Practice Weapons: Practice versions of all of the weapons made out of wood, rattan etc.

All of the swords and weapons used may be made plain/ utilitarian in design or decoration i.e., with no decorations or non-structural, non-utilitarian embellishments at all. However, they were also manufactured with style. We have examples of artful and incredibly ornate designs with this intention of imbuing a unique character into the weapon from its foundation, forging and construction. Carved and embellished handles, scabbards covered in carvings, brass, mother of pearl inlays, gems, crystals exotic woods. This includes customization of the business ends of the weapons as well. A great example is in some of the Buddhai Sawan collection of War Axes, where the base or neck of the axe is cast as a demon's head with the blade itself being the breath or wind blowing out from the mouth of the Demon!

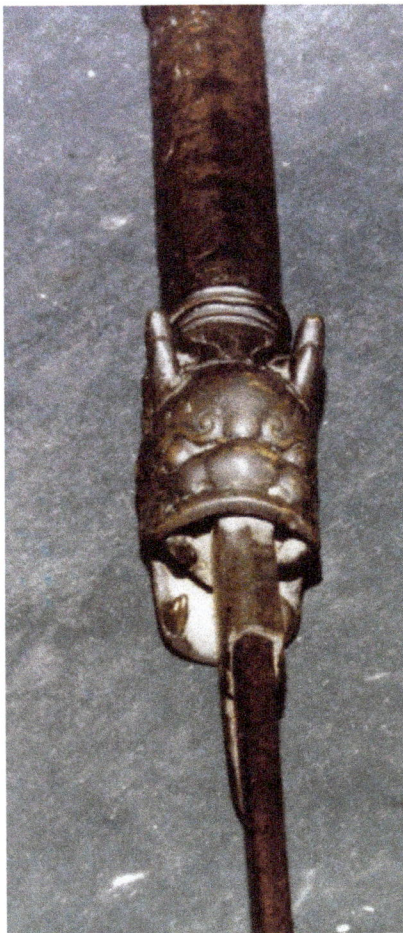

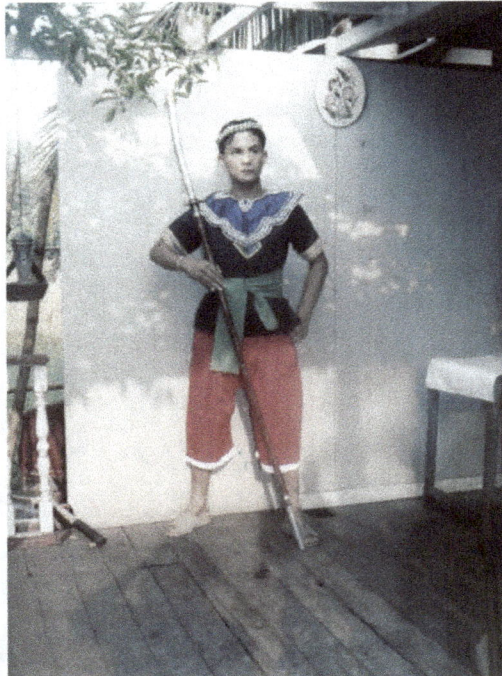

Kong Ngao

Another example being the long-poled weapons such as the *"Ha Kwan"* where the blade is cast in the appearance of "waves of water" flowing out from the pole/ handle or cast to appear as if the blade is a flame of fire. In the south we see the ornate Thai Kris styles which have intricate shapes, snake like blades with the handles and scabbards also being intricately carved and embellished and or also made from exotic and attractive woods.

After the swords are constructed, they may be additionally etched, stamped or hammered to further add embellishments of sacred characters and magic symbols added for assistance, blessing and or protection of the wielder. We also see some of the same symbols and characters in the sacred tattoo designs often adorned by monks (*Sak Yant*).

In the past the warriors would themselves tattoo these same designs found on their weapons on their bodies… sometimes covering their whole body. You never know when or where you might get hit! (Don't try this at home!).

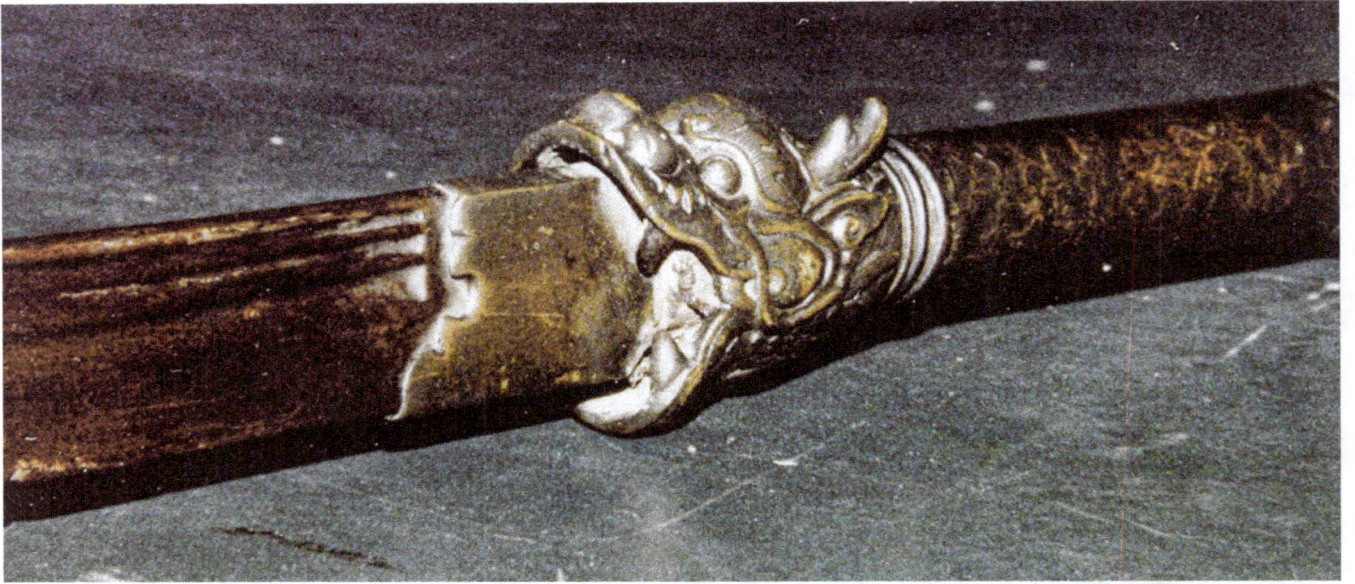

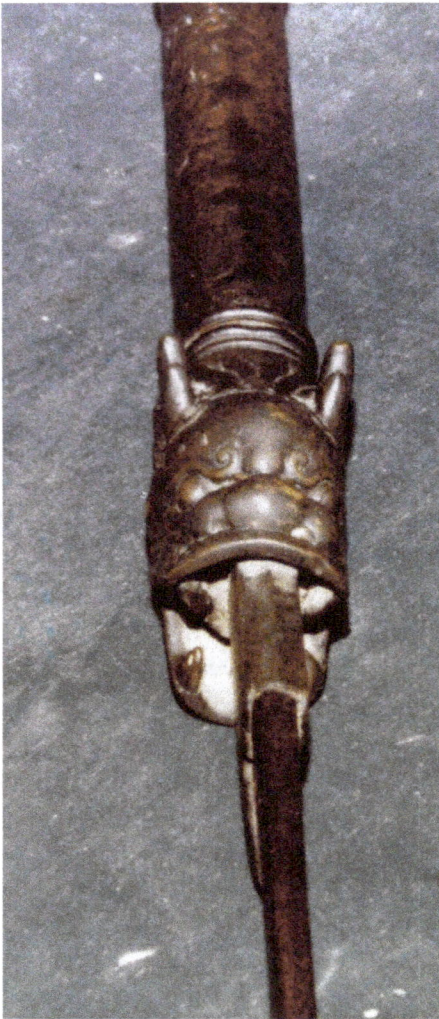

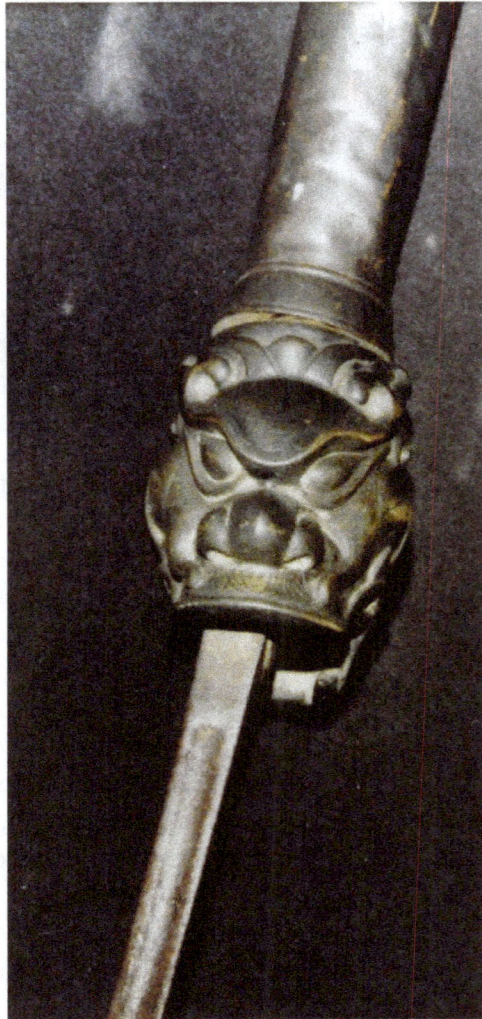

Examples of Buddhai Sawan Long Weapons (Krabong)

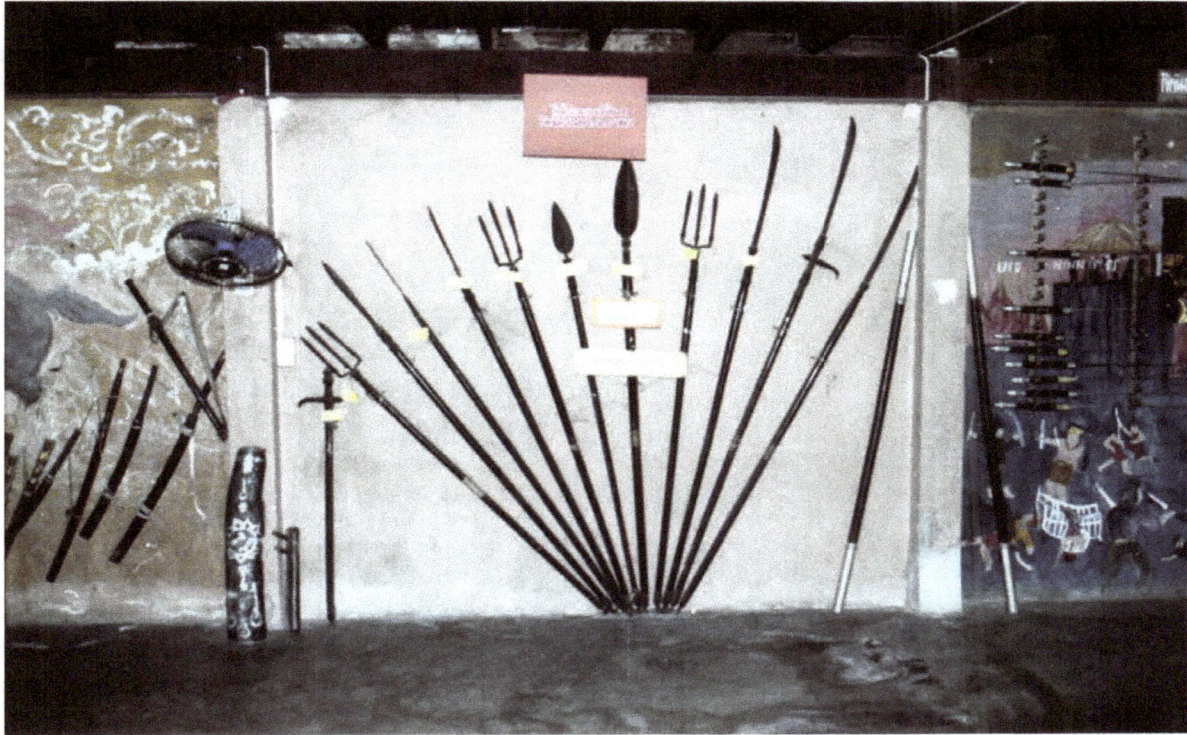

One of the BS Krabi Krabong Antique and historic weapon displays. Nongkam

The fine weapons collection of the Buddhai Swan Institute is considered a national treasure.

Many of the long weapons were primarily designed for use from the back of trained war elephants. There are hooks and or key shaped additions on the ends to secure them to the basket while transporting. These weapons are quite heavy. When fighting armor from a height this weight was advantageous.

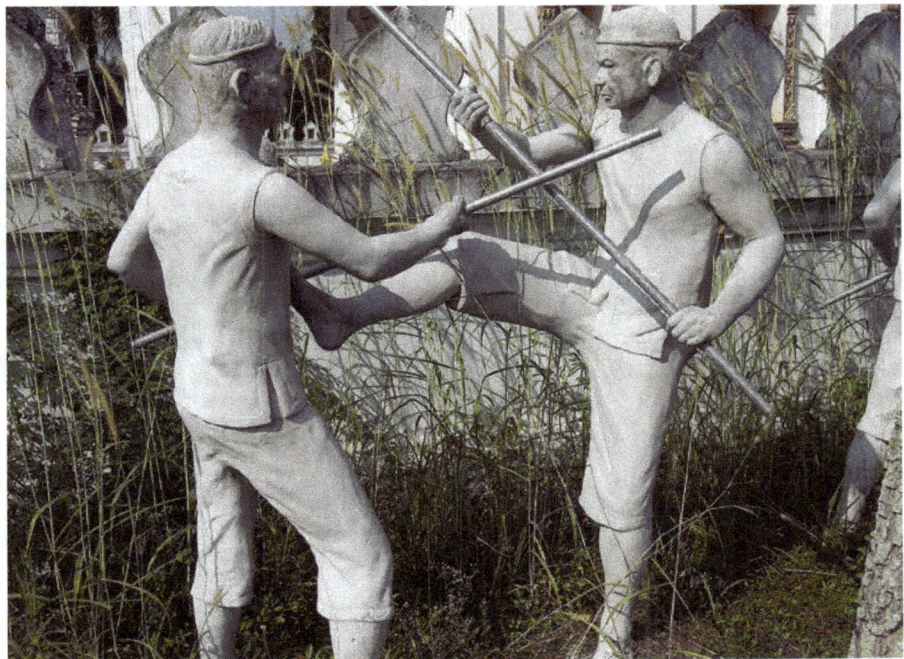

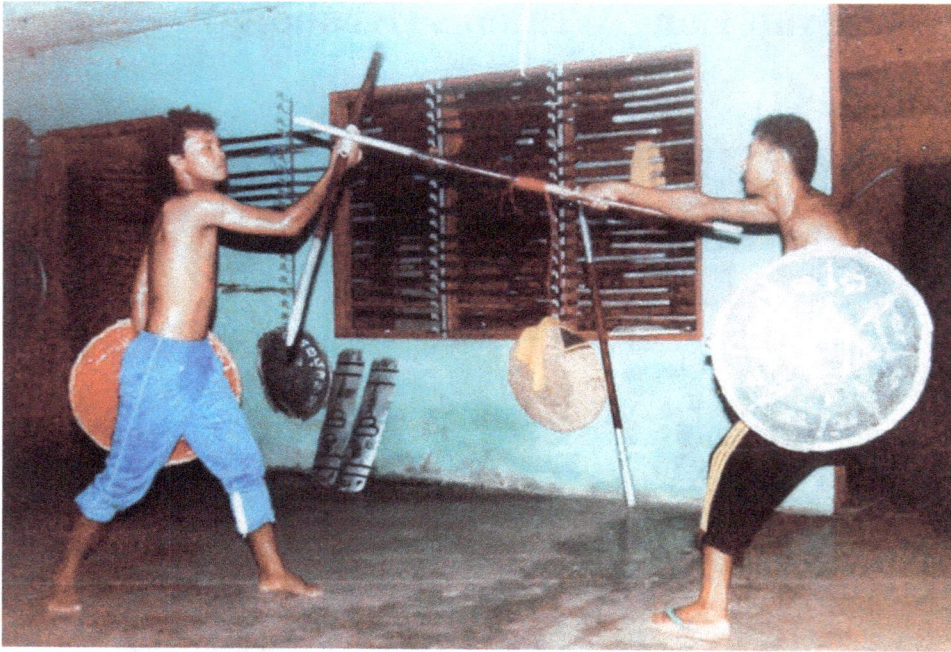

Today these heavy and long weapons are used as conditioning tools as much as anything. The Krabi Krabong equivalent of isotonic/ isokinetic exercise conditioning.

The quality and attention to detail in the traditional weapons of Buddhai Swan are equal to that seen anywhere. Notice the forged and finished mountings on these example polearms.

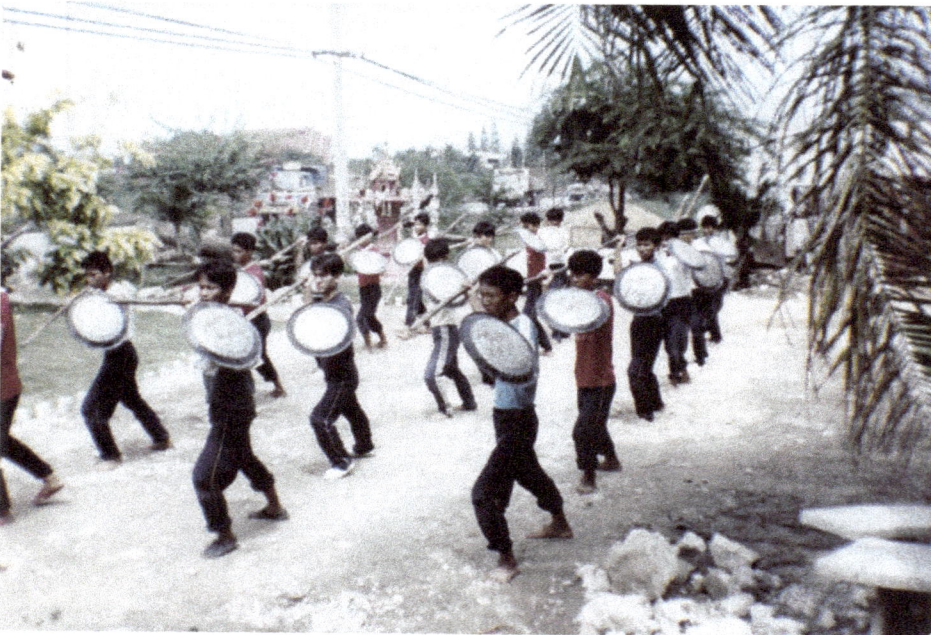

Additionally, notice the thickness and heaviness of the blade! This is the difference between a weapon made for daily use in battle and a decorative or show piece.

Examples of "Got tuan Lo Deo" Short lance and round shield.

Group practice Wai Kruu with "Got tuan Lo Deo" Short lance and round shield.

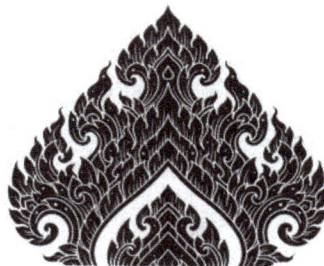

Examples of Buddhai Sawan Long *"Krabong"* Weapons

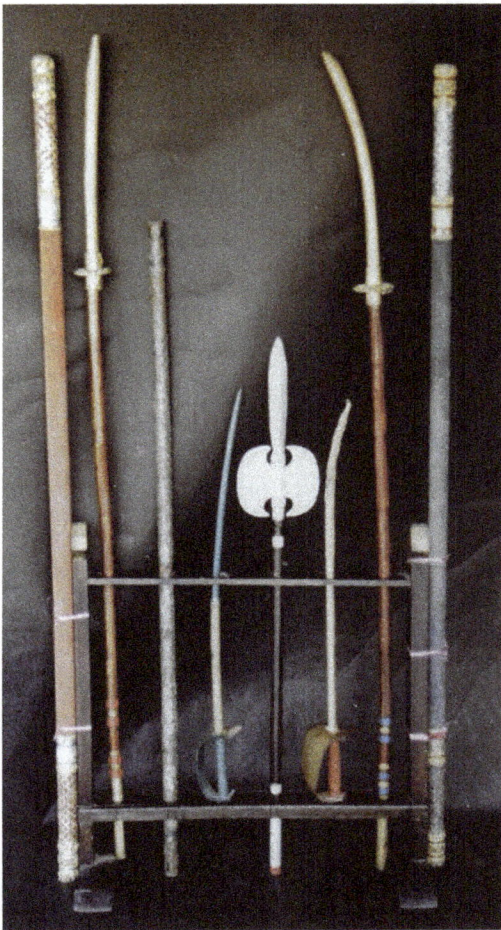

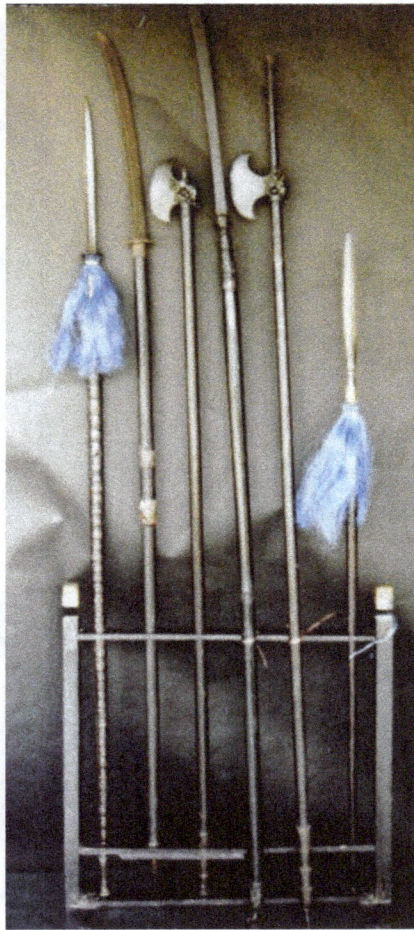

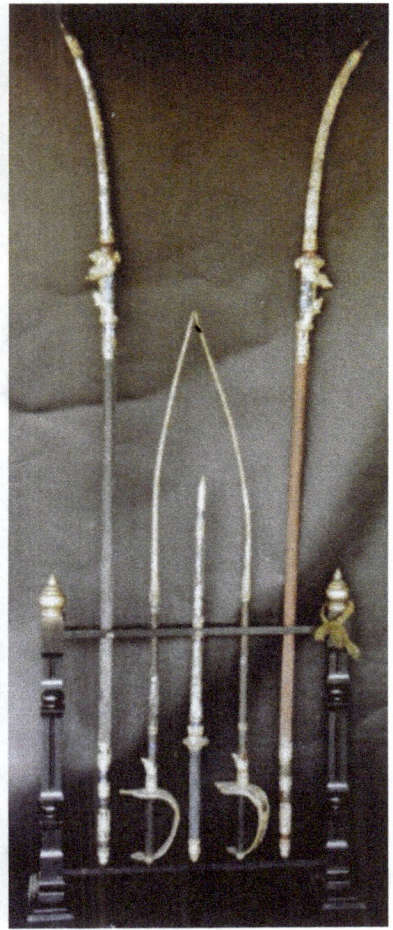

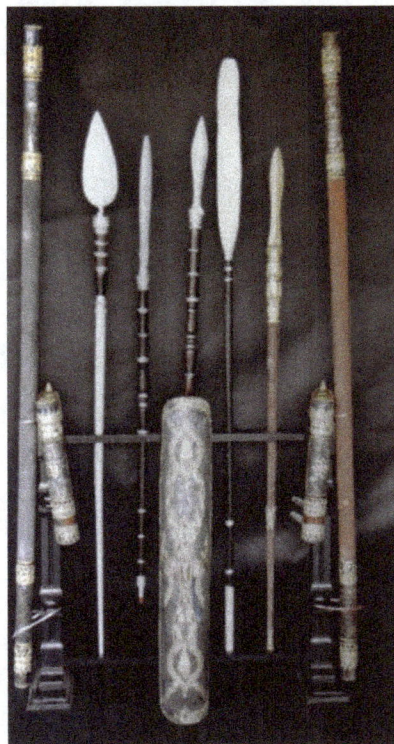

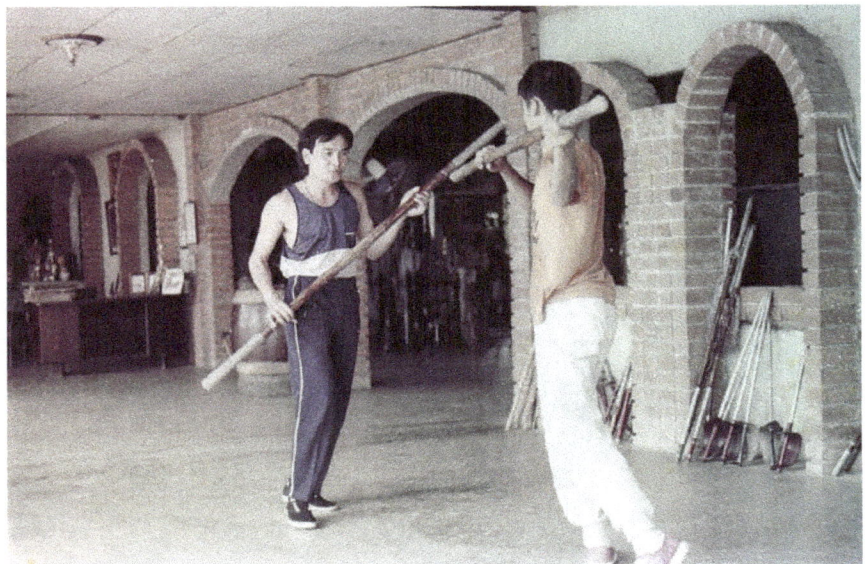

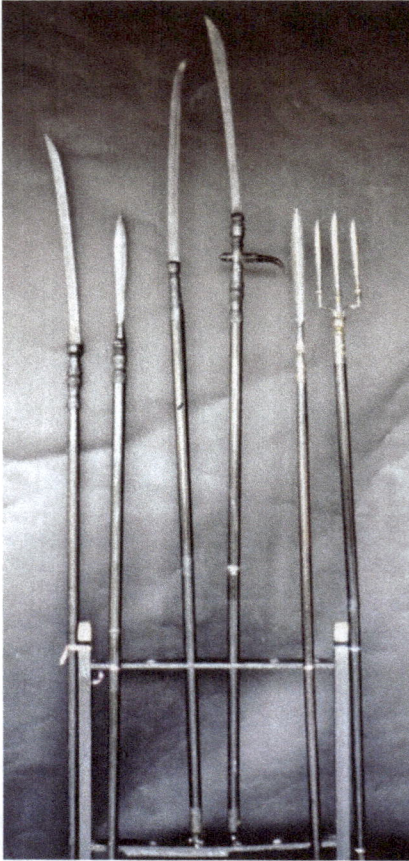

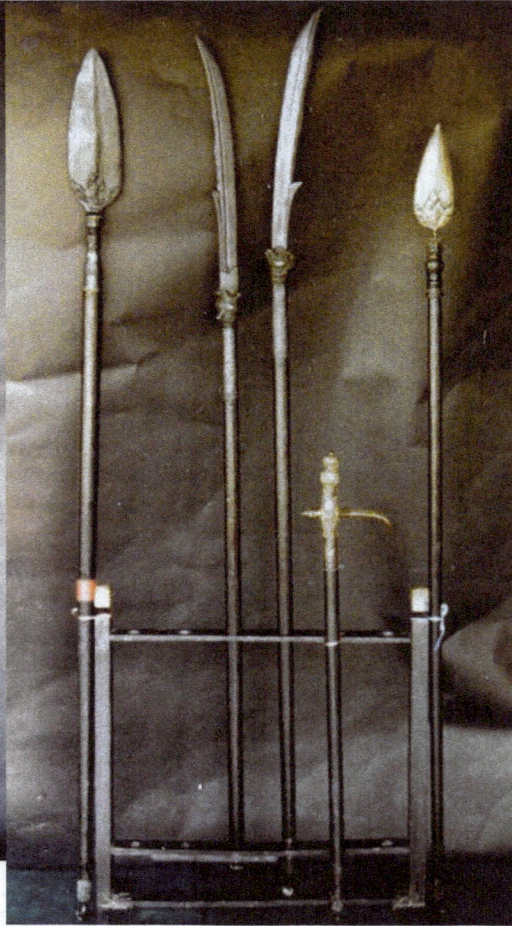

"*Bai Oi*", ("*Samnan*" or "*Chakri*" spear three bladed) and "*Nao Ciin*" (Chinese style broad Bladed Spear) with "*Kong Ao*" (Broad spear with Elephant hook), again demonstrate the hand forged artistry, and lethality of these hardy weapons. These weapons are from the collection of Buddhai Swan Sword Fighting Institute, Nongkam.

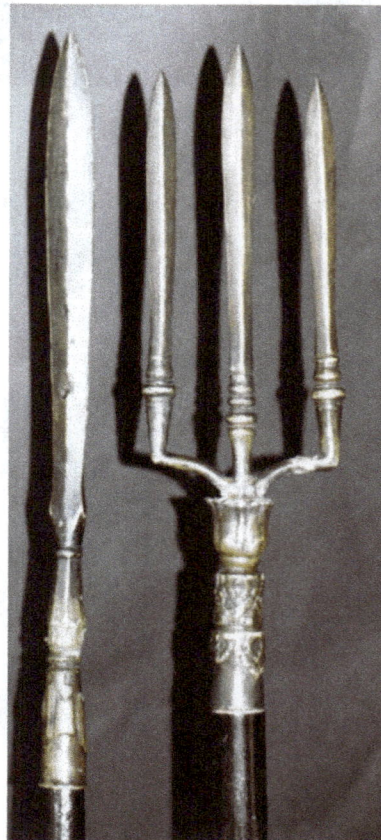

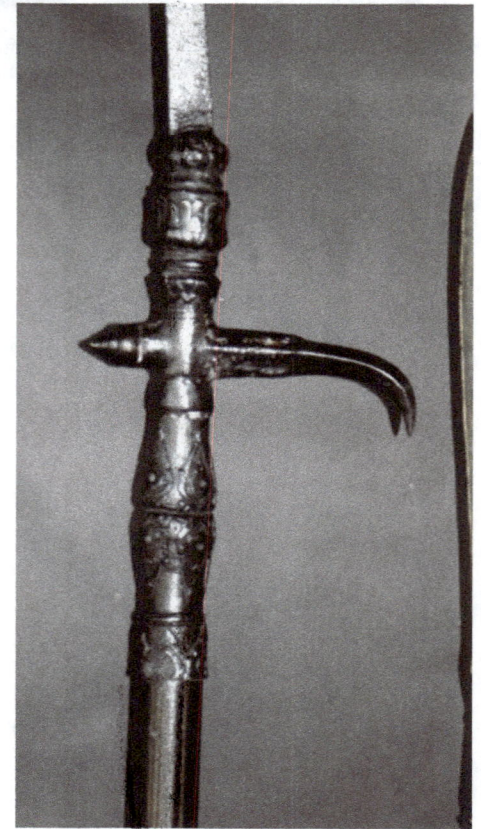

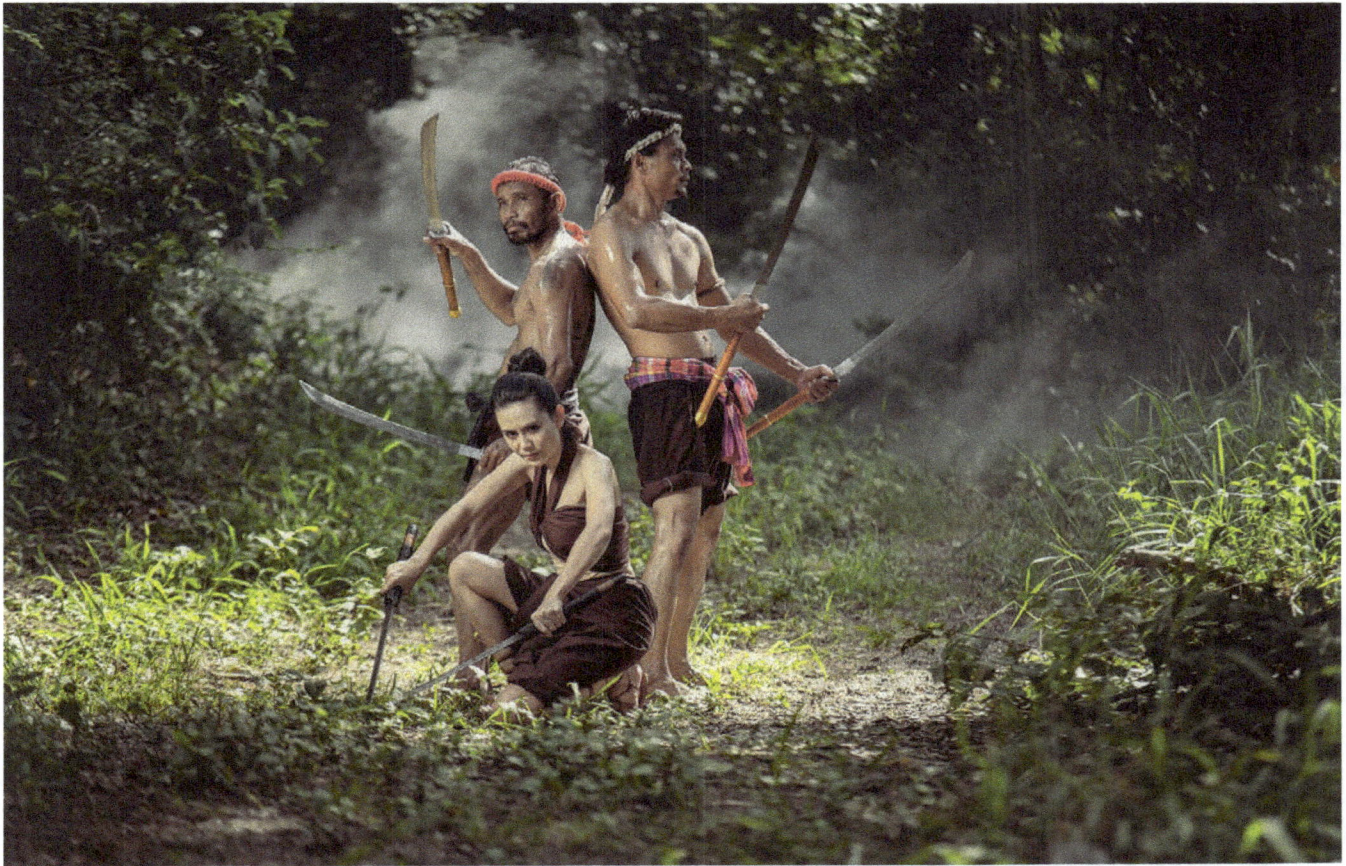

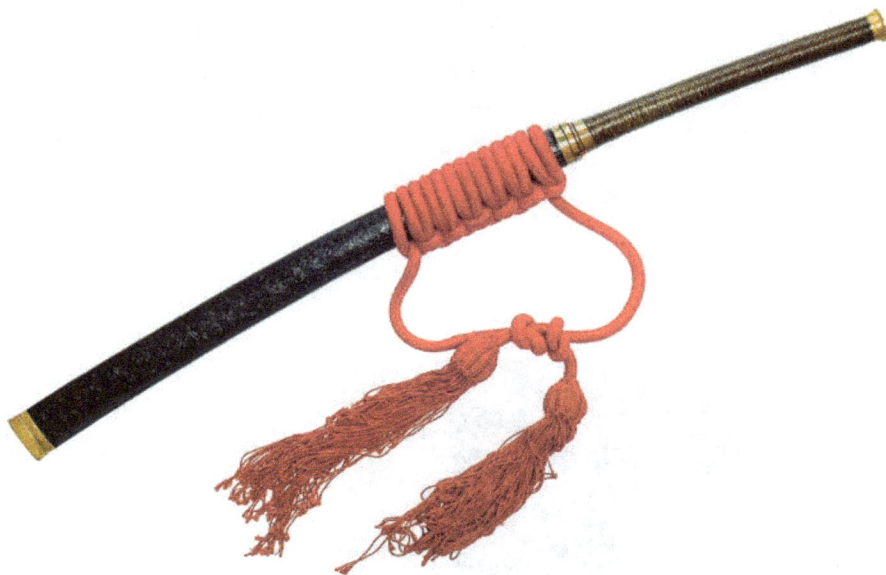

The Classic Thai Traditional"Dha/ Deo or Daap" is unique, elegant, well crafted by hand and deadly.

Dap Song Myrr Deo, Paired swords from Buddhai Sawan Collection.

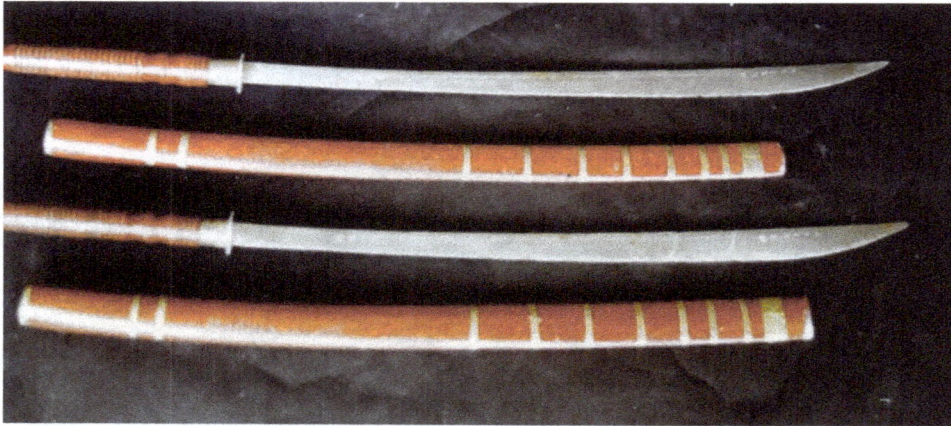

Below pict: With Phaa Kruu watching, Buddhai Sawan Kruu and seniors spar with steel swords.

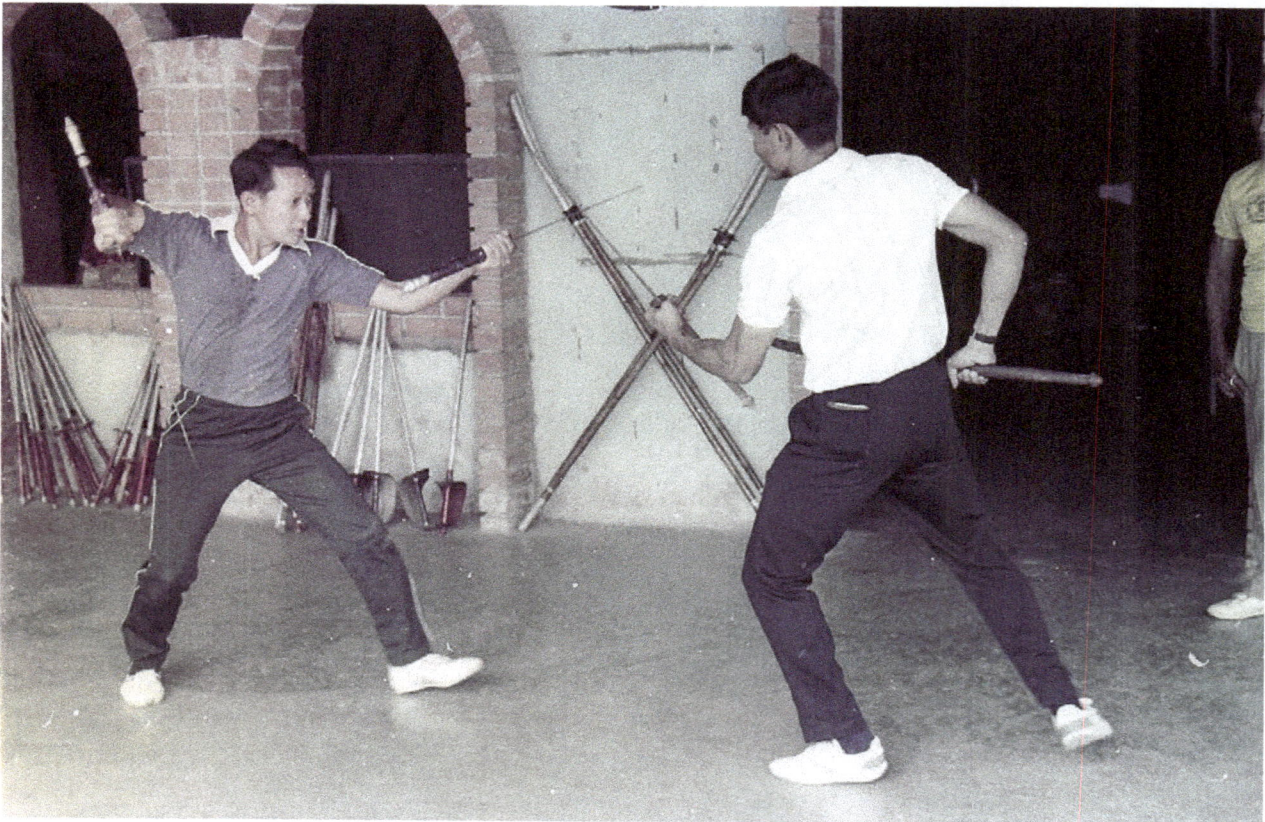

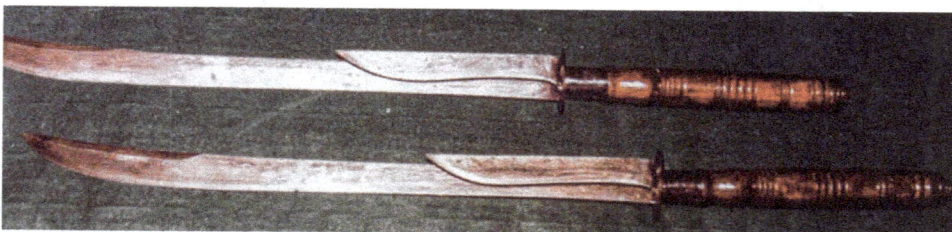

Rare Sword and Knife Comination, heavy Deo.

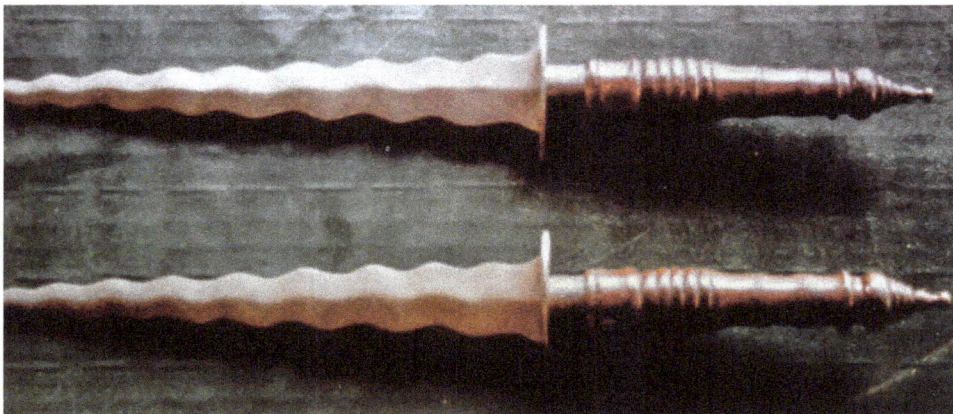

Thai Double "Kris" or Flame edged daggars. Southern style according to Phaa Kruu.

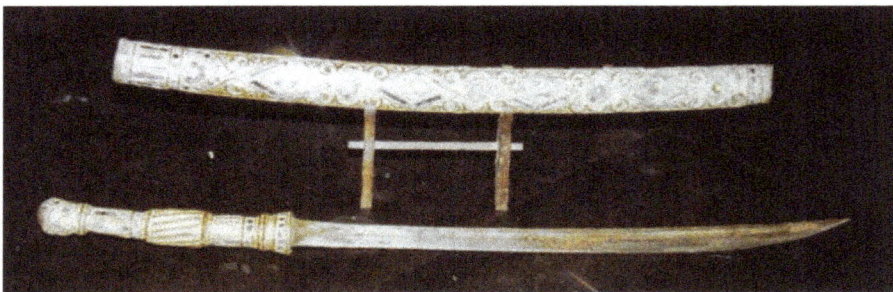

Decorative short Dhap-Dep

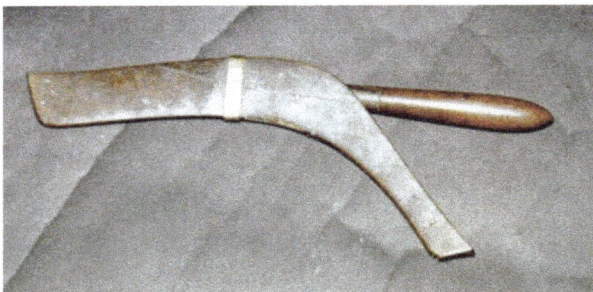

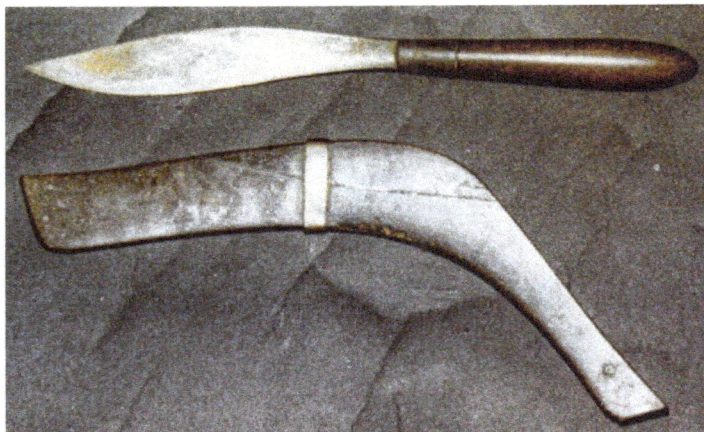

Traditional Leaf shaped Knife "Puab Meet" with fitted scabbard. Note shape of scabbard to secure or give purchase when tucked into or worn in the sash or belt.

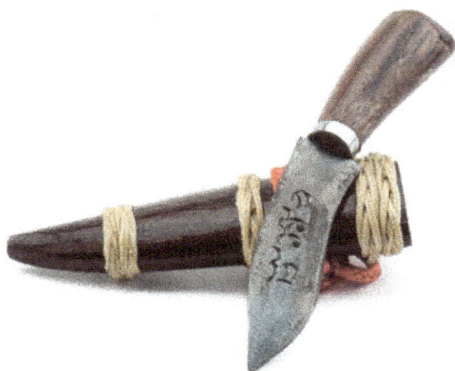

Another traditional Thai knife "Meet" with fitted scabbard.

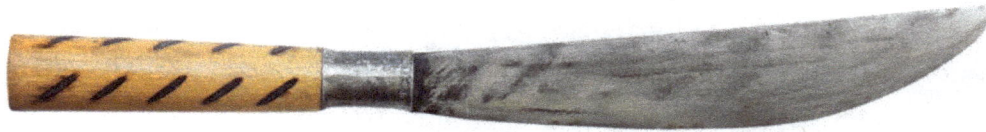

*Common Thai style 11"
Machete "Eee-knep" used
for farming and fighting.
Heavier than it looks at first
pass.*

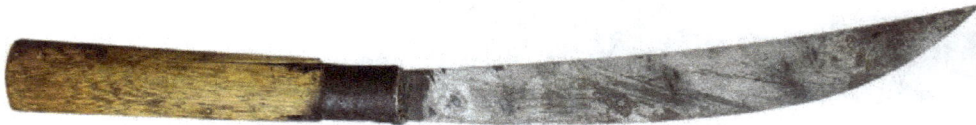

*Thai 11" to 14" Farmers
Knife. All pourpose*

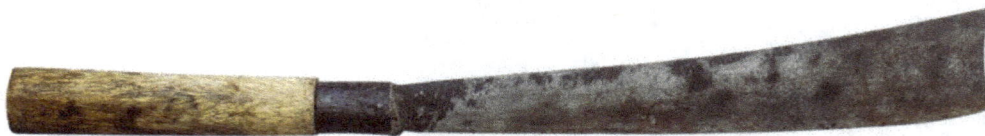

Machete variant: 11" to 14"
Thai "*Larp- Laap- laab*" is
more common in the north
and popular with Hill Tribe
people.

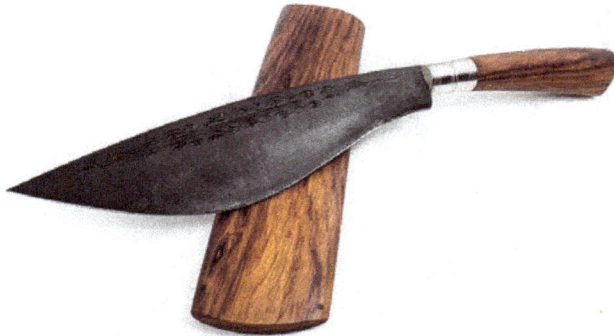

11" Blade Eee-knep with fitted scabbard

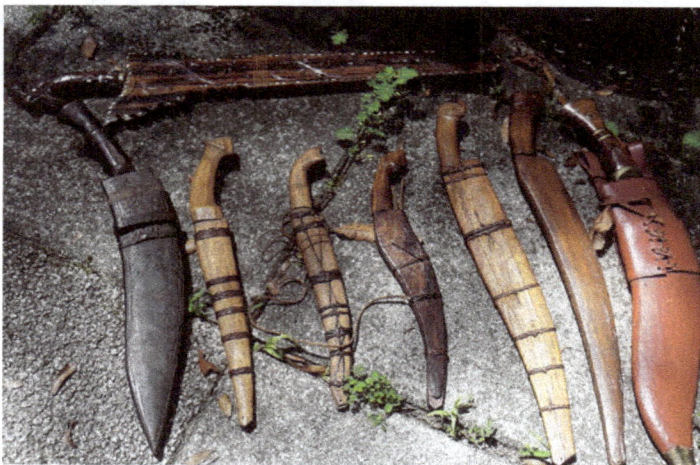

These weapons were obtained in Thailand, but their
designs and manufacture are clearly originating in Nepal,
Myanmar (Burma), Malaysia, Indonesia and Phillipines.
We see the Kukri, Kalis and Parang variations from 20"
to 11". Most are pre. 20th. Century origin except for the
"Officers Kukri" which was given to me by GM Dr. U
Maung Gyi is 1986.

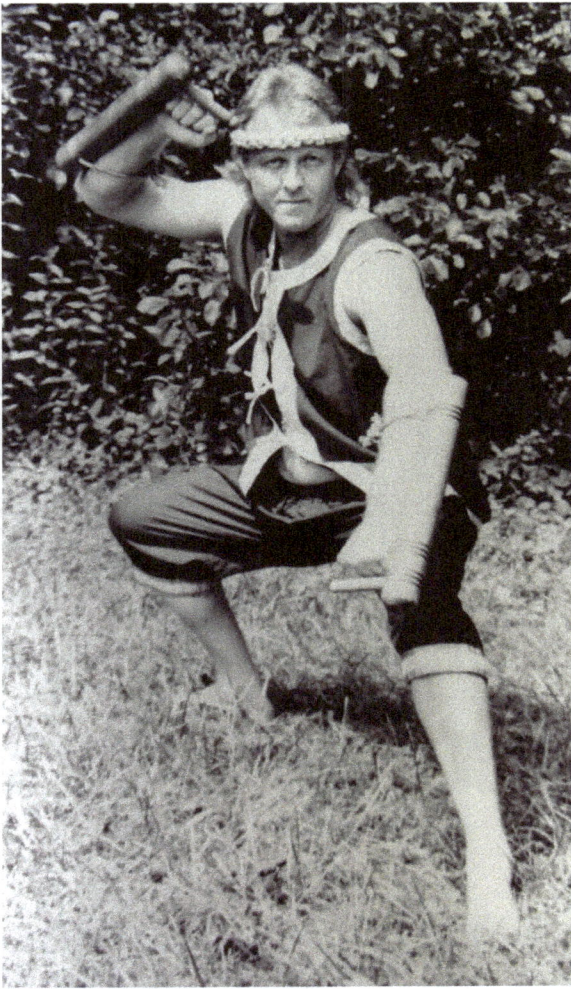

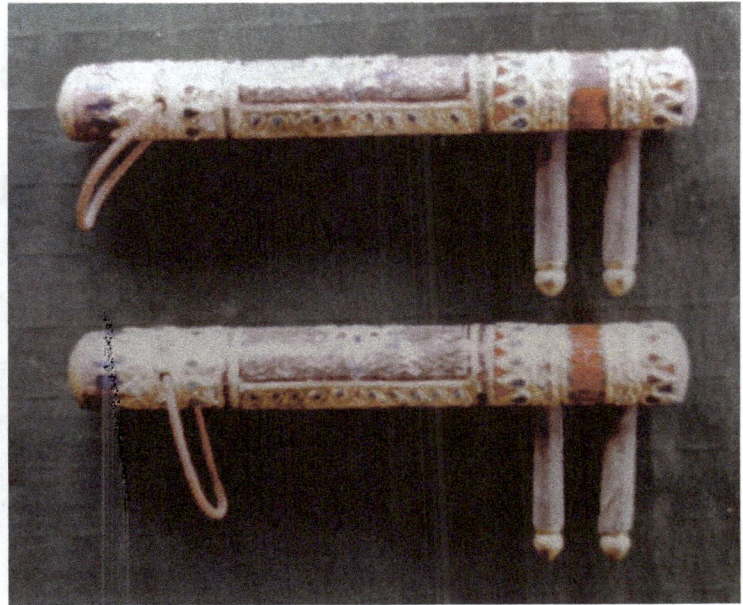

Mae Sowk, versitile and functional!

Buddhai Sawan Thailand, Kruu Jira Mesamarn wearing period appropriate attire for fighting. Light leather armor, forearm protection, lower leg protection holding a large Dhap-Deo. Photo courtesy Jira Mesamarn ©2022

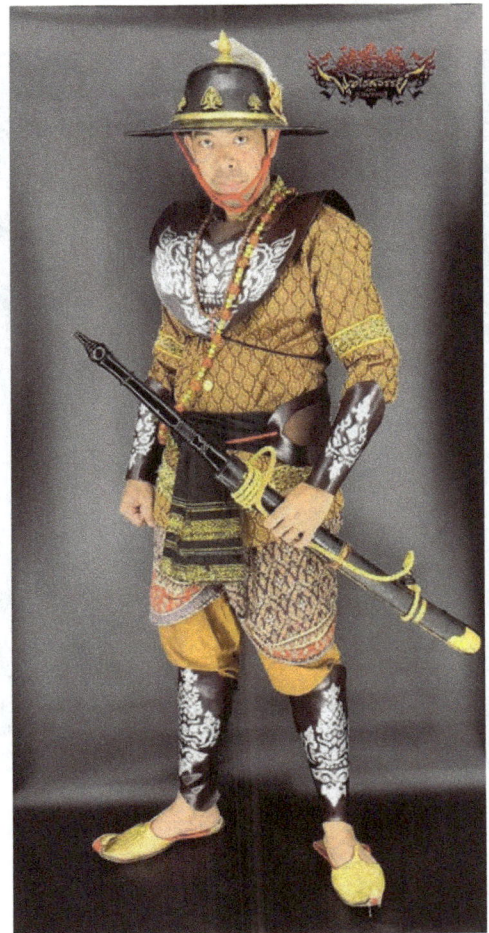

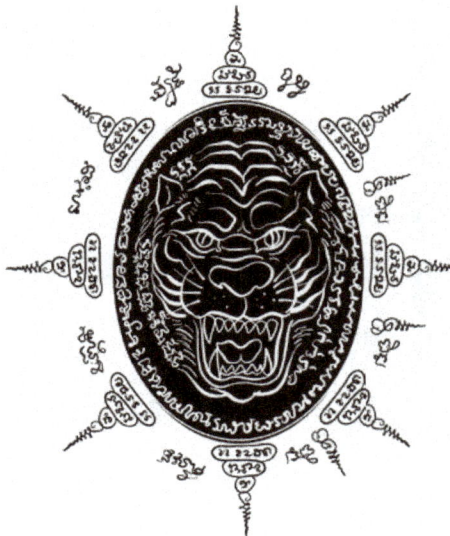

Shields and Helmets

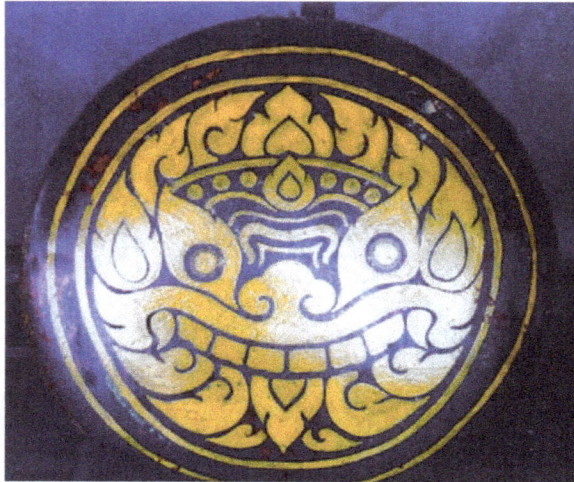

Buddhai Sawan Large Round Shield "Lo" and narrow rectangle shield "Ken"

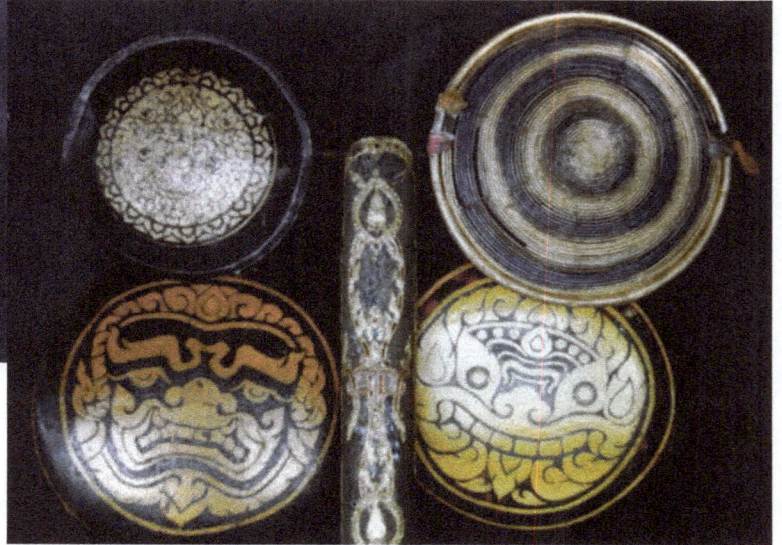

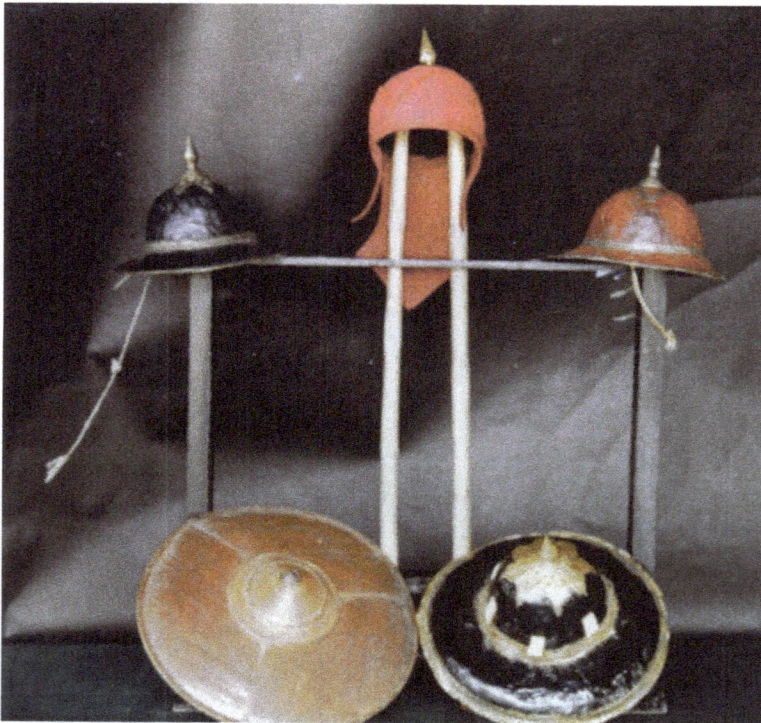

Buddhai Sawan collection of traditional head wear... Phaa khruu used to call them "Fighting Hats"!

Miscellaneous Traing Equipment

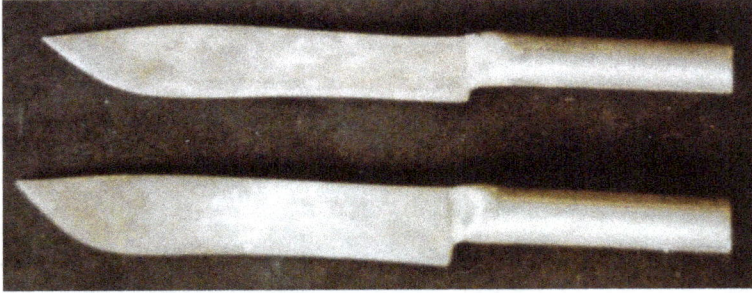

The infamous Thai Throwing Knife-Knives!

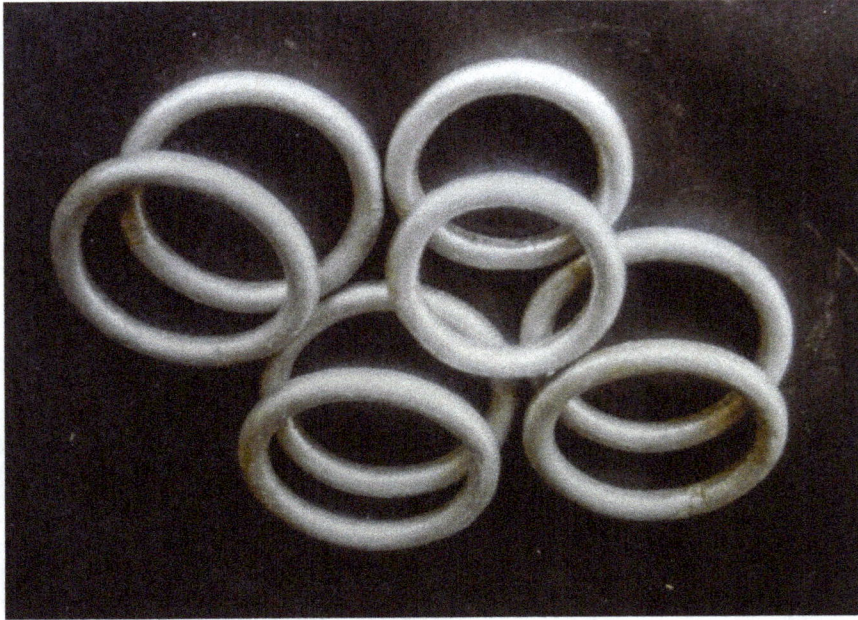

Heavy Steel Rings, worn on the arms during drills to build strength and control.

They also have a conditioning effect on the forearms and shoulders. Try it!

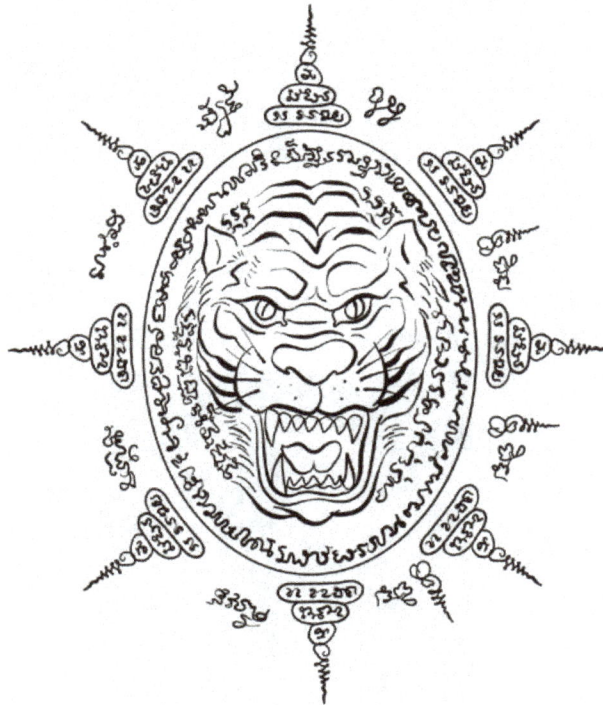

Imported Weapon Styles

Burmese

Burmese "*Dha*" – Popular on the border as it is easy to find!

Burmese "*Kukri*" – Favored short sword or long leaf shaped knife of the Burmese Hindu Gurkha warriors from Northern Burma. with a sharp point with scabbard. (Wood or Rattan)

Cambodian *Dao* – Similar to Burmese "*Dha*" but with no separate guard (Japanese "*Tsuki*") for the hand. The handle simply flares a bit to offer some additional protection. Generally carried in a set of one long and one short as in the Japanese style.

Chinese - All! Too many to list! See Thai History.

Japanese - *Tachi, Katana (Uchigatana), Wakizashi, Tanto, Nakiwara, Yari, Naginata, Nagamaki, Tsurugi, Tsukubo, Bo, Joken,* Spears, throwing, threshing weapons etc. Basically anything a Japanese Samurai (Elite Warrior / Soldier) would or could use.

Javanese (Malay, Indonesian) "*Kris*" (wavy blade), "*Kalis*" (Wavy on handle end and straight from the middle forwards)

Lao "*Dha*", similar to both Cambodian and Thai Swords

Phillipines- Filipino - Any and all as imported or traded through the archepelego's. "*Barong, Parang, Ginunting, Pinute, Talibong, Dahon Palay, Garab, Dagga, Sansibar, Panabas, Kampilan, Gayang, Janap, Binakuko, Pinsawali, Balasiong, Utak, Puyal*" etc.

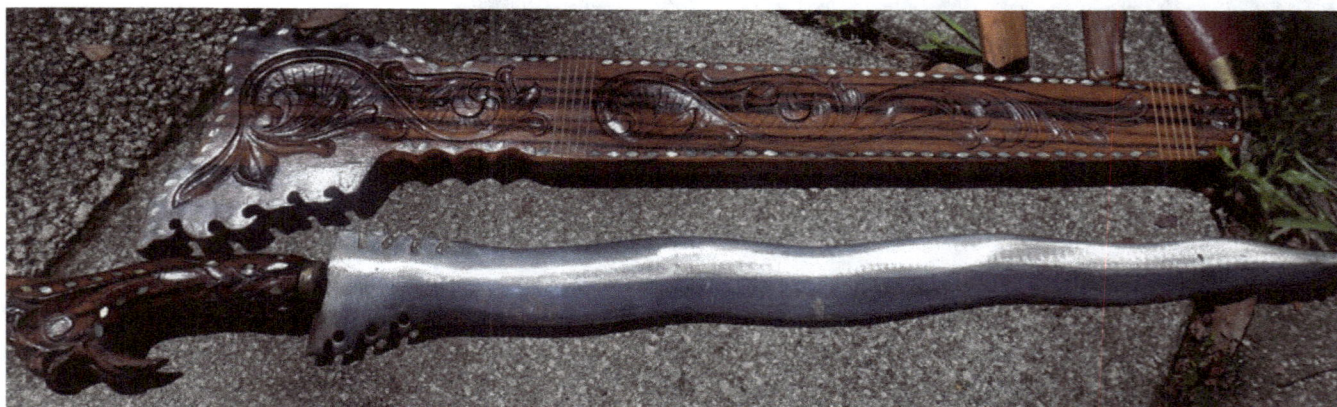

Above Photo: From my collection. Antique Moro Filipino "Kalis" with detailed blade and ornate, carved perl inlaid, stylistic handle with perl inlaid, intricately carved rare wood scabbard. Found in Thailand! The ,25 by 20" steel blade is deceptively heavy. The over all design is made to be "fast", close quarter, double edged, weapon with thrusting and close quarter use the base of the blade for deflection and or "raking" the opponent extremeties.

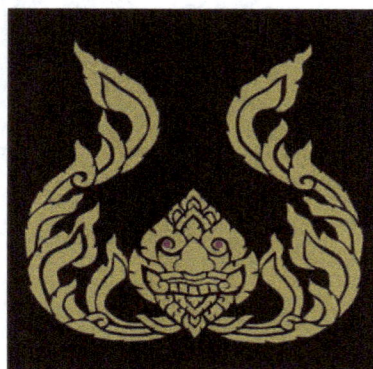

Thai Customs

The watch words for customs in Thailand, or do's and don'ts if you will, are courtesy and respect for others. You cannot be too polite. Thai people are polite, cheerful, and alert. Friendliness and honest expression are national characteristics. "Wealth in Thailand is measured by the number of your friends." Older people receive respect and deference.

Instead of the handshake, the Thai have the "wai." It is the traditional Buddhist greeting. It means "the spirit within me greets or pays respect to the spirit that is within you." Place the hands together in a praying attitude and bow the head. Touch the forehead with your fingers. This may signify respect, thanks, or apology. Failure to return a "wai." is similar to refusing to shake hands.

As a culture, the Thai people revere their religion. Do not make fun of their Buddha's or unnecessarily touch or even photograph them without permission.

The head of the Thai is a sacred part of the body. Do not touch the head! It is best to stay away from the shoulders and upper back as well. The head is where they say the spirit dwells. It is an insult to bring a lower part of the body--say your hand--into contact with a higher part of a Thai's. Back-slapping and head-rubbing are out except among close family and friends. It is also improper to stand over a seated Thai when speaking to him.

The feet are the lowest part of the body and have the least spiritual significance. It is improper to touch someone with your feet, even to sit with your legs crossed and pointed toward them. It is rude to stomp your feet or move something with them.

The doorway or entrance to a Thai household is guarded by a spirit, they say. Step over the sill, not on it. Thais, like the Japanese, do not wear shoes in their house so remove yours just outside or inside the door as appropriate for where you are. If you are not sure whether to wear or take off your shoes? Simply pause a moment, look to see where others place their shoes, and then do likewise.

Boisterousness, yelling, loud and obnoxious behavior, and swearing are looked upon as crude by all but the lower class.

Never give a Thai a knife or edged weapon as a gift. It is considered bad luck. You may, however, exchange it for some token.

The Royal Family, especially the King and Queen, are highly revered. Criticism of them in a disrespectful manner is the quickest way to lose friends.

Thai Krabi Krabong/ Muay Boran/ Muay Chaiya/ Muay Thai Vocabulary

(Thai to English: This list is Not inclusive!)

Ao - Elbow

Ayudhya - Old-time Capital of Thailand

Bai Oi - Long straight spear, double edged

Bai Pai - Small broad bladed spear

Bangkok - Modern Capital of Thailand

Bata - Cross or "x" block

Bplong/ Plong - Staff or long pole

Buddhai Swan - Buddha's Heaven

Buok - Inward shin block

Chai - Okay, "Got it!", Yes!

Chakri - Three-pointed spear; name of famous Thai Dynasty

Chat Lay Yak - Fighting distance or measure

Ching - Finger cymbals

Chok - Straight punch (Jab or Cross) with one hand

Dang - Narrow rectangular shield held with one hand

Dap Myrr Deo - Thai Sword, Single sword, long handle

Dap Song Myrr Deo - Double Thai Sword (One in each hand)

Diichan Sa Bye Dee - I am fine… Female

Diichan Chua - My name is. . . .

Djab Ko – Grappling (Similar to Combat Japanese Jiu-Jitsu)

Djong Yan - Round kick to thighs

Dtaa - Eye

Dtee - Hitting

Dtee Mat - Punching with the fist

Dtoi Lorn - Boxing with the wind; shadow boxing

Dtoi - Boxing

Fan Sa Pai Lang - Double sword sweeps

Fet Rao - Knockout; KO

Gai Luang Sai - Bird Bites the Stomach

Got Tuan - Short lance for horseback (Mongolian Lance- spear with rope)

Haw Kwan - Pole axe with spike

Haw Phoo - Long lance for horseback

Hok Sak Myrr - Short lance with tassel

Hok Bai Pai - Big broad-bladed spear

Hong Peek Hak - Bird with broken wing

Hua - Head

Huab Pan Lak - Buffalo passes the tree

Huang - Iron rings

Hy - Back; to rear

Jara Ka Kwan Klong - Crocodile Stops In River

Join Kao - Jumping knee

Ka - Knee joint

Kaak - Outward shin block

Krabi – Saber, Long arms, Pole arms, Long sticks, Spears, or any similar weapon.

Krabi Krabong - Nine Weapon Systems, Sword and spear, short and long weapons and the empty-hand arts that go with them.

Kao - Knee attack or technique

Kaw - Neck

Kaw Sap Chang - Elephant mace, Erewan Hammer, a type of club.

Kaw Tot - Excuse me

Ken - Rectangular shield

Khrap - (Thai slang: Male-Khrap, Yes) (Kaa… Yes, Female)

Khrap Khun - Thank you

Kruu - Teacher

Khun Chia Ari - What is your name?

Khun Sa Bye Dee Rue? - How are you?

Klong Kack - Seated drum

Kong Ao - Elephant spike

Kradot Kao - Flying knee

Kradot - To jump

Kradot-te - Jump round kick

Kruang Rang – Tiny Buddha image worn on bicep by Muay Boran / Muay Thai fighters.

Kruan Kratoop Fuan - Wave rolling or flowing

Ksum - Fighting stance

Kwan- Spirit or spiritual entity, your spirit, or the spirit of your Knee etc.

Kwang Puab - Diagonally Cut the Lotus Kwan - Long-handled ax

Len Chen - Sparring; controlled fighting with wood or steel swords.

Lerd Rit - Combat empty-hand; extreme power

Lo - Small round shield Loke - Advance

Lokewan - Spinning advance

Lu Rom - Street fighting, not nice… no rules, quick disable

Mai - No

Manora - Thai classical dance

Mat Aat - Uppercut punch

Mat Deo - Punch with the sword

Mat Drong - Straight punch or cross

Mat Tong - Hooking punch, Similar to Western Boxing Hook

Mon Kon Chon Gao - Little animal cuts the jewel

My Sok – Wooden short with handle and finger guard, Forearm shield with rope loop, used for blocking or striking

My Tat Dot - Hand stick, "*Yakiwara*". May be pointed or blunt, various lengths, sometimes carved and decorated.

Nakrian - Student

Nao Ciin - Chinese-style broad spear

Nao Krabong - Thai spear

Phaa Kruu - Master; Father/teacher… The "Old Man"

Phom Sa Bye Dee - I am fine… Male

Phom Chua - My name is. . . .

Pi - Javanese flute

Pii- Spirit

Pii Baan – Thai Spirit House, God's House, Belongs to spirits of the land.

Plong – Staff… A long pole

Puab Pang Pai - Lotus shield

Puab Salaat Baaj - Flower of the leaf blown in the wind.

Ranat-ek - A xylophone-type musical instrument played during BSKK performances.

Rap - Wall defense

Rongrian - School

Sak Yant- Sacred, Magic Tattoo

Samnan - Three-knife spear, Triangle shaped blade.

Sa Wat Dii Khrap – Hello! Wai and nod head when speaking to be polite.

Sok - Elbow strike

Sok Kun - Rising elbow strike

Sok Lun - Downward elbow strike

Sok Trong - Hook or side elbow

Tai Hon/ Yai Tai Hon - Elephant drum, Giant double headed Chinese style War drum, also used on back of Elephants to guide and cadence infantry- cavalry on the battlefield. Used today in BSKK practice and performance.

Te - Thai round kick

Thum - Throwing/sweeping techniques

Tiip - Front kick, side kick

Ting - Throw

Toi - Retreat

To Mon - Three-pointed Thai spear, Chakri spear

Ying Ded - Bow and arrow for archery

Wang - Inward swing

Wat - Temple or church

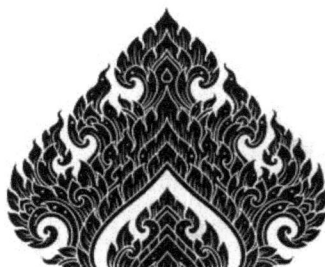

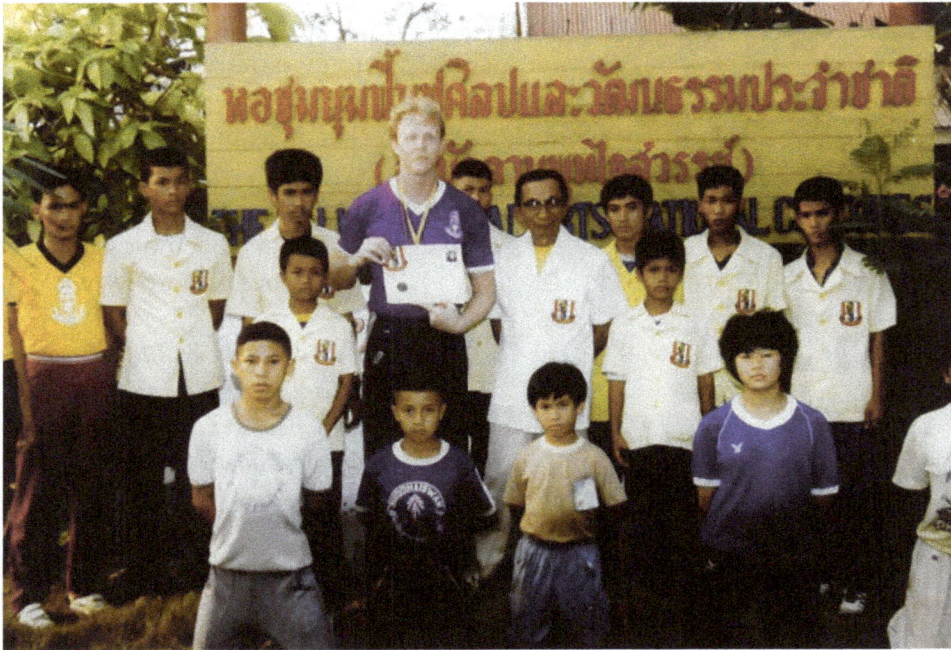

Miscellaneous Photo with "The Gang" and I standing in front of Buddhai Sawan Cultural Center sign, Nongkam, Thailand.

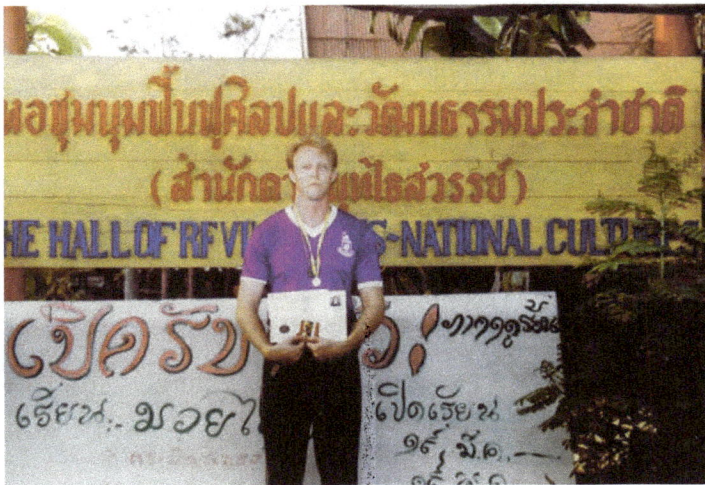

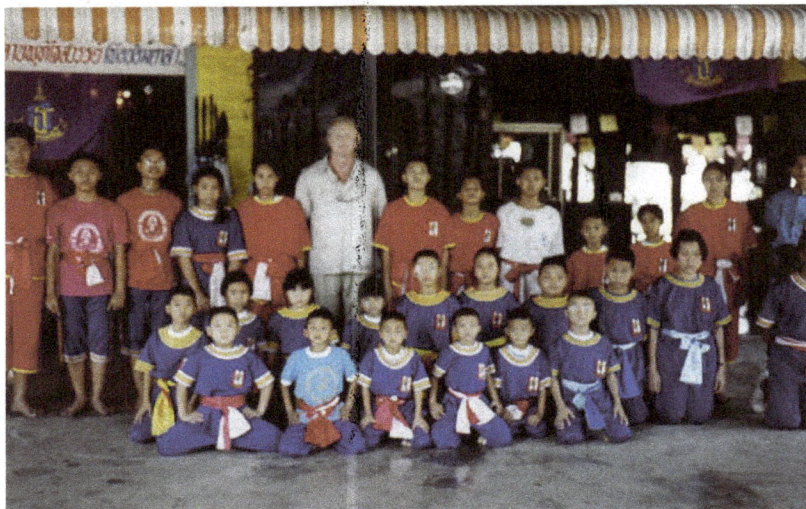

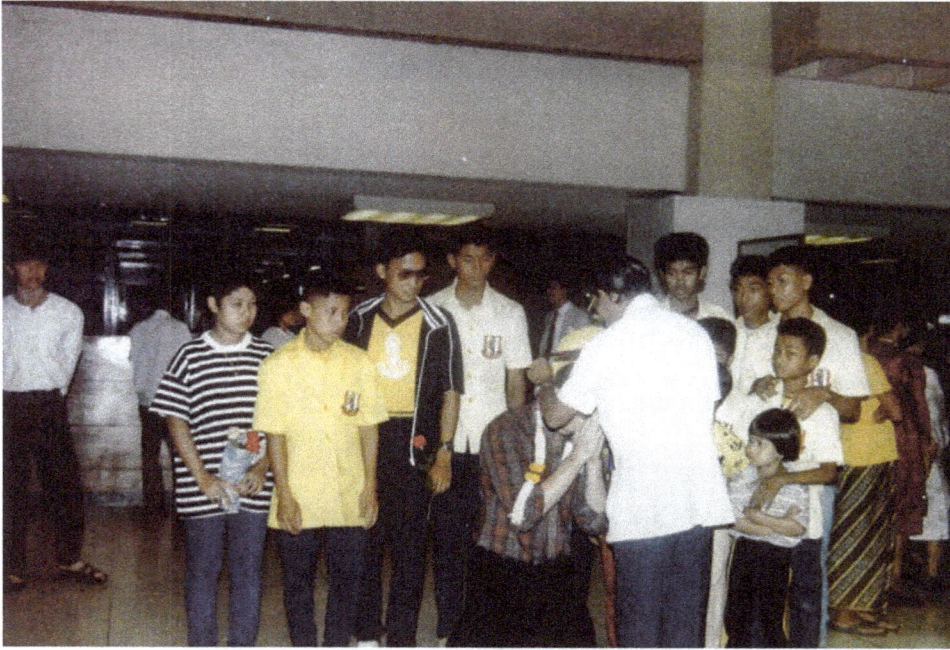

GM Phaa Kruu Samaii and fellow students escorted me to airport. Phaa Kruu wanted to give me a formal blessing on my departure to USA. This was the las time I was with him before he passed. I treasure this moment and truly have been blessed since that time in so many ways!

Below: My room. After I became a "Kruu" I was upgraded to a corner suite! Later I heard a flushing toilet was added! I was soo jealous!

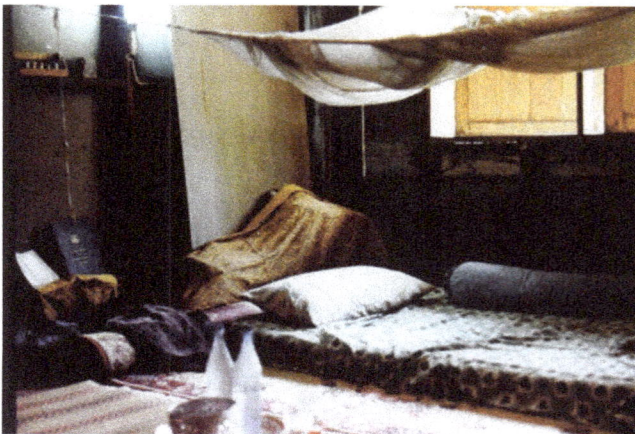

I was quite happy and comfortable to share space with the interesting alter. It was facinating and an honor to be thought of to sleep next to it. After having spent time in the community "Dorm" it was a luxery.

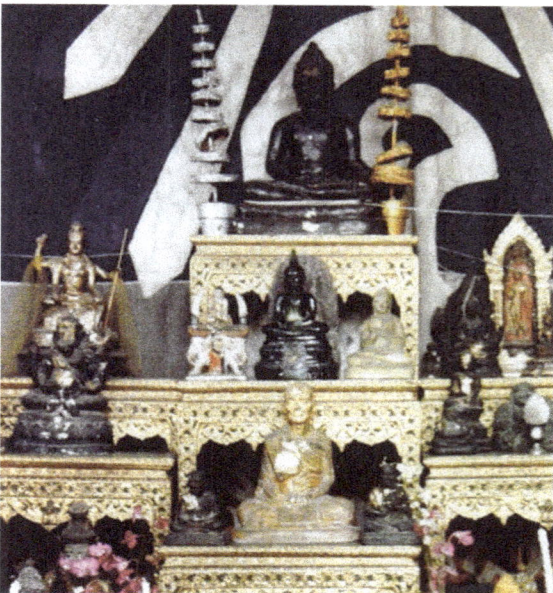

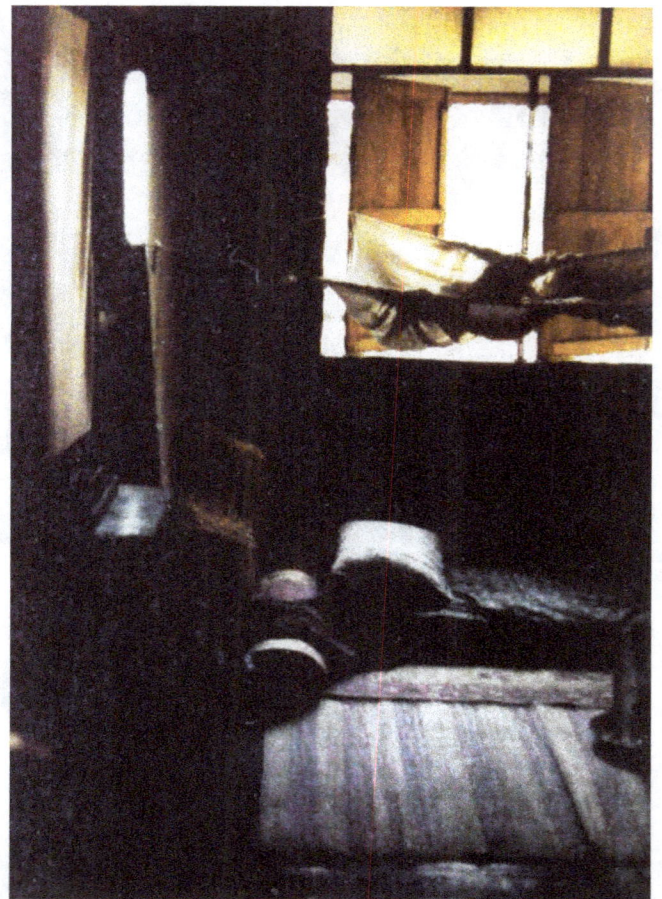

Medicine Teachings of Buddhai Sawan Traditional Krabi Krabong

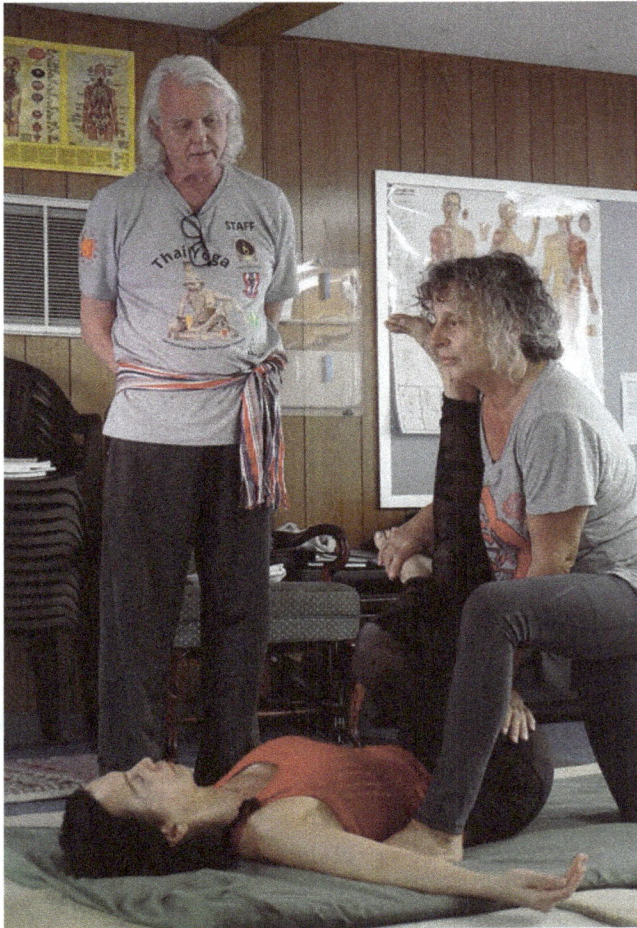

Nuad Phaen Boran Thai: Ayurveda, Indigenous Traditional Thai Medicine and Yoga Therapy is strongly based on Classical Indian Ayurveda. The Indigenous medicine systems of India (Ayurveda, Yoga) have been practiced in one form or another in the land we call Thailand longer than the land has been called Thailand. This comprehensive textbook covers the fundamental theories and philosophy of Traditional Thai Medicine.

The specific *"Ryksaa Thang Nuad Phaen Boran Thai"* style practiced at Buddhai Sawan, Nongkam was based heavily on the style of traditional Thai Ayurveda and Medicine as taught at the Pra Wat Chetuphon Traditional Thai Medical Massage school centrally located at Wat Po in Bangkok. However, this so-called "Royal" or "Southern" style was taught in many temples from North to far South.

Today in Thailand, it could be that of the nearest Budhist and or traditional medicine center to the schools current location.

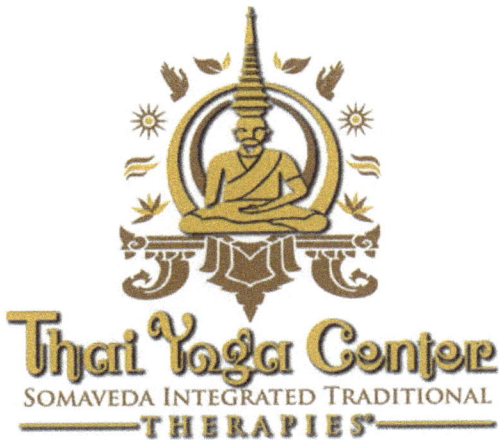

US Thai Yoga Center...
https://thaiyogacenter.com

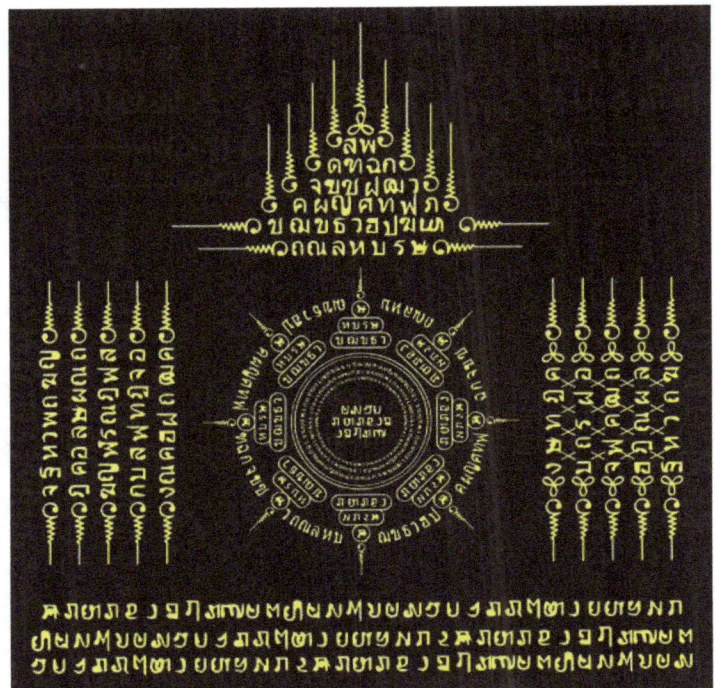

Where can I learn or train in Buddhai Sawan Krabi Krabong?

Buddhai Sawan USA (BSANA): https://buddhaisawan.org
Monsoon Society http://monsoonsociety.org/

Ajahn's & *"Kruu"* Currently Teaching: USA

1)	Ajahn, Dr. Anthony B. James (BSKK classes are usually part of ongoing SomaVeda® Thai Yoga & Ayurveda Certification Programs at The Thai Yoga Center in Brooksville, Florida… https://thaiyogacenter.com
2)	Ajahn, Steve Wilson: Mount Vernon, WA USA
3)	Ajahn Arlan Sanford: Santa Fe, NM USA
4)	Ajahn Jason Webster: Austin, TX USA : Ambush Muay Thai: https://www.ambushmuaythai.com
5)	Guro Kruu, Danny Inosanto: Inosanto Academy, Los Angeles, CA USA … https://inosanto.com/
6)	Ajahn Michael DeLio: Combative Fighting Arts: Hunting Beach, CA USA. http://www.combative-fightingarts.com/index.html
7)	Kruu Pat Gagnon, Ass. Kruu Rob Farr: Burlington, VT. USA Green Mountain Martial Arts. https://greenmountainmartialarts.com
8)	Ass. Kruu Jeff Ippolito: Boston, MA USA https://www.newenglandwarriorarts.com/
9)	Kruu Pablo Sanchez: Santa Fe, NM USA
10)	Kruu Eric Wong: Albuquerque, NM USA

Canada:

1) Khruu Loki Jorgenson, Ass. Khruu Gary "Pat" Gagnon, Ass. Khruu Nathalie Prevost, Asst. Khruu Chris Goard, Asst. Khru Brett Simms, Asst. Khruu Stuart Hill, Asst. Khruu Taran Rallings: Maelstrom Martial Arts: https://maelstromcore.com/

United Kingdom

Ajahn Tony Moore: Sitisiam Camp: Manchester, England: http://buddhai-swan.com/
Kruu Steven Moore / Kruu Gian Leganegro
Germany
1)	Ajahn Ralf Kussler: Thai Achira in Dülmen, near Münster: http://www.muay-chaiya.de/

Thailand

Original Temple Wat Buddhai Sawan (Wat Phuttai Sawan):
Buddhai Sawan Chapel: https://artsandculture.google.com/streetview/buddhaisawan-chapel/mQGW2A3j-3KwLA?sv_lng=100.4922203646394&sv_lat=13.7578684980997&sv_h=272.9781731048455&sv_p=-1.4653956267422217&sv_pid=3lMyB0h4yQ4AAAQrDW_eig&sv_z=0.7562044306354595

1)   Ajahn Pedro Solana: Muay Thai Sangha, Chiangmai, Thailand, https://muaythaisangha.com/, Muay Thai Sangha located just outside of Chiangmai City in Northern Thailand host instruction for both Thai and foreign students. Weekly and extended training, both live and Online are offered to visiting and or residential students. All levels are welcome. Muay Thai Sangha also offers Affiliate schools in Spain, Greece, Switzerland & USA.

2)   Yutha Phop Training Center: https://yuthaphop.com/buddhaisawan/
                Ajahn Khruu Nut and Jira Mesamarn, Ajahn Khru Sila Mesamarn

3)   Ajahn Kruu Kung: Samnak Sri Ayutthaya Chiang Mai Fencing Club

4)   Kruu Pol: (Yaowadee Paramee Snyder), who's also certify Kruu in Muay Chaiya from Baan Changthai, Bangkok, Thailand. Kruu Pol offers an interesting On-line training path. (https://krupolmuay-thai.com/)

Krabi Krabong & Related Books and Video's

1)   Documentary: "*Krabi Krabong: The Buddhai Sawan Path*" by Kruu Vincent Giordano: https://www.imdb.com/title/tt4015684/

2)   Textbook: "*Way of the Ancient Healers*" by Guro Virgil Apostle

3)   Textbook: "*Muay Boran: Pra Jao Seua, The Legendary Tiger Style: Volume 1*" by Ajahn Stuart Hurst and Kruu Neck Sema

4)   Old footage - Krabi-Krabong in Bangkok (1960): https://youtu.be/TuwXeK9qYeA

Where To Locate Krabi Krabong Swords and Weapons for Training

Of course, you can still find and purchase swords and traditional weapons of every type and price range in Thailand today. There are areas where the manufacture of such weapons, both genuine and for decorations, have been ongoing for several generations. Previously I mentioned the "*Wienlak*" neighborhood of Ayudthaya. "*Thunquian*" Market in Chiangrai has in the past had quite a good collection of unique handmade weapons for many years.

There is also now due to the increased popularity of Krabi Krabong martial art worldwide, an increase in access and availability of good quality practice weapons including wood, Rattan, steel, and not composite materials such as nylon.

Even large US manufacturers such as Cold Steel make "Thai" weapons such as the "*Dhap/ Daab*". They call them "All-purpose Tactical Machete" and the "Thai Machete with Sheath". They also offer a "Medieval Buckler" small round shield which is suitable for training as well.

Check out Amazon.com for Thai weapons, including decorative replicas and practice weapons of various quality.

1.	Siam Blades: Made by Ajahn Boontan Sitipaisal (High Quality): https://siamblades.com/blogs/news/the-last-ancient-swordsmith-of-thailand
2.	Reliks: Banshee Sword: By Paul Chen: Hanwei: Thai Krabi/ Burmese Dha Style (High Quality) https://www.reliks.com/functional-japanese-swords/banshee-sword/
3.	Caslberia: Banshee Sword: Many weapons: Paul Chen Designs: (High Quality): https://casiberia.com/product/banshee-sword/sh2126
4.

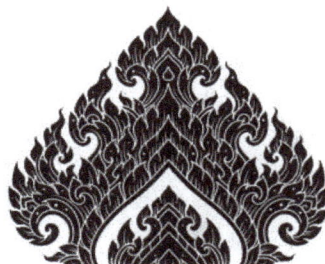

Appendix: Thai and Ayurveda Specific Bibliography

(Courtesy of "Ayurveda and Thai Yoga: Religious Therapeutics Theory and Practice" by Author Ajahn Dr. Anthony B. James, Meta Journal Press: 2017, Brooksville, FL USA ISBN: 978-1-886338-28-9)

[1] James, Anthony B.1983, Nuat Thai, Traditional Thai Medical Massage, Meta Journal Press, Atlanta Georgia, USA 140 pgs.

[2] Brun and Schumacher: "Traditional Herbal Medicine in Northern Thailand": 1994 edition, White Lotus, Bangkok, Thailand.

[3] Barbara Andaya, "Political Development between the Sixteenth and Eighteenth Centuries" in The Cambridge History of Southeast Asia, Volume One, Part Two, from c.1500 to c.1800 (Singapore: Cambridge University Press, 1992), 66-67.

[4] Anthony Reid, Southeast Asia in the Age of Commerce 1450-1680—Volume Two, Expansion and Crisis (New Haven and London: Yale University Press, 1993), 69.

[5] David Wyatt, Thailand: A Short History (New Haven and London: Yale University Press, 1982), 104.

[6] William A. R. Wood, A History of Siam (Bangkok: Chalermnit Bookshop, 1959), 146.

[7] http://www.samurai-archives.com/jia.html

[8] Seiichi Iwao, editor, and translator. Jeremias van Vliet Historiael verhael der Sieckte Ende (Tokyo: The Toyo Bunko, 1958) vii-viii.

[9] Kennon Breazeale, "Thai Maritime Trade and the Ministry Responsible" in From Japan to Arabia: Ayutthaya's Maritime Relations with Asia (Bangkok: Printing House of Thammasat University, 1999), 7.

[10] Barbara Andaya, "Political Development between the Sixteenth and Eighteenth Centuries" in The Cambridge History of Southeast Asia, Volume One, Part Two, from c.1500 to c.1800 (Singapore: Cambridge University Press, 1992), 66-67.

[11] Khien Theeravit, "Japanese-Siamese Relations 1606-1629: in Chavit Khamchoo and Reynolds Thai-Japanese Relations in Historical Perspective (Bangkok, Innomedia Co. Ltd., 1988), 19.

[12] Jivaka-Komarabhacca in Pali Cannon: http://www.palikanon.com/english/pali_names/j/jiivaka

[13] Jivaka called "*Komarabhaca*": "The treatment of infants", VT.ii.174; in Dvy. (506-18)

[14} Jivaka: http://nalanda-insatiableinoffering.blogspot.com/2010/06/jivaka-amravana.html

[15] Jivaka name documented in Pali Cannon: Studies in Traditional Indian Medicine in the Pāli Canon: Jīvaka and ayurveda", (Kenneth G. Zysk, Journal of the International Association of Buddhist Studies 5, pp. 309–13, 1982)

[16] Jivaka: "Giving of Robes" (Vin.i.268-81; AA.i.216)

[17] Jivaka treats Buddha's ailments: Buddha reads Jivaka's thoughts and bathed as required: Vin.i.279f; DhA. (ii.164f)

[18] Jivaka declared by the Buddha chief among his lay followers loved by the people (aggam puggalappasannānam) (A.i.26)

[19] Jivaka included in a list of good men who have been assured of the realization of deathlessness (A.iii.451; DhA.i.244, 247; J.i.116f)

[20] Jivaka and Vejjavatapada: In the seven articles, excerpts from four passages in the Pali canon, the Buddha lays down the attitudes and skills which would make "one who would wait on the sick qualified to nurse the sick." "Doctors Code of Conduct": Anguttara Nikaya III, p.144 (The Vejjavatapada likely predates the Greek Hippocratic Oath.)

[21] Provide for the sick: Brahma Net Sutra, STCUSC, New York, 1998, VI,9.

[22] Traditional Medicine in Kingdom of Thailand: http://www.searo.who.int/entity/medicines/topics/traditional_medicines_in_the_kingdom_of_thailand.pdf?ua=1

[23] Traditional knowledge and traditional medicine:

https://www.wto.org/english/tratop_e/trips_e/trilatweb_e/ch2d_trilat_web_13_e.htm

[24] Ministry of Public Health also controls the curricula of the institutions which provides teaching and practicing of Thai traditional medicine.: http://www.thailawforum.com/articles/Thai-traditional-medicine-protection-part1-3.html#64

[25] The efficacies of trance possession ritual performances in contemporary Thai Theravada Buddhism, p. 120: https://ore.exeter.ac.uk/repository/bitstream/handle/10871/15758/ChamchoyP_TPC.pdf?sequence=3&isAllowed=y

[26] The Use of Traditional Medicine in the Thai Health Care System: P. 146: http://thaiyogacenter.com/wp-content/uploads/2017/05/Thai-Healthcare.pdf

[27] Ayurveda of Thailand: Anthony B. James, Meta Journal Press, Brooksville, FL 34602, 2016

[27] The Role of Thai Traditional Medicine in Health Promotion: Vichai Chokevivat, M.D., M.P.H. and Anchalee Chuthaputti, Ph.D. Department for the Development of Thai Traditional and Alternative Medicine, Ministry of Public Health, Thailand

[28] Ban Chiang Archaeological Site: http://whc.unesco.org/en/list/575

[29] Kennon Breazeale, "Thai Maritime Trade and the Ministry Responsible" in From Japan to Arabia: Ayutthaya's Maritime Relations with Asia (Bangkok: Printing House of Thammasat University, 1999), 7.[30] Legal Status of Traditional Medicine and Complementary/ Alternative Medicine: A Worldwide Review: Thailand: Kennon Breazeale, "Thai Maritime Trade and the Ministry Responsible" in From Japan to Arabia: Ayutthaya's Maritime Relations with Asia (Bangkok: Printing House of Thammasat University, 1999), 7.

[31] Vichi Chockevivat and Anchalee Chuthaputti, 'The Role of Thai Traditional Medicine in Health Promotion' (Paper presented at the 6th Global Conference on Health Promotion, Bangkok, Thailand, 7-11 August 2005) 2.

[32] Angkor influenced Architecture in Thailand: http://www.hellosiam.com/html/Thailand/thailand-history.htm

[33] Traditional Thai Medicine: https://en.wikipedia.org/wiki/Traditional_Thai_medicine

[34] Ratarasarn, Somchintana. The Principles and Concepts of Thai classical medicine. Bangkok: Thai Khadi Research Institute, Thammasat University, 1986

[35] Beyer, C. 1907, Journal of the Siam Society, vol. 4, part 1:1-9 Bangkok, Thailand. The Siam Society. 9p.

[36] Hofbauer, Rudolf 1943 (Lecture delivered before the Thailand Research Society on 13 December 1942) Journal of the Siam Society, vol. 34, part 1:183-201 Bangkok, Thailand. The Siam Society. 19p.

[37] Bruce, Helen 1960 Nine Temples of Bangkok, Bangkok, Thailand. Progress Book Store Publishers. 93p

[38] Cunningham, Clark E, 1 970 Antibiotic Mediators In: Social Science & Medicine, vol.4, pp.1-24 England. Pergarnon Press. I 4p.

[39] Hinderling, Paul, 1972 Mit traditionellen Arzten Uber ErkIarungssysteme und Therapien. Aspekte der lnteraktion zwischen Arzten und Patlenten.[Folk medicine in Thailand - Interviews with traditional doctors about explanatory systems and therapies. Aspects of interaction between doctors and patients] Saarbrucken, Germany. Sozialpsychoi. Forschungsst. d. Univer. S. 140p

[40] Larr, Stephen, 1984 Bangkok's Other Massage Is an Euphoric Experience, If a Little Painful Bangkok Post, Bangkok, Thailand. Pp.

[41] Krungkrai Jenphanid, 1986 Traditional Thai Massage Therapy [in Thai]: • Lak phueen thaan kha'awng kaan nuad thai [Basics of Thai massage, Sp.] • Khunatham 16e jaryatham khaawng maaw nCiad thai [Qualities and ethics of the Thai massage doctor. 1p.] - In: A compilation of pirated text material Chiang Mai, Thailand. Old Medicine Hospital. Gp

[42] Krungkrai Jeenphaanid, 1986 Noad thai phua chiiwid mai [Thai Massage for a New Life, Status of Thai Massage Today] In: Raangkaai khawng rao: ph0uen thaan kaan nuad thai. [Our body: Basics of Thai massage; pp. 19-22], Bangkok, Thailand. Thai Massage Revival Programme. 4p.

[43] Krungkrai Jeenphaanid, 1986, Lak phuuen thaan lae jariyatham kha'awng kaan nuad thai. [Basic Rules and Ethics of Thai Massage] In: Raangkaai khaawng rao: phuen thaan kaan nuad thai. [Our body: Basics of Thai massage; pp. 42-50], Bangkok, Thailand. Thai Massage Revival Programme. 9p.

[44] Krungkrai Jenphanid Somboon Kidniyom 1988 Traditional Thai Massage Therapy [in Thai]: • Kham nam rueng kaan na'e naaew kaan jab sen phaaen boran [Introduction to traditional massage] • Bot wa' Kruu kaawn long mooe tham kaan jab sen [Paying respect to the teacher before starting massage] • Lak ph0een tha'an kha'awng kaan nuad thai [Basics of Thai massage] • Khunatham lae jariyatham khawng ma'aw nuad thai [Qualities and ethics of the Thai massage doctor] [A compilation of pirated text material] Chiang Mai, Thailand. Old Medicine Hospital. 126p.

[45] Thai Massage Revival Programme, 1986 Raangkaai khawng rao: phuen thaan kaan nuad thai. Eekasaan prakawb kaan obrom khaawng khroongkaan kaan nuad thai [Our body: Basics of Thai massage. Document complementing training by the Thai Massage Revival Programme], Bangkok, Thailand. Thai Massage Revival Programme. 165p. Thai Massage Revival Programme

[46] 1986 Khroongkaan fuek obrom kaan ndad thai sa'mrab chaaw ba'an [The training program in Thai massage for villagers] In: Ra'angkaai khaawng rao: phduen thaan kaan nuad thai. [Our body: Basics of Thai massage; pp. S-Il] Bangkok, Thailand. Thai Massage Reviva(Programme. 7p.

[47] Lorentzen, Fridtjof H- 1988 Traditional Thai Massage - A Handbook, [An independent study project, College Semester Abroad Program] Chiang Mai, Thailand. School for International Training. 51 p

[48] Meyer, Walter 1988 Beyond the Mask Toward a Transdisciplinary Approach of Selected Social Problems Related to the Evolution and Context of International Tourism in Thailand [Traditional Thai Massage: 327-329] Saarbrucken, Germany. Verlag Breitenbach Publishers. 533p.

[49] Prayood Bunsinsuk, Lukas Earnst , Peng Sarnkam, 1988 Kruu muue kaan nuad thai (nai kaan saatharana suk muun Tha'an) [Thai Massage Handbook (for Public Health], 2nd ed.(1985) Bangkok, Thailand. Thai Massage Revival Programme. 139p

[50] Somboon Kidniyom, 1988, Traditional Thai Massage Therapy [in Thai]: • Kham nam rueng kaan nae nasew kaan jab sen phaen boran [Introducing traditional massage. 2 p.] • Bot "wai Kruu kaawn long mooe tham kaan jab sen" [Paying respect to the teacher before starting massage, 1 p.] -In: A compilation of pirated text material Chiang Mai, Thailand. Old Medicine Hospital. 3p.

[51] Sharpe, Elizabeth A., 1989 Traditional Thai Massage (Man An Independent Study Project Paper. School for International Training. College Semester Abroad Program. Chiang Mai, Thailand. Personal copy. 31p.

[52] Krungkrai Jeenphaanid, 1989 Kaan nuad thai. Nuad dotton eeng dai - ma tawng phueng yaa. Thai Massage. You Can Massage Yourself - No Need to Depend on Medicine. By: KIum su.eksa'a panha'a yaa & Khrongkaan fuenfuu ka-an -nuad thai: Muulanjthi saathaaranasuk kab kaan phaflhanaa. [By: Drug Study Group & Thai Massage Revival Project.], Bangkok, Thailand. Foundation for Public Health & Development. 16p.

[53] Krungkrai Jeenphaanid, 1989 Kaan nuad. Thanaawm raksaa sa'aftaa ddai ton eeng & Kod jtid yud aakaan Massage. Conserve Eyesight by Yourself & Point Pressure to Stop Symptoms By: Klm sueksaa panha'a yaa & Khropgkaan fciuenfuu kaan nuad thai. Muulanithi saathaaranasuk kab kaan phaflhanaa. [By: Drug Study Group & Thai Massage Revival Project.] Bangkok, Thailand. Foundation for Public Health & Development. 12p.

[54] James, Anthony B., 1 991 Nuat Thai, Traditional Thai Medical Massage, Revised. 1995; Chicago,

IL, USA. Meta Journal Press. 140p.

[55] Phatraa Saengdaanuch & Mongkhon Plianbaangcha'ang, 1991Hiip nuad baaeb booraan thai [Traditional Thai Massage As a Profession] Bangkok, Thailand. Tdn Aaw Co. Ltd. 64 p.

[56] Phatraa Saengdaanuch & Mongkhon Plianbaangcha'ang, 1991 Aachiip nad baaeb booraan thai [Traditional Thai Massage As a Profession] Bangkok, Thailand. Tdn Aaw Co. Ltd. 64 p.

[57] Roullet, Claude & Foury, Patrick, 1 991 Le Massage Traditione. Les formationsem (1) [Presentation of the Wat Pho Thai traditional massage school: The setting, techniques, and teaching] In: KA Sant 6 Magazine, no. 390, France. 1p.

[58] Roullet, Claude & Foury, Patrick, 1991 [Presentation of the Old Medicine Hospital in Chiang Mai, Thailand], In: KA Sante Magazine, no. 391; 27 Sept.; rePlace: n. a., France. 1p.

[59] Kannika Piyapong & Uthai (Illustrations), 1992 Traditional_Thai...Massage. - A Handbook Bangkok, Thailand. Wat Pho Traditional Thai Massage School. 27p.

[59] Gaurier, Thierry, 1992 Pratique médicale du massage traditionnel thaïlandais; (I3.nd.ai.s. Paris, France. Encre/Ste Ary. 83p.

[60] James, Anthony B, 1993 Nuat Thai Traditional Thai Medical Massage- The Northern Style, Chicago, IL, USA. Metta Journal Press. 144 p.

[61] Sawaeng Thaenthaisong, 1993 Book 1 [A bilingual handbook] Khu'u muue kaan nuad phaaen booraan. Lm 1, Bangkok, Thailand. Chulalongkorn Rajavithayalai, Wat Mahathat. 79p.

[62] Yantra Tatooing: WIkipedia: https://en.wikipedia.org/wiki/Yantra_tattooing

[64] Jon Wetlesen, Did Santideva Destroy the Bodhisattva Path? Jnl Buddhist Ethics, Vol. 9, 2002 (accessed March 2010)

[65] AN 4.125, Metta Sutta. See note 2 on the different kinds of Brahmas mentioned.

[66] Metta Sutta: https://en.wikipedia.org/wiki/Metta_Sutta

[66] James, Anthony B., Ayurveda of Thailand, Indigenous Traditional Thai Medicine and Yoga Therapy, Meta Journal Press, Brooksville, FL, 2016 (https://www.amazon.com/Ayurveda-Thailand-Indigenous-Traditional-Medicine/dp/1886338051/ref=sr_1_1?s=books&ie=UTF8&qid=1495727024&sr=1-1&keywords=ayurveda+of+thailand)

[67] Prakriti and Vikruti, http://ayurveda.iloveindia.com/ , Blog Post, http://ayurveda.iloveindia.com/prakruti-vikruti/#d9P0hIzxYiEk2zCs.99

[68] Amazing Thai Yoga for the Hands: Reusi Dottan Based Restorative and Regenerative Yoga for Hands, Shoulders and Heart. Meta Journal Press, Brooksville, Florida https://www.amazon.com/Amazing-Thai-Yoga-Therapy-Hands/dp/1886338159/ref=sr_1_1?s=books&ie=UTF8&qid=1496266190&sr=1-1&keywords=amazing+thai+yoga+for+the+hands

[69] ***Wat Phra Chetuphon Wimon Mangkhalaram Ratchaworamahawihan***[1] (Thai: วัดพระเชตุพน วิมลมังคลารามราชวรมหาวิหาร; pronounced [wát pʰráʔ tɕʰêːt.tù.pʰon wíʔ.mon.maŋ.kʰlaː.raːm râːt.tɕʰá.wɔː.ráʔ.má.hăː.wíʔ.hăːn]).[3] The more commonly known name, Wat Pho, is a contraction of its older name, *Wat Photharam* (Thai: วัดโพธาราม; RTGS: *Wat Photharam*).[4]) (Wiki: https://en.wikipedia.org/wiki/Wat_Pho#:~:text=Wat%20Pho%20%28Thai%3A%20%E0%B8%A7%E0%B8%B1%E0%B8%94%E0%B9%82%E0%B8%9E%E0%B8%98%E0%B8%B4%E0%B9%8C%2C%20pronounced%20%5Bw%C3%A1t%20p%CA%B0%C5%8D%CB%90%5D%20%28listen%29%29%2C,Rattanakosin%20Island%2C%20directly%20south%20of%20the%20Grand%20Palace.)

THE AUTHOR

Ajahn, Dr. Anthony B. James, who began Martial Arts training at an early age, stands out as an example of the dedicated, hardworking, positive-thinking image demonstrated by his schools, classes, and students. Director and Chief Instructor of The Thai Yoga Center in Brooksville, Florida USA. He has authored more than ten books and award winning textbooks and educational documentaries on Traditional Thai Culture and his articles have been published in numerous magazines, such as Inside Kung Fu, Inside Karate, Black Belt, and Soldier of Fortune. John Metzger, of Soldier of Fortune magazine, called him a "Master of Defense..." (SOF Fight Back Special Issue/ Focus Issue, May1986)

Ajahn, Dr. James, one of only six U.S. Ajahn instructors of Krabi Krabong in USA and Canada, received this prestigious honor in Thailand from Grand Master Phaa Kruu Samai Mesamarn, his personal instructor. While training, Dr. James completed two levels of the FSI (Foreign Service Institute) American University Thai Language for Foreign Service Diplomats and Business course. Of course, GM Phaa Kruu Samaii, and GM Promote Mesamarn spoke excellent English!

Ajahn Dr. James is actively involved in promoting Thai Arts of Krabi Krabong, *Muay Boran* and *Muay Thai,* Thai Traditional Medicine, *Nuad Boran Thai*, Thai Ayurveda and Thai Traditional Yoga and Physical Therapy with the Thai Cultural Association U.S.A, and the Buddhai Sawan USA by doing many demonstrations and exhibitions since 1984.

Ajahn, Dr. James has received several prestigious awards for his work in promoting Thai culture over the years: Friend of Thailand "Ghinari" Award September 27, 2002 (https://thaiyogacenter.com/friends-of-thailand-award-2002/), Ajahn and Master Teacher Ajahn (Aacharn) professor - Special Instructor of Traditional Thai Massage Knowledge and Master Thai Traditional Medicine: Thai Yoga/ Thai Massage Teacher status through the Anantasuk Thai Massage School of Prajuab Khiri Khan Province, Wat Po Association of Thai Traditional Medical Schools (Hua HinThailand) (https://www.thaimassage.com/itta/images/aj/award06/), Lifetime Doctor of Traditional Medicine Membership Recognition with Union of Thai Traditional Medicine Society (UTTS) #520121896, (Ministry of Public Health, Thailand from President Aram Amaradit, December 2009).

In addition to Buddhai Sawan… Ajahn, Dr. James is "*Guro*" and certified to teach various systems of Filipino *Escrima*, *Arnis de Mano*, *Pekiti Tersia*, Vysian style *Lastra Maharlika* & Inosanto style *Kali* with traditional rank of Guro having trained extensively with both US and Filipino Masters: GM Tuhon Leo T, Gaje Jr. GM Guro Danny Inosanto, Guro Tom Bisio, Guro Nick Serrada, Guro Jorge Lastra, Guro Edwin Villarta, Additional Teacher certification in *Pencak Silat* by Indonesian Pendakar Suyadi Jaffri (Eddie). Black Belt rank in Go Budo Jiu-jitsu (Seishin Kai- Phillip Ballergeron, Daeshik Kim), "*Tang Soo Do Mu Duk Kwan*" (Master Hong Shik Chung & GM Chuck Norris style) and American Karate (PKA Style) (GM Lloyd Garrard, GM Joe Corley, GM Bill Wallace, GM Jeff Smith, GM Sam Chapman) & GM Sijo Francis Fong Wing Chun.

See extensive bio on the ThaiYogaCenter.com website at (https://thaiyogacenter.com/aachan-anthony-b-james-martial-arts-bio/)

Other Related Books by Dr. Anthony B. James

1) Learn "*Amazing Thai Yoga Therapy for the Hands*" By Ajahn Dr. Anthony B. James! New comprehensive textbook! (https://beardedmedia.com/product/amazing-thai-yoga-for-the-hands-reusi-dottan-based-restorative-and-regenerative-yoga-for-hands-shoulders-and-heart/)

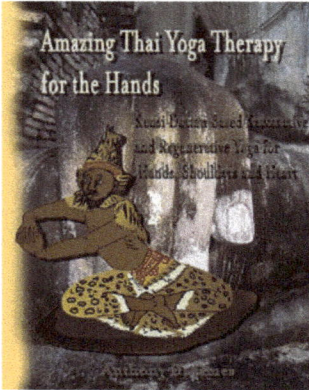

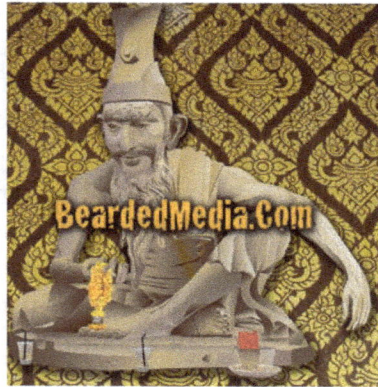

BeardedMedia.Com

Official source for SomaVeda Integrated Traditional Therapies® Educational Materials, Media, Books, Video's and More!

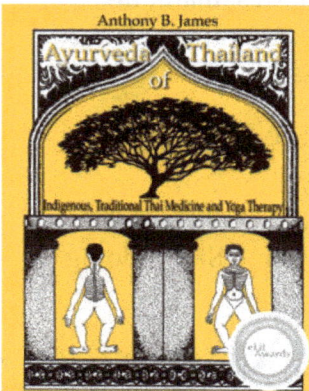

2) "*Ayurveda of Thailand: Indigenous Traditional Thai Medicine and Therapy*": Meta Journal Press, eLit Silver Award: September 2016: (https://beardedmedia.com/product/ayurveda-of-thailand-book/)

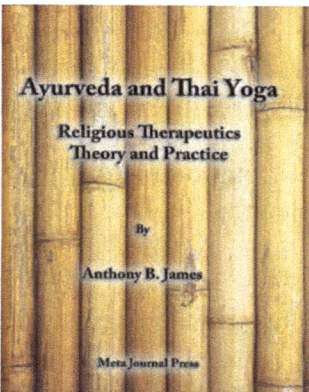

3) "*Ayurveda and Thai Yoga: Religious Therapeutics Theory and Practice*" : Meta Journal Press: Veda Vyasa Award: Best Ayurveda Textbook: June 2017: (https://beardedmedia.com/product/ayurveda-and-thai-yoga-religious-therapeutics-theory-and-practice/)

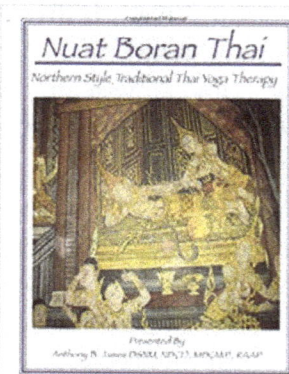

4) "Nuat Boran Thai, Traditional Thai Medical Massage": Meta Journal Press: January 2006 (https://beardedmedia.com/product/122/)

Krabi Krabong Tiger Sword Index

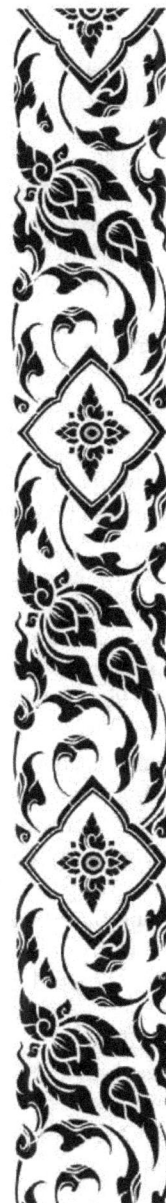

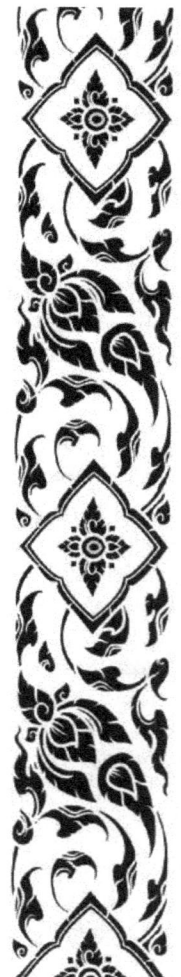

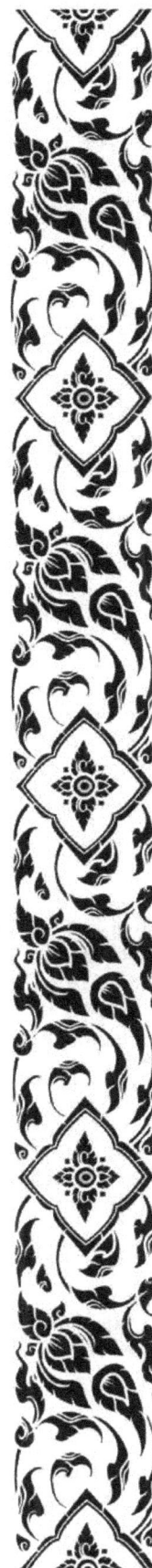

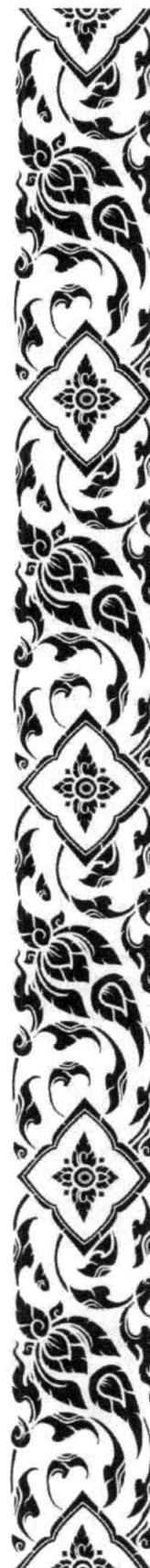

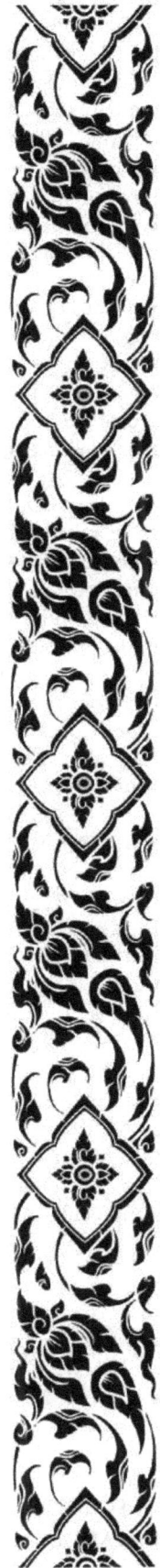

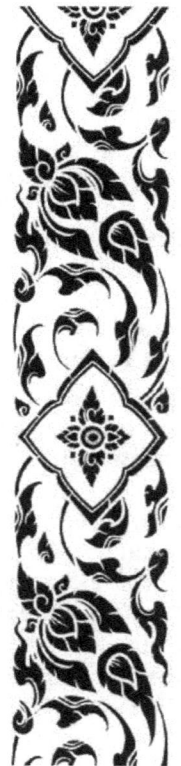

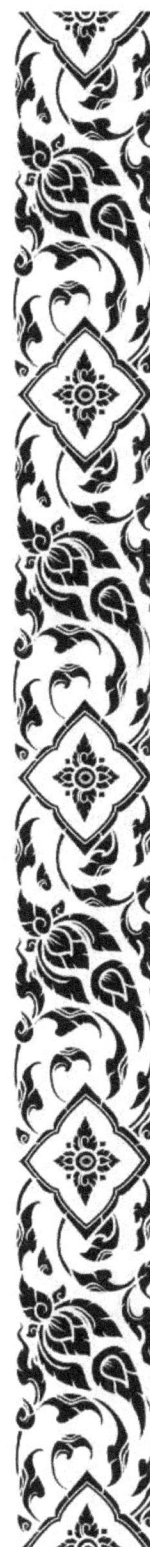

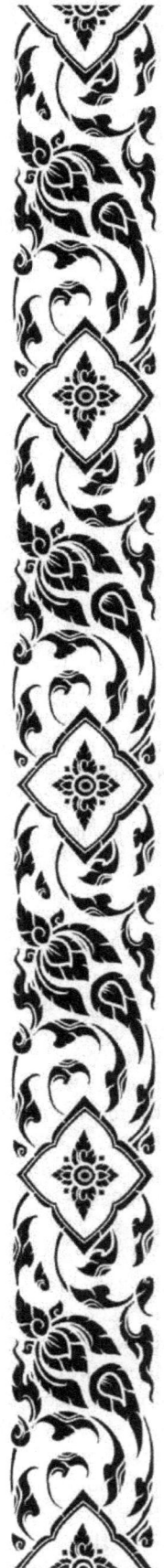

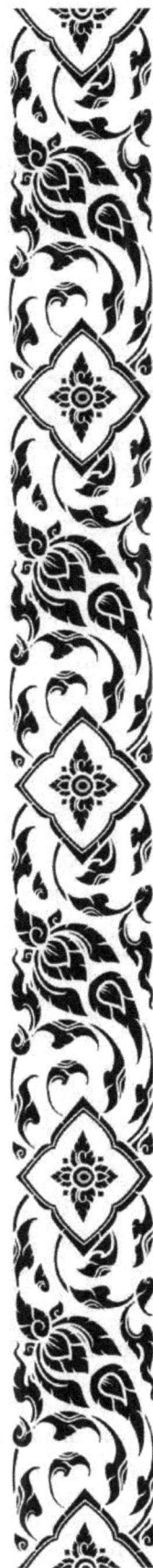

S

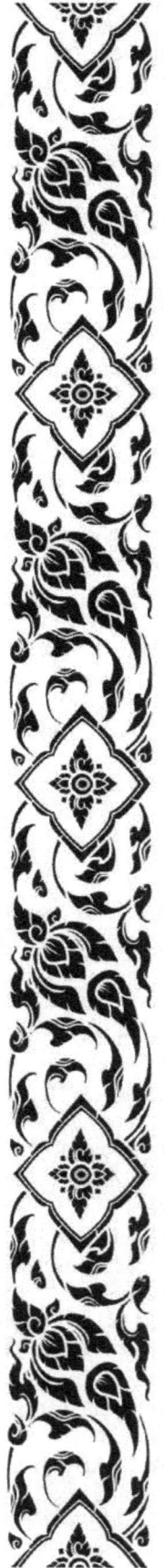

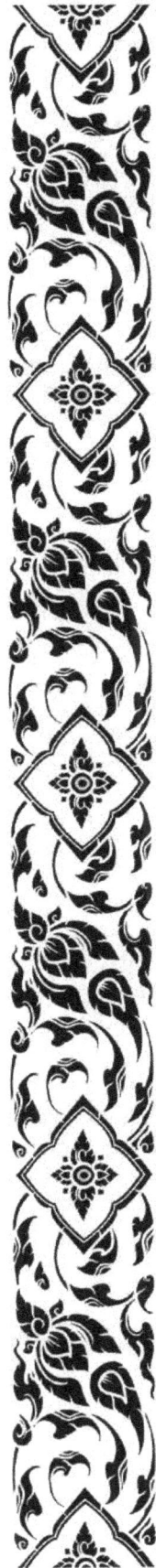

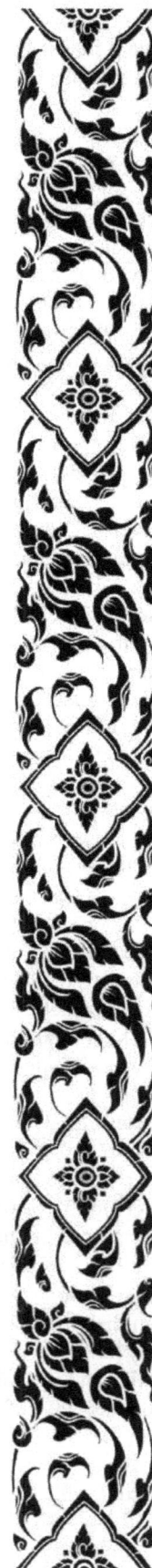

Honoring the Hero's Before Our Time

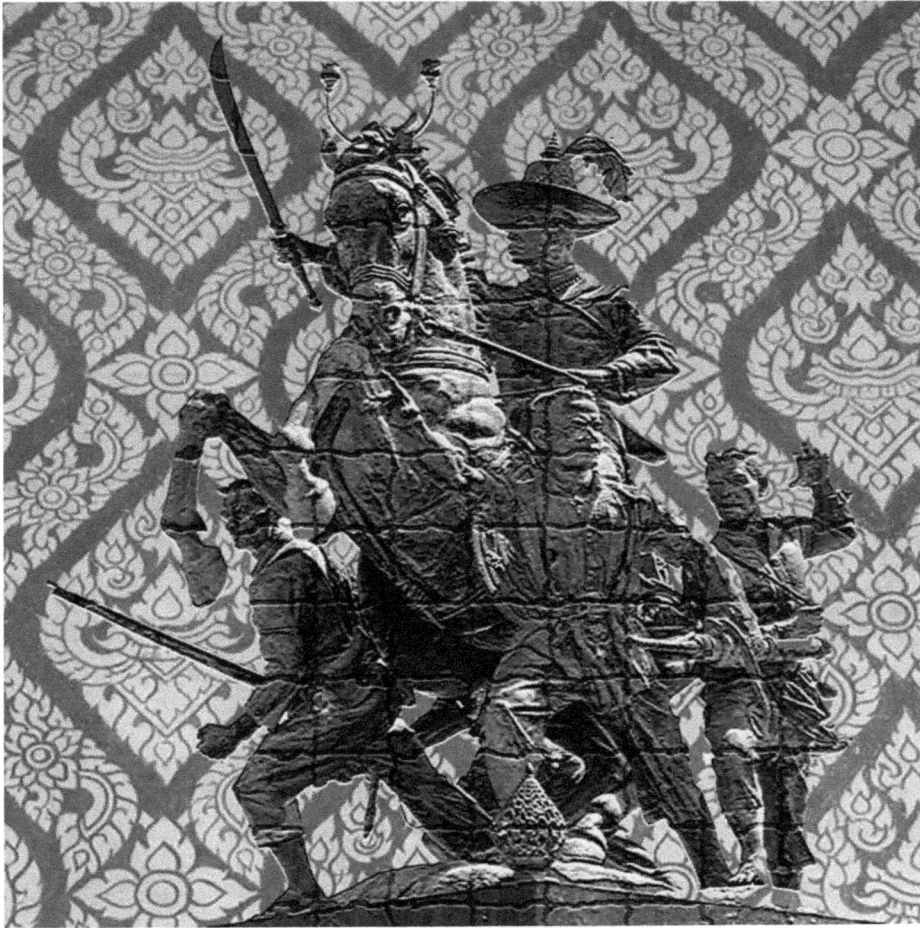

I have strived to pay respect where ever possible to the people, our elder's, our older brothers and sisters, fathers and mothers, Grand father's and Grand mother's, going back many generations... who lived and fought fiercely to create, preserve and protect the freedoms they believed they and their families and communities were all entitled to. The lineage of our schools and the sacrifices of our elders... those we know of and those we don't, bought and brought the "freedom" arts and sciences to us today.

For this reason and so many more, I give respect, honor, and gratitude to the great Thai Buddhai Sawan Krabi Krabong cultural heritage. For centuries, the Thai have given us examples of cultivating character, discipline and strength to be able to stand strong and fight for freedom and sovereignty against oppression and to create a space for the focus and cultivation of the sacred aspects of life.

To be "Thai" is to be FREE. This is truly a world heritage. These ideas and the practical expressions of them, the values of rights to self defense and self determination for ones self, family, city and nation are human rights and role models for us all. I hope by working to see these Ttraditional Martial Arts and their counterparts remain intact for posterity, to see always the dreams they support to remain alive for ourselves, those who know and practice, and for all good people. Despots and Tyrants beware.

Sincerely, Ajahn, Dr. Anthony B. James

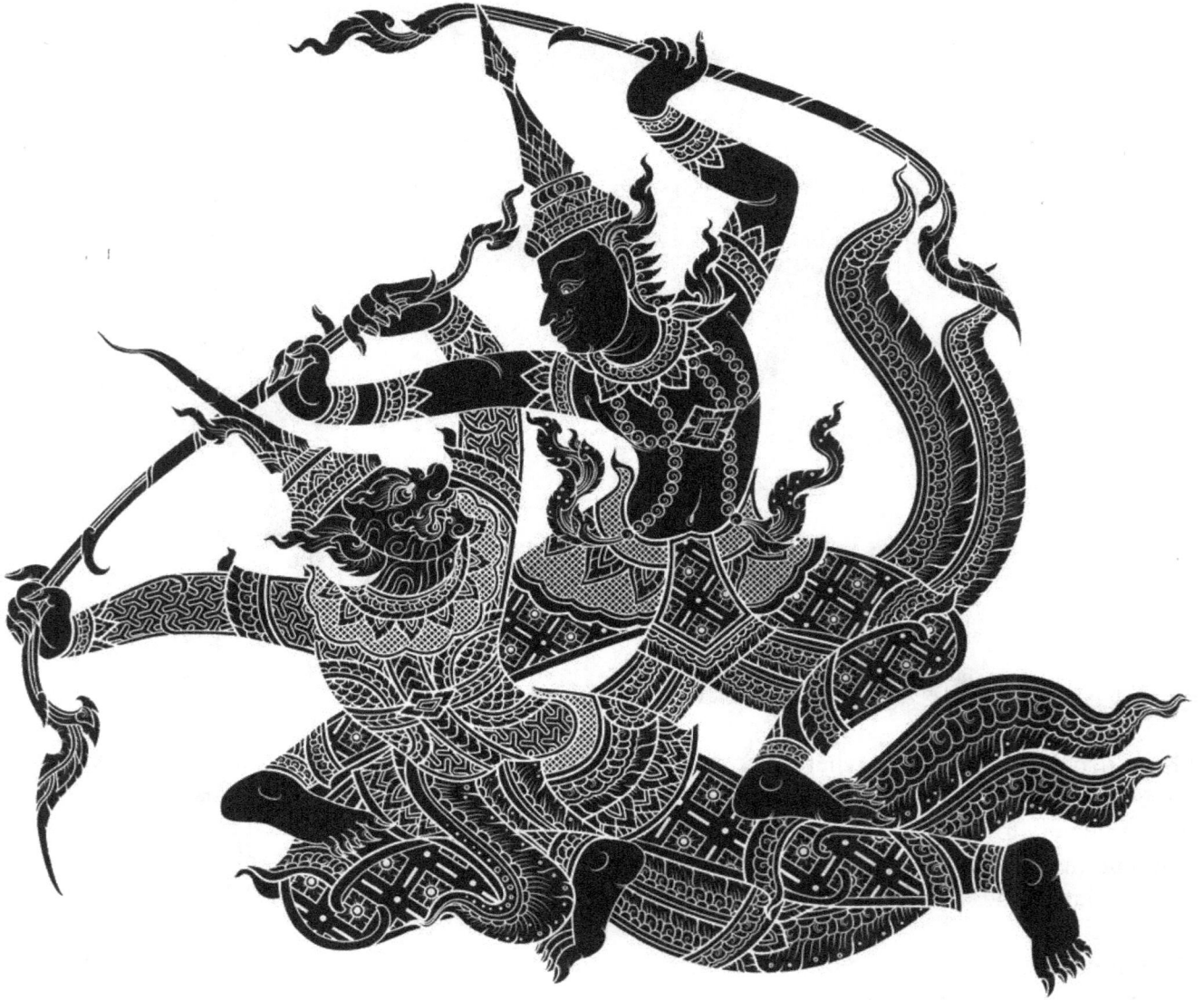

www.ingramcontent.com/pod-product-compliance
Lightning Source LLC
Chambersburg PA
CBHW080611270326
41928CB00016B/3002